Applications of RNA-Seq and Omics Strategies - From Microorganisms to Human Health
http://dx.doi.org/10.5772/66063
Edited by Fabio A. Marchi, Priscila D.R. Cirillo and Elvis C. Mateo

Contributors
Hetron Mweemba Munang\'Andu, Øystein Evensen, Masaaki Oyama, Hiroko Kozuka-Hata, William Seffens, Vahap Eldem, Melike Erkan, Gökmen Zararsiz, Yakup Bakir, Izzet Paruğ Duru, Tunahan Taşçi, Shui Ye, Daniel Heruth, Xun Jiang, Most Islam, Li Qin Zhang, Ding-You Li, Min Xiong, Uzma Qaisar, Tanzeela Rehman, Samina Yousaf, Anila Zainab, Asima Tayyeb, Vladimir Zhukov, Olga Kulaeva, Alexey Afonin, Igor Tikhonovich, Aleksandr Zhernakov, Eveline Ibeagha-Awemu, Duy Do, Bridget E. Fomenky, Michele Araújo Pereira, Eddie Luidy Imada, Rafael Guedes, Masayuki Machida, Toshitaka Kumagai, Frederico Malta, Maíra Cristina Freire, Patrícia Couto, Reshmi G, Bijesh George, Vivekanand Asokachandran, Aswathy Mary Paul, Sabhyata Bhatia, Chandra Kant, Subodh Verma, Vimal Kumar Pandey, Manish Tiwari, Santosh Kumar

Published by InTech
Janeza Trdine 9, 51000 Rijeka, Croatia

Publishing Process Manager Maja Bozicevic
Technical Editor SPi Global
Cover InTech Design team

First published September, 2017
Printed in Croatia
Legal deposit, Croatia: National and University Library in Zagreb

Additional hard copies can be obtained from orders@intechopen.com

Applications of RNA-Seq and Omics Strategies - From Microorganisms to Human Health, Edited by Fabio A. Marchi, Priscila D.R. Cirillo and Elvis C. Mateo
p. cm.
Print ISBN 978-953-51-3503-6
Online ISBN 978-953-51-3504-3

Meet the editors

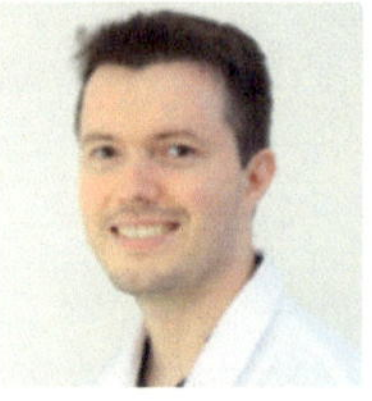

Fabio A. Marchi is a Scientific Researcher at A.C.Camargo Cancer Center in Sao Paulo, Brazil. He holds a PhD in Bioinformatics at Institute of Mathematics and Statistics, University of São Paulo, Brazil, and completed a postdoc in oncology investigating multidimensional data analysis. Dr. Marchi is actively involved in cancer research projects associated with big data, especially in systems biology area.

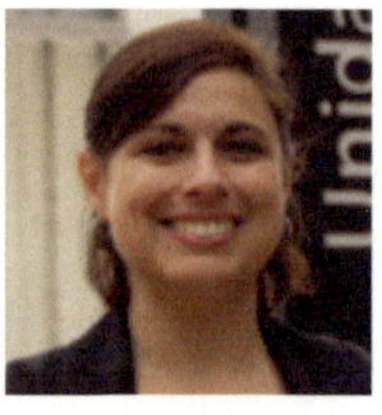

Priscila D. R. Cirillo is a biologist and S enior Researcher at Hermes Pardini Institute, R&D Division, Belo Horizonte, Brazil. She started her career at the Institute of Biosciences of Botucatu, São Paulo State University, Brazil, where she concluded her master's and PhD degrees in the field of cancer genetics. As postdoc at the Center for Translational Research in Oncology, São Paulo State Cancer Institute, Brazil, she has involved mainly in fundamental aspects of tumor biology, focusing on mechanisms of chemoresistance. She published many articles about cancer genomics and also is a reviewer of Oncotarget journal (USA).

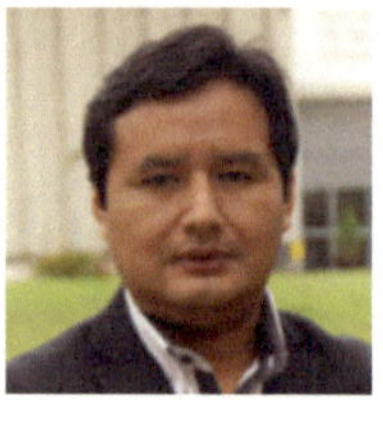

Elvis C. Mateo is a Scientific Coordinator of Research and Development Division (R&D) at Hermes Pardini Institute in Belo Horizonte, Brazil. He concluded his master's and PhD degrees in Human Genetics and Medical Science, all at the University of São Paulo, São Paulo, Brazil. Dr. Mateo is involved in the development of new diagnostic strategies using various molecular techniques.

Contents

Preface

This book is an overview about transcriptome analysis and how other "omics" could be applied in different fields, from microorganisms to precision medicine. The content of each chapter was designed to encourage three types of readers. First, this book will benefit those interested in learning about the most powerful and cost-efficient methods applied for a broad analysis of gene expression regulation of a single cell, a tissue, or the whole living organisms. We aim to offer a wide view of these applications in distinct areas, from agriculture to human diseases, introducing and revising advanced concepts of RNA-Seq technology. In addition, some particularities of the vast world of RNAs were investigated. Most researchers would agree that the memorable event in the RNA area over the last 20 years has been the discovery of the driver functions of noncoding RNAs, such as siRNA and miRNA. These new findings allowed new extensive researches on the control of RNA levels. Besides the contribution to uncover the multitude of small RNAs regulating gene expression, the development of high-throughput sequencing technologies also allowed the investigation of mechanisms related to RNA modifications. Unlike the well-established role of DNA modifications in gene regulation, little is known about modifications in RNA and their influence on gene expression. Mechanisms of RNA modification were addressed here, discussing future challenges and perspectives of studies that attempt to unravel the processes related to the regulation of several stages of the biological system. In spite of the numerous initiatives with animal model investigation, the study of gene expression in plants was also assessed in this book. We point out tools and methodologies for those who are interested in transcriptome analysis in this area, considering the most diverse aspects involved in this challenge. Some points discussed were the influence of transcriptome regulation and mechanisms associated to the responses of environmental stresses, plant-pathogen interactions, and resistance, which in many aspects are closely related to studies performed in the agriculture field to improve, for example, the productivity.

Second, this book will also benefit those who are interested in developing an RNA-Seq study, from the experimental design to the exploration of the most varied algorithms available, following the best practices currently recommended. We present an overview of state-of-the-art methods including experimental design, library preparation, quality check, and preprocessing of raw reads. The particularities involved in differential expression analysis and an accurate investigation of data for specific biological questions aims to show the different approaches that could be found by researchers during the development of the most varied experiments using this technology. Besides presenting a description of concepts and tools, the chapters also offer *in silico* mechanisms to initiate an experiment and to perform a good quality data analysis. Numerous options of bioinformatics tools were presented considering users with limited access for computational resources or little experience with com-

mand-line execution. Also, free online and commercial platforms that can be very helpful and intuitive were discussed, once as important as having the methods available is to fully understand each step in which this method could be used. A good prior planning to choose the correct algorithms and statistical criteria that best fit the different conditions and types of data results in a pleased journey toward success.

Third, it is also for those who are interested in an idea about other omics and the different areas where the big data could be applied. Widely known for having a crucial role in biological systems, post-translational modifications contributed to the recent explosion of proteomic data. Remarkable technological advances in mass spectrometry-based proteomics have resulted in a large quantity of information obtained with great sensitivity in different aspects. We also introduce high-resolution shotgun proteomics technology in combination with bioinformatics platforms to better understand the crucial network structures based on phosphorylation dynamics, as well as global protein expression profiles. Another powerful tool to study the hidden microbial treasure, the metagenomics field, has accelerated the investigation of emerging pathogens, thereby contributing to the design of disease control strategies. Here, we also present the most current knowledge about this technology in scientific studies and commercial application in aquaculture. Regardless of the omics investigated, the large amount of data generated requires the development of new and efficient tools to deal with such information and then to contribute to several studies worldwide. Regarding genomics field, we discuss many molecular tools that have been developed to allow a better understanding of the biology of some diseases, their particularities and variabilities concerning the sequencing of genomes of different species. These tools allow medical and scientific groups to improve patient management, providing personalized prevention and treatment of diseases with more specific and accurate approaches. The potential use of next-generation sequencing in personalized medicine is enormous and the comprehension of this technique is necessary for an effective implementation in the clinical workplace.

In general, there are a great number of books dealing with transcriptomics or other omics in several areas, but our intention was to offer the readers the opportunity to have all this content in one book. Here, the readers can find an overview of different areas of knowledge and take advantage of such knowledges to develop their own pipelines and be in touch with the most current algorithms and platforms used for the scientific community.

Fabio A. Marchi
A.C.Camargo Cancer Center
São Paulo, Brazil

Priscila D.R. Cirillo
Hermes Pardini Institute
Belo Horizonte, Brazil

Elvis C. Mateo
Hermes Pardini Institute
Belo Horizonte, Brazil

Section 1

Getting Started with RNA-Seq Data Analysis

Chapter 1

RNA-seq: Applications and Best Practices

Michele Araújo Pereira, Eddie Luidy Imada and
Rafael Lucas Muniz Guedes

Additional information is available at the end of the chapter

http://dx.doi.org/10.5772/intechopen.69250

Abstract

RNA-sequencing (RNA-seq) is the state-of-the-art technique for transcriptome analysis that takes advantage of high-throughput next-generation sequencing. Although being a powerful approach, RNA-seq imposes major challenges throughout its steps with numerous caveats. There are currently many experimental options available, and a complete comprehension of each step is critical to make right decisions and avoid getting into inconclusive results. A complete workflow consists of: (1) experimental design; (2) sample and library preparation; (3) sequencing; and (4) data analysis. RNA-seq enables a wide range of applications such as the discovery of novel genes, gene/transcript quantification, and differential expression and functional analysis. This chapter will encompass the main aspects from sample preparation to downstream data analysis. It will be discussed how to obtain high-quality samples, replicates amount, library preparation, sequencing platforms and coverage, focusing on best recommended practices based on specialized literature. Basic techniques and well-known algorithms are presented and discussed, guiding both beginners and experienced users in the implementation of reliable experiments.

Keywords: RNA-seq, next-generation sequencing, transcriptome, data analysis, best practices

1. Introduction

A transcriptome represents the entire repertoire of RNA content from an organism, a tissue or a cell and it is dynamic, changing in response to genetic and environmental factors. Several approaches have been developed for transcriptome analysis: hybridization-based (DNA microarray [1]) or sequence-based (ESTs—Expressed Sequence Tags [2], SAGE—Serial Analysis of Gene Expression [3], CAGE—Cap Analysis of Gene Expression [4] and MPSS—Massively Parallel Signature Sequencing [5]). The first sequence-based methods relied on

Sanger sequencing [6], but with advances in next-generation sequencing technology (NGS), transcriptomic studies have evolved considerably and RNA-seq [7, 8] became the state-of-art for transcriptome analysis.

RNA-seq consists of the direct sequencing of transcripts by NGS. Several NGS platforms [9–11] are commercially available nowadays. In general, an RNA set of interest is converted to a library of complementary DNA (cDNA) fragments and sequenced in a high-throughput manner. Compared to ESTs, RNA-seq provides better resolution and representativeness, whereas when compared to microarrays, the independence of reference sequences facilitates the discovery of novel genes and isoforms [8].

RNA-seq experiments harbors challenges from the experimental design to data analysis. Since a complete comprehension of each step is critical to make right decision, this chapter will encompass essential principles required for a successful RNA-seq experiment, focusing on best recommended practices based on specialized and recent literature. Basic techniques and well-known algorithms are presented and discussed, guiding both beginners and experienced users in the implementation of reliable experiments.

2. Experimental design

In order to obtain a successful RNA-seq experiment, it is critical to have a good experimental design. Despite its importance, a proper planning is not always done. There are many experimental options available, and to fully comprehend each step, it is essential to make right decisions, avoiding inconclusive results. These choices depend on extrinsic (e.g., cost, time, samples availability) and intrinsic (e.g., experimental design complexity, transcriptional variability among tissues, samples and organisms) factors. The amount of available resources is usually the main extrinsic limiting factor driving researchers' decisions. First, it is necessary to identify the main goal of an RNA-seq experiment in order to be able to choose the best approach. Qualitative (e.g., annotation) and quantitative (e.g., differential gene expression—DGE) data analyses have some different requirements such as those related to the starting RNA amount, the number and type of replicates, library type and preparation, sequencing platforms, throughput, coverage and depth, and read length. Scotty [12], RNASeqPower [13] and RnaSeqSampleSize [14] are statistical tools designed to aid in the conception of the experimental design, adjusting many of these variables to the main objective and taking into account the financial limitations. A detailed workflow from experimental design to library sequencing is presented in **Figure 1**.

2.1. Starting sample amount

The necessary starting amount of an RNA sample varies between kits and platforms, and the amount of available RNA is one of the limiting factors for an RNA-seq experiment. The majority of library construction kits require micrograms of RNA, sometimes limited to high-quality samples. Takara Bio USA Inc presents some kits for low quantity and/or quality RNA samples: SMARTer Ultra Low mRNA-seq kits (as little as 1 cell or 10 pg of total RNA), SMARTer

http://dx.doi.org/10.5772/intechopen.69250

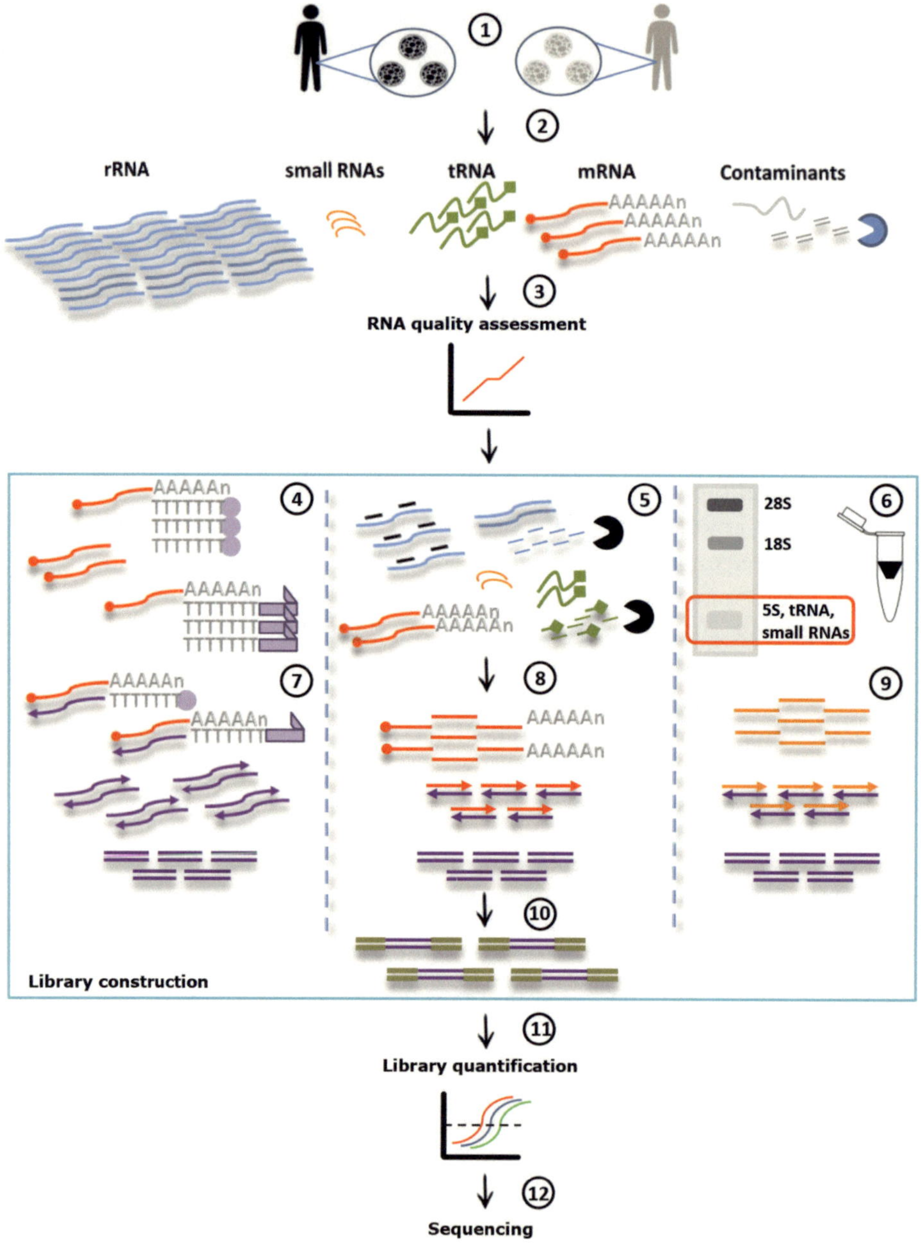

Figure 1. A typical RNA-seq workflow. (1) Experimental design definition of qualitative and quantitative goals. Differential gene expression among different conditions is exemplified; (2) Sample selection, RNA extraction and elimination of contaminants such as genomic DNA; (3) Assessment of RNA integrity; (4-6) RNA enrichment. (4) mRNA enrichment using magnetic or cellulose beads coated with oligo(dT) molecules or oligo(dT) priming; (5) mRNA enrichment through rRNA depletion with conserved probes or Selective Depletion of abundant RNA (SDRNA); (6) Small RNA size-selection through electrophoresis or based on solid phase extraction; (7-9) cDNA single/double strand synthesis. (7) cDNA synthesis followed by fragmentation; (8) mRNA fragmentation followed by cDNA synthesis; (9) cDNA synthesis for small RNA without fragmentation; (10) Adapters ligation; (11) Library quantification and (12) Library sequencing with NGS technology.

Stranded kits (100 pg, regardless of RNA quality) and SMARTer Universal kits (200 pg, regardless of RNA quality). These kits are compatible with both Illumina and Ion Torrent platforms. NuGEN company has also some kits with input RNA levels of 10 pg (Ovation Ultralow Library System V2 and Ovation SoLo RNA-Seq System) available only for Illumina. For a comparison study of four commercially available RNA amplification kits using low-input RNA samples, see Ref. [15].

2.2. Replicates

The variability of an RNA-seq experiment depends on the organism, the biological question under investigation and the available laboratory techniques, and it can be measured by technical and biological variances. Technical replication consists on the repeated analysis of the same sample to infer the variance associated with the technology, that is, equipment and protocols [16]. If only experimental errors analysis is desired, technical replication is satisfactory. Otherwise, biological replicates are necessary [17]. Three biological replicates are the minimum suggested for any inferential analysis [18], although the minimum amount required for a reliable RNA-seq experiment depends on the desired statistical power. For example, in DGE analysis, performing more biological replication is recommended over increasing the sequencing depth [19, 20], and from 6 to 12 biological replicates have been suggested [21]. Biological replication is often preferable to enrich the inferential analysis and increase your statistical power. Statistical knowledge helps to understand the different statistical analysis methods required for different levels of replication [16, 17, 22].

2.3. Sequencing platforms

There are several sequencing platforms available with diverse data formats, throughputs and qualities [9–11]. Two commonly used approaches are sequencing by synthesis (e.g., Illumina, Helicos and PacBio) and ion semiconductor sequencing (Ion Torrent). They can also be classified as clonal amplification-based sequencing (e.g., Illumina and Ion Torrent) or single-molecule-based sequencing (e.g., Helicos, PacBio, Nanopore). For RNA-seq experiments, the most popular platform is Illumina due to its high throughput and low-error rates. PacBio has gained attention due to read length increases since its reads can be long enough to recapitulate a full-length cDNA transcript [23–26]. RNA-seq approaches can also be combined to take advantage of each method benefits. Further information and comparison studies are available in Refs. [11, 27–29].

2.4. Sequencing depth

The required sequencing depth for RNA-seq experiments varies over several degrees. Transcripts are expressed at different levels within the cell, and their coverage differs considerably in any RNA-seq experiment. A deeper sequencing is required to detect low abundance transcripts and rare splicing events, but their relevance can only be assessed with a good biological replication [30]. However, deeper sequencing may increase the detection of off-target RNA species and the number of false positives in differential expression calls [31]. A

correlation between sequencing depth and accuracy demonstrated that as low as one million reads can provide similar information of transcript abundance as more than 30 million reads for highly expressed genes. This result was consistently shown in all six widely used model organisms (*Arabidopsis thaliana, Caenorhabditis elegans, Drosophila melanogaster, Homo sapiens, Mus musculus* and *Saccharomyces cerevisiae*) that represent a wide range of genome sizes [32]. For the majority of human tissue genes, the amount required was about 15–50 million reads [33]. It is noteworthy that there is a point of sequencing depth saturation where a deeper sequencing results in only a small gain of information. More about the impact of sequencing depth on gene detection, gene expression quantification and structural variants discovery can be found in Ref. [33].

2.5. Read length

Short-read sequencing is cheaper than long-read sequencing. RNA-seq experiments usually make use of short-reads; however, longer reads can be helpful and more informative. Reads are usually shorter than full-length transcripts, and a single read may map to multiple positions in the genome stickling expression analysis and transcriptome assembly. Longer read length reduces mapping bias and ambiguity in assigning reads to genomic elements [34] and improves splicing detection [35, 36] and complex transcriptome analysis [37, 38]. However, some studies question the advantages of long reads sustaining that for humans, there are no substantial improvements in transcriptome assembly quality with reads over 150 base pairs [39] and in differential expression analysis with reads over 50 base pairs [35].

2.6. Library type

Standard RNA-seq library protocols do not retain the strand orientation for each original transcript, making it difficult to discriminate gene expression from overlapping genes. Therefore, it is often desirable to construct strand-specific libraries [40–42]. There are several strand-specific protocols available, and they can be performed by two main alternatives. One method consists of marking the second strand by chemical modification, preventing it from being amplified by PCR and leading to the amplification of the first strand only. The deoxy-UTP (dUTP) approach [43] is a well-known example, and it is one of the leading protocols. The other method involves adapter's ligation in a known orientation in the RNA molecule such as Illumina RNA ligation method [44]. A comparison between seven library-construction protocols reveals strong differences and substantial variation in the experimental complexity [40]. Stranded RNA-seq provides more accurate downstream expression analysis, and it is the recommend approach for RNA-seq studies [40, 42]. Moreover, the dUTP and the Illumina RNA ligation methods were identified as the best overall protocols [40, 45].

2.7. Spike-in

The External RNA Control Consortium (ERCC) [46] has developed a set of 92 polyadenylated synthetic spike-in controls for normalization and noise reduction of gene expression. ERCC spike-ins mimic eukaryotic mRNAs and can be added ('spiked') equally to each sample prior

to library construction [47]. Ambion ERCC spike-in control mixes (Thermo Fisher Scientific) are commercially available. Sequins, another set of spike-in RNA standards, can also be used as internal controls and are freely available for non-profit research upon request [48]. Normalization methods should be carefully chosen to ensure that spike-in will behave as expected. The R package *erccdashboard* [49] and Anaquin [50] can be used for spike-in analysis.

3. Sample preparation and library construction

After defining the experimental design, a typical RNA-seq experiment workflow consists of (i) RNA preparation, (ii) cDNA library construction, (iii) sequencing and (iv) bioinformatic analysis. Each step will be briefly discussed below.

3.1. RNA preparation

Since RNA is more labile than DNA and RNases are ubiquitous and very stable enzymes, special precautions and more stringent working practices should be taken to obtain pure and high-quality RNA. Best practices can be found at [51] or spread on diverse companies' websites such as Thermo Fisher Scientific, Qiagen and Ambion.

In an RNA-seq experiment, the RNA preparation consists basically of isolation/extraction and enrichment. Many RNA sample preparation techniques and commercial kits are available. No unique method is optimal for every application, and combination of methods may vary depending on the sample type and the study goals. It is always recommended to carefully follow manufacturer's instructions.

3.1.1. RNA isolation and extraction

In order to isolate high-quality RNA, the samples need to be processed immediately after harvest. If an immediate isolation is not possible, samples can be stabilized in an intermediary solution to preserve RNA integrity and allow storage. Commonly used stabilizers are RNA*later* (Thermo Fisher Scientific and Qiagen) and RNAstable (Sigma-Aldrich). RNA isolation and extraction methods can be manual (e.g., TRIzol–Thermo Fisher Scientific) or automated (e.g., RNeasy—Qiagen), and different types of samples require different approaches, although all of them comprise: (i) sample solubilization in the presence of detergent and chaotropic agents, (ii) sample homogenization for complete cell disruption and (iii) RNA recovery from the lysate with organic or solid-phase extraction. It is also important to have a final RNA free of genomic DNA (gDNA) contaminants. Some protocols can carry over some gDNA into total RNA samples that can be removed by a DNAse treatment. gDNA contamination can lead to a counting bias in downstream analysis and can be detected by reads background over the whole genome (false positive signal). Further information about sample preparation techniques and some commercial kits available can be found in Ref. [52]. Different commercial kits demonstrated satisfactory RNA yield, but differences in the quality of extracted RNA were observed, which can interfere on the downstream analysis [53].

RNA quality can be assessed by gel electrophoresis (agarose or polyacrylamide) or through Agilent Bioanalyzer. RNA quantity can be assessed using spectrophotometer (e.g., Nanodrop), fluorometer (e.g., Qubit) or Agilent Bioanalyzer. No single RNA quantification and quality control method are ideal, and it is necessary to know the limits of each method. We recommend Bioanalyzer since it measures the RNA integrity and level of degradation by the RNA Integrity Number (RIN) score that allows sample quality comparison by a scale with a range from 1 (most degraded) to 10 (most intact) [54, 55]. There is no consensus about the RIN cut-off for sample inclusion or exclusion in a study, but RIN ≥ 6 are commonly acceptable. DGE analysis could be performed even with RIN scores around 4 [56], but non-degraded RNA is preferred for a successful transcriptome analysis. It is also important to highlight that some organisms do not present typical rRNAs peaks and cannot be evaluated by RIN value. Most insect RNA shows a cleavage of 28S rRNA into two similar fragments (28Sα and 28Sβ) that comigrate with 18S rRNA depending on pretreatment and electrophoresis conditions. This comigration is due to the disruption of the hydrogen bonds responsible for maintaining the two 28S fragments together. This profile should not be misinterpreted as low integrity and degradation [57]. In these cases, check the overall Bioanalyzer trace. More information about each method and a comparison study can be found in Refs. [58, 59], respectively.

3.1.2. RNA enrichment

The type of the desired RNA molecule drives the RNA enrichment approach. Selection of mature mRNAs by their poly(A) tails is the most common application and can be carried out with magnetic or cellulose beads coated with oligo(dT) molecules or through oligo(dT) priming for reverse transcription (RT). Therefore, since RNAs from formalin-fixed and paraffin-embedded (FFPE) are degraded and mRNA-seq poorly captures degraded mRNAs, it is not an appropriate method to use with FFPE samples [42], unless adapted protocols are applied such as the recently described protocol based on *in vitro* T7 transcription for linear amplification of mRNA [60]. In order to surpass this limitation, rRNA depletion protocols have been developed based on hybridization in highly conserved ribosomal regions, including the selective depletion of abundant RNA (SDRNA) with RNase H [61, 62], Ribominus (Thermo Fisher Scientific), Ribo-Zero (Illumina), GeneRead (Qiagen) and RiboGone (Takara). Another approach is the duplex-specific nuclease (DSN) normalization by depletion of abundant transcripts, such as rRNAs and tRNAs [63, 64]. Samples can be also enriched of small ncRNAs (e.g., miRNA, siRNA and piRNA) via size-selection through electrophoresis or based on solid phase extraction with commercial kits such as mirVana (Thermo Fisher Scientific) and miRNeasy (Qiagen). For comparison studies between these methods, see Refs. [42, 65]. rRNA depletion is recommended rather than oligo(dT) because it can capture a complete view of the transcriptome and can be used for low-quality RNA samples [65].

3.2. cDNA Library construction

The library construction includes four steps: (i) RNA/cDNA fragmentation, (ii) cDNA synthesis, (iii) adapters ligation and (iv) quantification. Some specific points will be briefly discussed below, but additional information can be found in Refs. [41, 45].

3.2.1. RNA/cDNA fragmentation

The length of your RNA insert is a key factor for library construction and sequencing. Since most current platforms sequence only short reads, most protocols incorporate an RNA or cDNA fragmentation step that allows amplification and sequencing. For short RNAs (under 200 pb), no fragmentation is required. There are three main ways to fragment the nucleic acid samples: physical (e.g., sonication, nebulization), enzymatic (e.g., RNase III, DNase I or Fragmentase) and chemical (e.g., heat, metal ion) shearing. Little information is known about which is the best method for each application. A comparison study of nebulization, sonication and enzymatic digestion showed that all three methods presented equal performance and that fragmentation is indicated [66]. In most cases, RNA is fragmented before conversion into cDNA. Furthermore, it is important to highlight that due to FFPE samples degradation, cDNA fragmentation must be performed instead of RNA fragmentation when using oligo(dT) priming for first-strand synthesis.

3.2.2. cDNA synthesis

After an adequate RNA preparation, RNA must be converted to double complementary DNA (cDNA) via RT, generating a cDNA:RNA hybrid. This process is known as first-strand cDNA synthesis and requires an oligonucleotide primer. Three options are available: oligo(dT) priming, random priming or gene-specific priming. The first two are the mainly used for RNA-seq. Oligo(dT) priming is one of the oldest methods for first-strand synthesis and involves oligo(dT) primer to capture the poly(A) tail of mature mRNA. Because of their specificity for poly(A) tails, oligo(dT) priming is not compatible with fragmented RNA, such as FFPE samples, nor for RNAs that lack poly(A) tails, such as non-mRNAs (e.g., microRNAs (miRNAs)). If using this methodology, cDNA fragmentation must be performed instead of RNA fragmentation. Besides that, RTs are not highly processive polymerases and can prematurely terminate the strand biosynthesis, leading to 3′ end bias and under-representation of the 5′ ends. Random priming involves oligonucleotides with random base sequences that prime at random positions along the RNA (i.e., no template specificity), and it is preferable to oligo(dT) priming. This approach allows recovery of non-poly(A) RNAs and prevents 3′ end bias, resulting in a more uniform transcript coverage. However, it was shown that random priming is not completely random leading to a nucleotide bias across the first reads positions [67, 68].

The first-strand cDNA is used as a template to generate double-stranded cDNA. Second-strand cDNA synthesis can be performed by (i) RNA nicking of the RNA template by RNase H and synthesis with *E. coli* DNA polymerase I and T4 DNA ligase [69], (ii) using an oligo that is complementary to an adapter located in the 5′ end of the RNA template or by (iii) Clontech's SMART (Switching Mechanism At 5′ end of RNA Transcript) technology [70]. RNase H method presented a better performance for low-quality RNA when compared to four other methods (Ribo-Zero, NuGEN, SMART and DSN-lite) [65].

3.2.3. Adapters sequences and ligation

Adapters sequences must be ligated at the ends of every single molecule during library preparation, and this process varies depending upon the sequencing platform. It can contain one

or more extra functional elements such as barcode/index to allow multiplexing and a second sequencing-priming site to allow paired-end sequencing. The addition of adapter via Y-adapter PCR is the most commonly used technique. Adapters can also be added via RT/PCR during the first- and second-strand synthesis process or via ligation.

3.2.4. Library quantification

To ensure the maximum yield (i.e., data output) and quality from your RNA-seq experiment, it is important to have a precise quantification of your NGS libraries. Inaccurate quantification may lead to lower throughput, lower sequences qualities and poor samples balance within your multiplex. There are many ways to quantify your libraries, but the most accurate and effective method is quantitative real-time PCR (qPCR). qPCR is more sensitive and only quantifies amplifiable DNA molecules (i.e., molecules that contain both adaptor sequence), providing a more precise estimation. Some commercial kits available are KAPA Library Quantification Kit (Kapa Biosystem), GeneRead Library Quant System (Qiagen), Ion Library TaqMan Quantitation Kit (Thermo Fisher Scientific), QPCR NGS Library Quant Kit (Agilent), PerfeCTa NGS Quantitation Kit (Quantabio) and NEBNext Library Quant Kit (New England BioLabs). Other methods are similar to the previously mentioned for RNA quantification: spectrophotometer (e.g., Nanodrop), fluorometer (e.g., Qubit) and Agilent Bioanalyzer. However, since these methods measure total nucleic acid concentrations, including non-amplifiable DNA, they can lead to inaccurate results. It is also recommended to verify the libraries fragment size distribution, which can be performed by electrophoresis, preferably Agilent Bioanalyzer. Bioanalyzer electropherogram needs to show a narrow distribution with a peak height of the average size fragmentation value. After quantification, the library must be sequenced with the platforms discussed in Section 2.3, and data must be analyzed through bioinformatic tools. RNA-seq data analysis will be discussed below.

4. Data analysis

RNA-seq data analysis involves many different strategies that depend on the goals and biological questions established at the time of the study design. A typical data analysis includes quality control, reads preprocessing, alignment to a reference or *de novo* assembly and downstream analysis such as transcripts annotation, DGE, gene fusion analysis and alternative splicing. In the following topics, we will emphasize common steps and applications of this technology. A detailed workflow for data analysis is presented in **Figure 2**. Bioinformatic tools discussed in this chapter are compiled at **Table 1**, and a more exhaustive list of available tools can be found in Ref. [71]. For those with limited access for computational resources or little experience with command-line execution of these bioinformatic tools, free online (Galaxy [72]) and commercial (Illumina BaseSpace [73] and Geneious [74]) platforms can be very helpful and intuitive.

4.1. Quality control and reads preprocessing

A complete pipeline for an RNA-seq analysis demands some checkpoints in order to ensure the quality of the results and elimination of noise from the biological samples. After sequencing,

the analysis starts with files containing the raw reads. The FASTQ [75] is the standard format used to store the nucleotide sequences along with a per base quality score in Phred log scale. The qualities, typically with scores from 0 to 40, are represented by single letters encoded with pre-defined ranges of characters from the American Standard Code for Information Interchange (ASCII) table. Currently, there are two patterns: Phred + 64, used in initial Illumina versions 1.3 + and 1.5 + and Phred + 33, the default encoding for Sanger and more recent sequencers. The FASTQ is widely accepted and used in most downstream software, although the unmapped BAM (uBAM) format has been recently encouraged as it is capable of storing important sequencing metadata not present in FASTQ, and for being binary, it demands less disk storage. Some sequencing platforms, like Ion Torrent, have already included uBAM as default output format in their pipelines. Both formats are interchangeable by using Picard [76], BamUtil [77] and BamTools [78].

The first step is to perform a quality control (QC) of the data, checking parameters like amount of reads per sample, general read and base qualities, mean reads length, G+C content, presence of unclipped adapters or PCR primers and unexpected repetitive sequences. This general overview will indicate if library construction and sequencing were properly performed, or if errors like contaminants, poor ribosomal RNA depletion or low sequencing output will demand a new round of experiments. The most common software used to retrieve these basic statistics is FastQC [79] and PRINSEQ [80]. The first was mainly designed for Illumina, while the later for 454/Roche technology and may be also used for preprocessing. Both programs are available with intuitive graphical user interfaces (GUI), accept other sequencing technologies input files and generate graphical reports, which are very useful for guiding the choice of filtering thresholds.

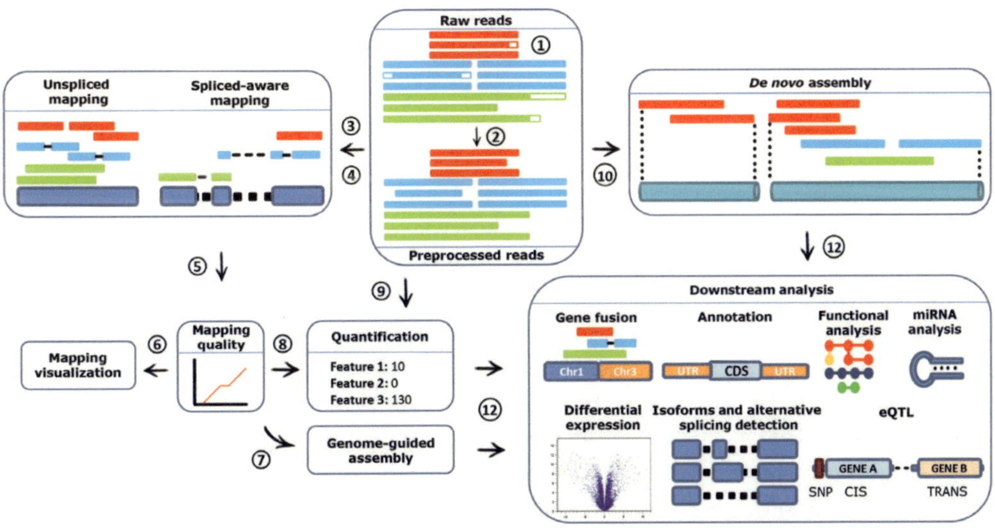

Figure 2. RNA-seq data analysis. (1) Raw single-end and paired-end reads obtained from NGS sequencing; (2) Adapters clipping and base quality trimming. Alternatively error correction can be performed; (3) Mapping without preprocessing using soft-clipping; (4) Unspliced or spliced-aware reads mapping; (5) Assess mapping quality and biases; (6) Mapping visualization; (7) Transcriptome genome-guided assembly; (8) Per feature quantification using mapped reads; (9) Per feature quantification using quasi-mapping approach; (10) Transcriptome de novo assembly; (11) Mapping reads to de novo assembled transcriptome; (12) Downstream data analysis.

Category		Tools
Experimental design		Scotty [12]
Raw reads quality control		FASTQC [75]
Reads preprocessing	Read clipping/trimming	Picard [72], BamUtil [73], BamTools [74], PRINSEQ [76], Cutadapt [78], FASTX-Toolkit [79], Trimmomatic [80]
	Paired-end reads overlapping detection	FLASh [84], PEAR [85]
	Reads error correction	SEECER [86], Rcorrector [87]
Unspliced mapping	Hash Table index based	BFAST [90], MAQ [92], Mosaik [93], Novoalign [94], RMAP [95], SHRiMP [96]
	FM-index based	Bowtie2 [97], BWA [100]
Spliced-aware mapping	Hash Table index based	GSNAP [91], RNASEQR [103]
	FM-index-based	TopHat2 [98], HISAT2 [99], SOAP-splice [101], STAR [102], RNASEQR [103]
Alignment quality assessment		Picard [72], BamUtil [73], BamTools [74], Samtools [106], Qualimap2 [107], BAMstats [108], SAMstat [109]
Assembly	Genome-guided	Cufflinks [111], Scripture [112], StringTie [113]
	De novo	Rnnotator [115], Trans-ABySS [116], Trinity [119], Oases [120]
Assembly quality assessment		Detonate [122], TransRate [123], BUSCO [124]
Alignment visualization		IGV [125], Tablet [126], UCSC [127]
Raw read counts	Mapped-based	featureCounts [129], HTSeq-count [130], RSEM [136]
	Pseudoalignment	Kallisto [140], Salmon [141]
Raw read counts quality assessment		NOISeq [131]
Differential expression		DESeq [132], DESeq2 [133], edgeR [134], CuffDiff2 [137], BitSeq [138], Ballgown [139]
Annotation		BLAST [145, 146], DIAMOND [147], InterProScan [148], tRNAscan-SE [149], RNAmmer [150], Blast2GO [151], Annocript [152], TRAPID [153], Trinotate [154]
Enrichment analysis		GSEA [155]
Alternative splicing		Cufflinks [111], Scripture [112], StringTie [113]
Differential alternative splicing		CuffDiff [111], Ballgown [139], DEXSeq [161], rMATS [162], SpliceR [163], MISO [164], DiffSplice [165]
Fusion genes		SOAPfuse [170], FusionCatcher [171], JAFFA [172]
miRNA		miRdeep2 [179], miReNA [180], miRanalyzer [181]

Table 1. Tools for RNA-seq data analysis.

The following preprocessing step is crucial and can greatly influence the data analysis [81]. Besides PRINSEQ, other tools like Cutadapt [82], FASTX-Toolkit [83] and Trimmomatic [84] are efficient in preprocessing reads, but FASTX-Toolkit cannot be used with paired-end reads. Generally, due to problems inherent in sequencing technologies, the bases in 3′end of reads have lower quality, and one may choose to filter off reads with low mean quality or trim only the low-quality ends. Trimming in most cases may improve mappability, although shorter reads have a higher probability of erroneous mapping. Therefore, it is recommended to remove short reads in conjunction with non-aggressive base-quality trimming to avoid spurious mapping and incorrect inferences [85, 86]. Adapter removal and trimming low-quality ends improve RNA-seq assembly, single nucleotide polymorphism (SNP) detection and gene-expression analysis.

Modern mapping tools (see next section) are capable of labeling the unaligned read ends, a process known as soft-clipping, without actually removing them (hard-clipping). There is no consensus on which approach is the best, but it has been considered that keeping as much as information as possible would be better for downstream analysis. For example, the soft-clipped reads are important for detection of genomic structural variants [87].

When the goal is to perform RNA-seq *de novo* assembly, supplementary tools can be used to join overlapping paired-end reads, like FLASh [88] and PEAR [89]. Additionally, base error correction can be applied as an alternative to read trimming and filtering, increasing the amount of useful data and consequently the contig sizes. SEECER [90] and Rcorrector [91] were specifically designed for this task. Both strategies will likely improve assembly qualities.

In summary, preprocessing is beneficial, but there is no best tool for any experiment or general rule for filtering thresholds. All software has its own standard parameters, advantages and limitations, being recommended a case-by-case analysis and a thorough software comparison.

4.2. Mapping, assembling and visualizing mapped reads

Now that the raw reads have been preprocessed, alternative approaches can be chosen according to the availability of a reference sequence. If present, reads can be mapped to the genome and the gene that originated the transcript from which the reads were derived may be inferred and expression quantified. The genome may also be used to guide transcriptome assembly, resulting in several contigs representing the genes and its isoforms. On the other hand, if the studied species still lacks a reference sequence, reads can be *de novo* assembled, and transcripts can now be used as a mapping reference.

4.2.1. Mapping to a reference

Mapping reads to a reference can be also seen as a traditional pair-wise sequence alignment, as observed in common Basic Local Alignment Search Tool (BLAST) [92], but with the main difference that a vast amount of reads are compared with a database composed of fewer and longer sequences instead of several thousand nucleotides/proteins. This is a field under constant development with plenty of tools available [93]. These tools have to deal with inherent mapping challenges, such as sequencing errors, natural sequence variability like SNPs and

indels, reads spanning exon junctions and repetitive regions or pseudogenes in references. To guarantee reproducibility, it is highly recommended reporting alignment parameter details, such as mapper and reference versions and sources, allowed seed mismatches, minimal alignment score and treatment given to multi mapping reads.

Mappers can be roughly divided by the algorithm chosen to create indexes and by the ability to recognize exon-exon junctions. Indexes have the purpose of making the alignments significantly faster and are mainly divided into Hash Table or compressed prefix or suffix array-like structures (FM-index). Their principle is to quickly find small local alignments representing substrings of whole reads—designated as seeds—in the reference and then extend those alignments surpassing a defined quality threshold toward the read ends, assigning a Phred-based mapping quality score for each read. Unfortunately, most mappers have developed their own mapping quality formulas, creating a non-uniform mapping qualification. Some well-known Hash Table-based algorithms are BFAST [94], GSNAP [95], MAQ [96], Mosaik [97], Novoalign [98], RMAP [99] and SHRiMP [100], while Bowtie2 [101], TopHat2 [102], HISAT2 [103], BWA [104], SOAP-splice [105] and STAR [106] are examples of FM-index based algorithms.

Regarding the splicing events, they can be divided into unspliced and splice-aware aligners. Most recent mappers are capable of using reference annotation files to deal with known exon-exon junctions and to predict new splice sites, which is essential when analyzing RNA-seq data from most eukaryotes. GSNAP, SOAP-splice, RNASEQR [107], STAR and TopHat2 are some recommended options for spliced alignments, but for intronless species, miRNA and transcriptomes, unspliced aligners can be used. Comparative evaluations showed that FM-index-based mappers are preferable [108] and that, again, no tool is the best for every performance parameters like speed, alignment yield, exon discovery and accuracy [109].

The standard alignment output is the Sequence Alignment/Map (SAM) format or its binary version BAM and they are essential inputs for many downstream applications. Picard [76] and Samtools [110] are frequently used to manipulate these files. It is advisable to assess the alignment quality from SAM/BAM files with tools like Qualimap2 [111], BAMstats [112] and SAMstat [113] for general characterization or for comparing mappers' performances.

4.2.2. *Genome-guided assembly*

Short RNA-seq reads represent only a small portion of most transcripts, and therefore, overlaps have to be detected in order to fully reconstruct the original molecules. Paralogous genes, alternative splicing, alternative transcription initiation and termination sites increase the complexity and impose computational challenges in Eukaryotic assembly analysis [114]. For Bacteria, Archaea and lower eukaryotes, the absence or smaller amount of introns makes the assembly more straightforward.

RNA-seq assemblers greatly differ from DNA-seq algorithms because a wide range of transcripts coverage is expected, and several gene isoforms can be observed resulting in thousands of contigs stead of ideally one per chromosome. When a good quality reference genome is available, the usual procedure is to use the coordinates of aligned reads to separate them into clusters and perform a *de novo* alignment individually for each locus, from which individual

isoforms can be inferred. Cufflinks [115], Scripture [116] and StringTie [117] are recommended tools, and their algorithm strategies have been reviewed [118], with StringTie [117] presenting better transcript reconstruction performance. Paired-end, strand-specific libraries and longer reads are highly encouraged for better assemblies and to allow distinction in overlapping transcripts from opposite strands for gene-dense species and antisense transcription. Genome-guided assembled transcriptomes can be used to improve gene structures annotation through detection of transcription boundaries and splice-sites.

4.2.3. *De novo assembly*

In the absence of a reference sequence or if only a fragmented draft genome is available, overlaps have to be detected from the complete read set in a *de novo* assembly approach. The independence from a good quality reference and mapping procedures can be also seen as an advantage. The counterpart is that sequencing depth must be obtained in a higher coverage, estimated around 30× [119], while genome-guided approach requires about 10× [120, 121] to find full-length transcripts. The higher throughput increases the processing requirements, so data digital normalization is recommended in order to remove redundancy without impacting the assembly outcome [122]. Although the *de novo* approach is usually more error prone and computationally intensive, it allows the discovery of novel splicing events, unpredicted genes and exons, chromosomal rearrangements and trans-splicing. Trinity [123], Oases [124], Rnnotator [119] and Trans-ABySS [120] are advised for this task. Whenever possible, a combined genome-guided/*de novo* strategy is recommended, as enhanced performance is observed [125]. A comprehensive overview of transcriptome assembly can be found in Ref. [121]. Evaluation of the assembly quality and transcriptome completeness can be assessed with Detonate [126], TransRate [127] and BUSCO [128].

4.2.4. *Visualization*

Alignment output SAM files are hard to be interpreted with common text editors, and therefore, a number of graphical browsers have been developed to inspect NGS sequencing data at any specific loci at nucleotide level. IGV [129], Tablet [130], Browser Genome [131] and UCSC [132] are extremely useful when validating novel transcripts and gene junctions, checking the coverage support for genomic variants and spot read piles, which may represent repetitive regions.

4.3. Downstream analyses

After conducting these general steps, the experiments can be directed to specific applications in order to address the scientific questions, designated as downstream analysis.

4.3.1. *Quantification and differential expression*

The primary goal of most RNA-seq projects is to quantify and compare the gene expression under different conditions and infer biological function to differential expression at gene or transcript level. Intra-sample abundance comparisons were commonly performed with

Reads Per Kilobase per Million (RPKM mapped reads) or Fragments Per Kilobase per Million (FPKM mapped reads) metrics. Their principle is to count the amount of raw reads mapped to each genomic feature and normalize considering the gene length and library depth. Although still widely applied, these normalization metrics should be avoided as RPKM has shown to be inconsistent and Transcripts Per Million (TPM) is preferable [133]. Raw reads counting can be obtained with feature counts [134] and HTSeq-count [135], which are capable of detecting multi-mapping reads, exon junctions and overlapping reference features. NOISeq [136] can be used to assess the count quality parameters, such as saturation and specificity, in a set of comprehensive plots.

DESeq [137], DESeq2 [138] and edgeR [139] packages are recommended for between-sample comparisons to detect differences in the relative abundances of genes [140]. Quantification at transcript level can be analyzed with Cufflinks [115] and RSEM [141] and compared with DESeq2, CuffDiff2 [142], BitSeq [143] or Ballgown [144]. Variations in expression between different conditions are usually measured in log2 fold-change units. DESeq2 can also perform pair-wise and time series analysis.

Generally, a control set of housekeeping genes should present non-differential expression and a high between replicates correlation (Spearman $R^2 \geq 0.9$) observable in Principal Component Analysis (PCA) plots [18]. For a set of 12 or less replicates, at gene level, edgeR or DESeq2 is recommended to detect differential expression and DESeq when more than 12 replicates are available [21]. Thresholds in log2 fold-change should be applied to increase the true positive and decrease the false positive rates, but this parameter is highly dependent on the amount of biological replicates, varying from 0.1 to 0.5 [21].

Recently, quasi-mapping (or pseudoalignment) approaches have been proposed for RNA-seq quantification, like Kallisto [145] and Salmon [146]. Their main difference is that reads are assigned to reference sequences without base-to-base alignment, making analyses usually considerably faster. They have shown comparable performance over complete mapping-based methods, can incorporate information from multi-mapping reads, and provide counts and abundances already as normalized TPM values, which can be used as input for differential expression analysis. These are promising although under development tools.

Although RNA-seq provides a precise and accurate estimation of RNA abundance, these findings are still widely required to be further validated through quantitative PCR, also known as qPCR or real-time PCR as it is still considered the gold standard for gene expression quantification. However, it is still questionable whether qPCR validation is still necessary for RNA-seq studies. High correlation between RNA-seq and qPCR results has been observed in previous studies [7, 147, 148]. Due to this high consistency, qPCR may be more useful when performed on different biological replicate samples from those already sequenced, confirming the DGE findings and validating the biological conclusions.

4.3.2. *Annotation*

In computational biology, annotation is the process of identifying the location and sequence of genomic elements and/or assigning biological function to them. Despite the annotation process

being mostly carried over genomic sequences, such as newly sequenced genomes, RNA-seq data can provide valuable information to improve existing annotations [149] or create novel transcript annotations for an unsequenced organism [123].

The major drawback of using genome sequences for annotation is that only features with patterns or conservation with annotated elements, such as open reading frames (ORFs), tRNAs and rRNAs can be inferred from it. On the other hand, RNA-seq data provide a new layer of information that allows precise identification of pattern less features such as untranslated regions (UTRs), non-coding RNAs and post-transcriptional events. Even though some features can be somewhat inferred through DNA sequences, for example, Transcription Start Site (TSS), TATA box/CpG islands and splicing sites, transcriptomic data still provide a more reliable annotation.

Transcriptome assembly, *de novo* or reference-guided, often reveals new potential transcripts whose functions are unknown. Before any further step can be made, it is crucial to gather information on these transcripts function in order to extract any meaningful answer.

The most common approach to annotate a transcript is to look for similar known transcripts or protein sequences in large databases. This is usually done using versatile tools like BLAST/BLASTX [150, 151] or DIAMOND [152] when looking for similar nucleotide or protein sequences. It is often better to perform searches at protein level since it is easier to find homology, as they tend to be more conserved than nucleotide sequences, especially if the study subject has no close species sequenced.

InterProScan [153] can be used to search for conserved protein signatures. This is especially useful when it is difficult to find full sequence homologs given that the study organism might be too divergent from species sequences available in the database. Protein families often present signature domains that are well conserved even among divergent species, so these signatures can give insights into the putative function of the protein. The process for annotating non-coding transcripts differs from protein coding transcripts. They usually present poor sequence conservation since their function relies on factors, such as secondary structure, rather than amino acid sequences. Therefore, their annotation process requires specialized software to detect those intrinsic characteristics of a given class of non-coding transcripts, for example, tRNAscan-SE [154] for tRNAs and RNAmmer [155] for rRNAs.

Given the importance of annotation, there are plenty of tools and pipelines developed to streamline this process. Some annotation tools like Blast2GO [156] are generic and very user-friendly, although it requires a paid license to use it. Others like Annocript [157], TRAPID [158] and Trinotate [159] are pipelines developed specifically for annotating transcriptomes. It is important to note that although automatic pipelines often ease and speed up the analysis, it comes at a cost of lesser control of the annotation process.

4.3.3. Enrichment analysis

Functional enrichment analysis is a computational method capable of determining whether a pre-defined set of genes shows significant differences between samples. The GSEA software from Broad Institute runs the original GSEA algorithm [160]. Although alternative algorithms

have been published since then, the original algorithm is still the most widely used. In order to perform an enrichment analysis from RNA-Seq data, the GSEAPreranked software is recommended and it requires two types of data: a gene set list and a ranked list.

A gene set is a set of genes related to the feature to be tested for enrichment. A variety of features can be tested from general features such as pathways and chromosome location, to more specific features such as cancer signatures or miRNAs targets. Gene sets can be obtained from the Molecular Signatures Database (MSigDB) that comprehends thousands of pre-defined gene sets, or it can be created by the user.

A ranked list of the genes needs to be provided to test if the chosen gene set is significantly enriched at either end of the ranking. The list can be ranked according to any quantitative feature such as gene expression or fold-change results from DGE analysis.

4.3.4. *Alternative splicing*

Alternative splicing (AS) is a post-transcriptional mechanism present in the majority of eukaryotes that greatly increases the diversity of proteins that can be encoded by a determined genome. This process occurs when particular regions of a gene are included or excluded, through splicing, from the final processed mRNA sequence. AS can occur in several ways, such as exon skipping, intron retention, alternative 5′ donor and 3′ receptor sites [161, 162], analysis of new AS events or patterns is relevant since many traits, especially genetic diseases such as cancers, are related with disorders in splicing patterns that generates aberrant variants [162, 163].

AS analysis by deep sequencing requires splice-aware programs capable of aligning transcripts reads to a reference genome while performing the difficult task of placing spliced reads across introns by determining the exon-intron boundaries. A systematic evaluation of splice-aware alignment programs for RNA-seq data performed by the RNA-seq Genome Annotation Assessment Project (RGASP) Consortium [109] tested 26 RNA-seq alignment protocols and concluded that, in general, GSNAP [164], MapSplice [165] and STAR [106] compared favorably to other methods. Still, two of this software (GSNAP and STAR) presented many false exons junctions in the output if they were not filtered based on the number of supporting alignments.

Following the alignment step, software like cufflinks [115], scripture [116] and StringTie [117] can be used to perform transcript reconstruction, which can reveal new splicing isoforms evidenced by the alignments. This step usually yields an updated GTF annotation file as output that can be used in subsequent steps.

If data from different conditions are available, differential AS analysis can be performed. With the alignment results (SAM file) and a GTF annotation file at hand, differential exon usage analysis can be performed with DEXSeq [166] and differential analysis of AS events, such as skipped exon, alternative 5′ and 3′ splice site, mutually exclusive exons, and retained intron events can be performed with rMATS [167]. There are plenty of other software specialized in performing differential AS analysis each one with their advantages and disadvantages, such as CuffDiff [115], Ballgown [144], SpliceR [168], MISO [169] and DiffSplice [170].

4.3.5. Fusion genes

Fusion genes or chimeras are aberrant alterations commonly found in tumor cells [171] that can be useful biomarkers or therapeutic targets [172]. They may originate from chromosomal rearrangements, insertions, deletions and inversions or even by trans-splicing events. The increasing throughput and reads length from NGS technologies have facilitated their detection and supported the development of several bioinformatic tools [173]. For fusion detection, most and more accurate methods rely on good quality read alignments supporting discordant mappings (read segments aligning to different genes) and both single- or paired-end sequencing, although paired data increase the probability of fusion detection [174]. A recent evaluation defined SOAPfuse [175], FusionCatcher [176] and JAFFA [177] the best tools among 18 options for real and simulated data, and their combination has shown increased performance, albeit high false-positive rates are still a reality in this field, with space for improvements [178].

4.3.6. miRNA

MicroRNAs (miRNAs) are a subset of small non-coding RNAs, usually 21–23 nt long that play a post-transcriptional regulatory role in several pathogenic and developmental processes [179]. These molecules are part of an RNA-induced silencing complex (RISC) containing Dicer, Argonaute and many associated proteins that can cause enhanced decay/cleavage of mRNA target, elongation and ribosomal binding inhibition, thus acting at transcriptional and translational levels [180].

A common miRNA pipeline follows the same steps as the conventional RNA-seq: (i) raw data must be preprocessed as previously described where adapters and low quality bases are trimmed with a minimum length filter (e.g., 18–21 nt for miRNAs), (ii) sequences are mapped to a reference (genome, RefSeq, miRBase) and raw counts are estimated, (iii) the raw count of mapped reads is normalized and (iv) downstream analysis is conducted to investigate biologically relevant questions. Due to its small nature, miRNA sequencing analysis has some caveats that require attention especially in steps (ii) and (iii).

The read mapping step is crucial for accurate miRNA abundance estimation, and therefore, the alignment algorithm must be carefully selected and adjusted to deal with its small size. Although a wide range of software are available to perform this task, some aligners are designed and optimized for specific tasks (e.g., SNP calling, splicing detection, gapped alignment) that might not be appropriate for the task at hand [181]. Compared with conventional RNA-seq, indels and splicing events are usually not relevant to miRNA alignment, and therefore, splice-aware aligners are not required for this task. To these extent general purpose aligners such as BWA-MEM, bowtie [182] and STAR [106] can be used. Most aligners default settings are set for conventional longer RNA-seq reads, and since miRNAs are very short, aligners' parameters should be tweaked. The default seed size for these aligners is longer than miRNA sizes and therefore should be set to a value that is at least shorter than the smallest read size. Given that sequencing errors might occur and the fact that many miRNAs often does not present an exact match with their target, it is recommended to allow at least one mismatch in the seeding and alignment process as well [183]. Also during the mapping step, it

is very common to find multi-mapping reads since we are dealing with very small sequences. Similarly to conventional RNA-seq, multi-mapping reads are usually not taken into account for the abundance estimation, since it is impossible to know from where the read was originated. As long as these aligners are properly set, they should yield similar results [181].

Please note that for the aforementioned pipeline, miRNA annotations or sequences are usually required for raw counting estimation. If annotations are not available for the study subject or looking for novel miRNAs candidates, algorithms such as miRdeep2 [184], miReNA [185] and miRanalyzer [186] can be used to annotate novel canonical and non-canonical miRNA.

After raw miRNAs abundances are estimated, a normalization step is required in order to remove bias of non-biological origin (e.g., sequencing depth, sample handling, library preparation). A good normalization technique should reduce those biases without generating noise, so that the remaining differences between samples are truly of biological origin. Previous comparative studies on normalization procedures for miRNA data resulted in conflicting results. A study from Garmire and Subramaniam [187] supported the use of quantile and Lowess normalization, while Tam et al. [181] and Dillies et al. [140] advocated for the use of Trimmed Mean of M (TMM) and Upper quartile (UQ) normalization. Nevertheless, the results from any of these methods and also DESeq2 normalization [138] method should be highly similar, while other normalization methods such as CPM, total count scaling and linear regression should be avoided since they tend to present higher variance and bias [181]. Several R/Bioconductor packages can be used to normalize the data and also run differential expression, such as edgeR [139] (TMM and UQ), DESeq2 [138] (DESeq normalization) and limma [188] (quantile and cyclic loess).

After all these processing steps, the resulting miRNA estimation is ready to conduct downstream analysis. This can be done with useful databases. Being the primary miRNA sequence repository, miRBase [189] contains several features that may help to investigate the roles for miRNAs of interest, such as annotations for a wide range of species, references links for studies and deep sequencing evidence.

4.3.7. eQTL

Quantitative trait loci (QTLs) are genomic regions that contain sequence variants that can affect any given trait. Since genome-wide association studies (GWAS) started [190], thousands of variants have been associated with complex traits and diseases. The process of assigning variants to a gene is relatively straightforward when variants are located in coding regions that can have a direct effect on a gene product; however, most variants are found in non-coding regions making difficult to identify the causal genes [191]. By integrating transcriptomic data, it is possible to identify causal genes for non-coding variants that affect its expression. When the trait in question is gene expression, they are referred as expression quantitative trait loci (eQTLs) that, similarly to other QTLs, are sequence variants capable of affecting the expression level of one or more genes that will ultimately result in different phenotypes. eQTLs can be classified according to the location of the QTL itself and its targeted gene, and according to the mechanism that affects the expression [192].

Regarding the eQTL-Gene position, when they are located close to the genes, they influence they are called local eQTLs. Local eQTLs can affect a gene in two ways: in *cis* (cis-eQTL) when the variant affects only the gene that is located on the same chromosome and not affecting the copy of the homologous chromosome, thus causing an allelic imbalance; and in *trans* (trans-eQTL) when the eQTLs do not affect the target expression directly, but instead affect an intermediate factor that will ultimately affect its target expression. Since the intermediate factor acts equally for both alleles, it does not cause allelic imbalance. On the other hand, eQTLs located further away from their target genes are referred as distant eQTLs, usually act in *trans* and are harder to find [192]. Several eQTL-mapping studies published in the past few years showed that many variants often affect gene expression levels of nearby and distant genes [193–197] highlighting the importance of integrating transcriptomic and genomic data.

Despite the mapping process for eQTL analysis being conceptually simple, since this analysis is dealing with allelic specific expression, some caution is required during its counting estimation. For the aligning process, general purpose aligners or variant aware aligners such as GSNAP [164] can be used. After the alignment, some steps are recommended for retrieving allelic-specific counts, such as removing duplicate reads that may arise from PCR artifacts. However, it is important that the choice for discarding a duplicate read is not done by mapping score as this might bias toward the reference allele [198]. Also, mapping bias should be controlled by filtering sites with likely bias [199]. Some tools like ASEReadCounter from GATK for allelic-specific expression implement these filters by default [200].

The GTEx portal is a valuable resource to study human gene expression and regulation related to genetic variation. It hosts data from several eQTL studies and much information on laboratory and analysis methods for eQTL [201].

5. Concluding remarks

In the past few years, recent advances in sequencing technologies allowed the cost-efficient generation of an unprecedented amount of biological information. Similarly, RNA-seq techniques are under continuous improvements allowing wide range applications and development of high level resolution experiments such as those based on the emergent single-cell RNA sequencing (scRNA-seq) field. To couple with this ever increasing data, several tools and pipelines have been constantly developed. The bioinformatics field changes in an astonishing pace, in a way that it is almost impossible to keep up with all the new tendencies, the overwhelming amount of available software and the controversial opinions in the scientific community. For some aspects, it is difficult to find a consensus on the best pipeline to be applied. This chapter goal was to guide RNA-seq users through its complex steps, providing a brief overview of the complete workflow, highlighting accessible protocols and currently available tools, most of which correlated with supporting benchmark studies.

http://dx.doi.org/10.5772/intechopen.69250

Author details

Michele Araújo Pereira[1*], Eddie Luidy Imada[2] and Rafael Lucas Muniz Guedes[1]

*Address all correspondence to: michele.pereira@hermespardini.com.br

1 Hermes Pardini Group, Vespasiano, Brazil

2 Federal University of Minas Gerais, Belo Horizonte, Brazil

References

[1] Ramsay G. DNA chips: State-of-the art. Nature Biotechnology. Jan 1998;**16**(1):40-44

[2] Adams MD, Kelley JM, Gocayne JD, Dubnick M, Polymeropoulos MH, Xiao H, et al. Complementary DNA sequencing: expressed sequence tags and human genome project. Science. 21 Jun 1991;**252**(5013):1651-1656

[3] Velculescu VE, Zhang L, Vogelstein B, Kinzler KW. Serial analysis of gene expression. Science (80-). 20 Oct 1995;**270**(5235):484-487

[4] Kodzius R, Kojima M, Nishiyori H, Nakamura M, Fukuda S, Tagami M, et al. CAGE: Cap analysis of gene expression. Nature Methods. 3 Mar 2006;**3**(3):211-222

[5] Brenner S, Johnson M, Bridgham J, Golda G, Lloyd DH, Johnson D. et al. Gene expression analysis by massively parallel signature sequencing (MPSS) on microbead arrays. Nature Biotechnology. Jun 2000;**18**(6):630-634

[6] Sanger F, Nicklen S, Coulson AR. DNA sequencing with chain-terminating inhibitors. Proceedings of the National Academy of Sciences. 1 Dec 1977;**74**(12):5463-5467

[7] Nagalakshmi U, Wang Z, Waern K, Shou C, Raha D, Gerstein M. et al. The transcriptional landscape of the yeast genome defined by RNA sequencing. Science (80-). 6 Jun 2008; **320**(5881):1344-1349

[8] Wang Z, Gerstein M, Snyder M. RNA-Seq: A revolutionary tool for transcriptomics. Nature Reviews Genetics. Jan 2009;**10**(1):57-63

[9] Goodwin S, McPherson JD, McCombie WR. Coming of age: Ten years of next-generation sequencing technologies. Nature Reviews Genetics. 17 May 2016 May;**17**(6):333-351

[10] van Dijk EL, Auger H, Jaszczyszyn Y, Thermes C. Ten years of next-generation sequencing technology. Trends in Genetics. Sep 2014;**30**(9):418-426

[11] Metzker ML. Sequencing technologies—The next generation. Nature Reviews Genetics. Jan 2010;**11**(1):31-46

[12] Scotty. Available from: http://bioinformatics.bc.edu/marthlab/scotty/scotty.php [Accessed: 3 February 2017]

[13] Hart SN, Therneau TM, Zhang Y, Poland GA, Kocher J-P. Calculating sample size estimates for RNA sequencing data. Journal of computational biology. Dec 2013;**20**(12):970-8

[14] Zhao S, Li C, Guo Y, Sheng Q and Shyr Y. RnaSeqSampleSize: RnaSeqSampleSize. R package version 1.8.0. 2017

[15] Shanker S, Paulson A, Edenberg HJ, Peak A, Perera A, Alekseyev YO, et al. Evaluation of commercially available RNA amplification kits for RNA sequencing using very low input amounts of total RNA. Journal of Biomolecular Techniques. Apr 2015;**26**(1):4-18

[16] Blainey P, Krzywinski M, Altman N. Points of significance: replication. Nature Methods.28 Aug 2014;**11**(9):879-880

[17] Fang Z, Cui X. Design and validation issues in RNA-seq experiments. Briefings in Bioinformatics. 1 May 2011;**12**(3):280-287

[18] Conesa A, Madrigal P, Tarazona S, Gomez-Cabrero D, Cervera A, McPherson A. et al. A survey of best practices for RNA-seq data analysis. Genome Biology. 26 Dec 2016;**17**(1):13

[19] Liu Y, Zhou J, White KP. RNA-seq differential expression studies: More sequence or more replication? Bioinformatics. 1 Feb 2014;**30**(3):301-304

[20] Ching T, Huang S, Garmire LX. Power analysis and sample size estimation for RNA-Seq differential expression. RNA. Nov 2014;**20**(11):1684-1696

[21] Schurch NJ, Schofield P, Gierliński M, Cole C, Sherstnev A, Singh V. et al. How many biological replicates are needed in an RNA-seq experiment and which differential expression tool should you use? RNA. Jun 2016;**22**(6):839-851

[22] Gu X. Statistical detection of differentially expressed genes based on RNA-seq: From biological to phylogenetic replicates. Briefings in Bioinformatics. Mar 2016;**17**(2):243-248

[23] Rhoads A, Au KF. PacBio sequencing and its applications. Genomics Proteomics Bioinformatics. Oct 2015;**13**(5):278-289

[24] Au KF, Sebastiano V, Afshar PT, Durruthy JD, Lee L, Williams BA. et al. Characterization of the human ESC transcriptome by hybrid sequencing. Proceedings of the National Academy of Sciences. 10 Dec 2013;**110**(50): E4821-E4830

[25] Love KR, Shah KA, Whittaker CA, Wu J, Bartlett MC, Ma D. et al. Comparative genomics and transcriptomics of *Pichia pastoris*. BMC Genomics. 5 Dec 2016;**17**(1):550

[26] Gao S, Ren Y, Sun Y, Wu Z, Ruan J, He B. et al. PacBio full-length transcriptome profiling of insect mitochondrial gene expression. RNA Biology. 16 Sep 2016;**13**(9):820-825

[27] Liu L, Li Y, Li S, Hu N, He Y, Pong R. et al. Comparison of next-generation sequencing systems. Journal of Biomedicine and Biotechnology. 2012;**2012**:1-11

[28] GLENN TC. Field guide to next-generation DNA sequencers. Molecular Ecology Resources. Sep 2011;**11**(5):759-769

http://dx.doi.org/10.5772/intechopen.69250

[29] Chu Y, Corey DR. RNA sequencing: platform selection, experimental design, and data interpretation. Nucleic Acid Therapeutics. Aug 2012;**22**(4):271-274

[30] Sims D, Sudbery I, Ilott NE, Heger A, Ponting CP. Sequencing depth and coverage: Key considerations in genomic analyses. Nature Reviews Genetics. 17 Jan 2014;**15**(2):121-132

[31] Tarazona S, Garcia-Alcalde F, Dopazo J, Ferrer A, Conesa A. Differential expression in RNA-seq: A matter of depth. Genome Research. 1 Dec 2011;**21**(12):2213-2223

[32] Lei R, Ye K, Gu Z, Sun X. Diminishing returns in next-generation sequencing (NGS) transcriptome data. Gene. Feb 2015;**557**(1):82-87

[33] Hou R, Yang Z, Li M, Xiao H. Impact of the next-generation sequencing data depth on various biological result inferences. Science China Life Sciences. 8 Feb 2013;**56**(2):104-109

[34] Cho H, Davis J, Li X, Smith KS, Battle A, Montgomery SB. High-resolution transcriptome analysis with long-read RNA sequencing. Buratti E, editor. PLoS One. 24 Sep 2014;**9**(9): e108095

[35] Chhangawala S, Rudy G, Mason CE, Rosenfeld JA. The impact of read length on quantification of differentially expressed genes and splice junction detection. Genome Biology. 23 Dec 2015;**16**(1):131

[36] Tilgner H, Jahanbani F, Blauwkamp T, Moshrefi A, Jaeger E, Chen F. et al. Comprehensive transcriptome analysis using synthetic long-read sequencing reveals molecular co-association of distant splicing events. Nature Biotechnology. 18 May 2015;**33**(7):736-742

[37] Sharon D, Tilgner H, Grubert F, Snyder M. A single-molecule long-read survey of the human transcriptome. Nature Biotechnology. 13 Oct 2013;**31**(11):1009-1014

[38] Tilgner H, Raha D, Habegger L, Mohiuddin M, Gerstein M, Snyder M. Accurate identification and analysis of human mRNA isoforms using deep long read sequencing. G3: Genes|Genomes|Genetics. Mar 2013;**3**(3):387-397

[39] Chang Z, Wang Z, Li G. The impacts of read length and transcriptome complexity for De Novo assembly: A simulation study. Papavasiliou FN, editor. PLoS One. 15 Apr 2014;**9**(4):e94825

[40] Levin JZ, Yassour M, Adiconis X, Nusbaum C, Thompson DA, Friedman N. et al. Comprehensive comparative analysis of strand-specific RNA sequencing methods. Nature Methods. 15 Sep 2010;**7**(9):709-715

[41] Head SR, Komori HK, LaMere SA, Whisenant T, Van Nieuwerburgh F, Salomon DR. et al. Library construction for next-generation sequencing: Overviews and challenges. Biotechniques. 1 Feb 2014;**56**(2):61-77

[42] Zhao W, He X, Hoadley KA, Parker JS, Hayes D, Perou CM. Comparison of RNA-Seq by poly (A) capture, ribosomal RNA depletion, and DNA microarray for expression profiling. BMC Genomics. 2014;**15**(1):419

[43] Parkhomchuk D, Borodina T, Amstislavskiy V, Banaru M, Hallen L, Krobitsch S. et al. Transcriptome analysis by strand-specific sequencing of complementary DNA. Nucleic Acids Research. 1 Oct 2009;**37**(18):e123-e123

[44] Illumina. Directional mRNA-Seq Sample Preparation Guide. Part # 15018460 Rev. A. Oct 2010. Available from: https://support.illumina.com/downloads/directional_mrna-seq_sample_preparation_guide.html [Accessed: 16 May 2017]

[45] van Dijk EL, Jaszczyszyn Y, Thermes C. Library preparation methods for next-generation sequencing: Tone down the bias. Experimental Cell Research. Mar 2014;**322**(1):12-20

[46] Baker SC, Bauer SR, Beyer RP, Brenton JD, Bromley B, Burrill J. et al. The external RNA controls consortium: A progress report. Nature Methods. Oct 2005;**2**(10):731-734

[47] Jiang L, Schlesinger F, Davis CA, Zhang Y, Li R, Salit M. et al. Synthetic spike-in standards for RNA-seq experiments. Genome Research. 1 Sep 2011;**21**(9):1543-1551

[48] Hardwick SA, Chen WY, Wong T, Deveson IW, Blackburn J, Andersen SB. et al. Spliced synthetic genes as internal controls in RNA sequencing experiments. Nature Methods. 8 Aug 2016;**13**(9):792-798

[49] Munro SA, Lund SP, Pine PS, Binder H, Clevert D-A, Conesa A. et al. Assessing technical performance in differential gene expression experiments with external spike-in RNA control ratio mixtures. Nature Communications. 25 Sep 2014;**5**:5125

[50] Wong T, Deveson IW, Hardwick SA, Mercer TR. ANAQUIN: A software toolkit for the analysis of spike-in controls for next generation sequencing. Bioinformatics. 27 Jan 2017;btx038

[51] Nielsen H. Working with RNA. Methods in Molecular Biology. 2011;**703**:15-28

[52] Thatcher SA. DNA/RNA Preparation for molecular detection. Clinical Chemistry. 1 Jan 2015;**61**(1):89-99

[53] Sellin Jeffries MK, Kiss AJ, Smith AW, Oris JT. A comparison of commercially-available automated and manual extraction kits for the isolation of total RNA from small tissue samples. BMC Biotechnology. 14 Dec 2014;**14**(1):94

[54] Mueller O, Lightfoot S, Schroeder A. RNA Integrity Number (RIN) -Standardization of RNA quality control. Agilent Technologies. 2004;1-8. 5989-1165EN

[55] Schroeder A, Mueller O, Stocker S, Salowsky R, Leiber M, Gassmann M. et al. The RIN: an RNA integrity number for assigning integrity values to RNA measurements. BMC Molecular Biology. 31 Jan 2006;**7**(1):3

[56] Gallego Romero I, Pai AA, Tung J, Gilad Y. RNA-seq: Impact of RNA degradation on transcript quantification. BMC Biology. 2014;**12**(1):42

[57] Winnebeck EC, Millar CD, Warman GR. Why does insect RNA look degraded? Journal of Insect Science. Sep 2010;**10**(159):1-7

[58] Wieczorek D, Delauriere L, Schagat T. Methods of RNA quality assessment. Promega Corporation Website. October 2012;1-14. Available from: http://www.promega.com.br/resources/pubhub/methods-of-rna-quality-assessment [Accessed: 16 May 2017]

[59] Aranda R, Dineen SM, Craig RL, Guerrieri RA, Robertson JM. Comparison and evaluation of RNA quantification methods using viral, prokaryotic, and eukaryotic RNA over a 104 concentration range. Analytical Biochemistry. Apr 2009;**387**(1):122-127

[60] Ferreira EN, de Campos Molina G, Puga RD, Nagai MA, Campos AHJFM, Guimarães GC. et al. Linear mRNA amplification approach for RNAseq from limited amount of RNA. Gene. Jun 2015;**564**(2):220-227

[61] Sinicropi D, Morlan J, City F. Methods for depleting RNA from nucleic acid samples. US20110111409. Vol. 1; 2011

[62] Morlan JD, Qu K, Sinicropi D V. Selective depletion of rRNA enables whole transcriptome profiling of archival fixed tissue. Dadras SS, editor. PLoS One. 10 Aug 2012;**7**(8):e42882

[63] Zhulidov PA. Simple cDNA normalization using kamchatka crab duplex-specific nuclease. Nucleic Acids Research. 13 Feb 2004;**32**(3):37e-37

[64] Yi H, Cho Y-J, Won S, Lee J-E, Jin Yu H, Kim S. et al. Duplex-specific nuclease efficiently removes rRNA for prokaryotic RNA-seq. Nucleic Acids Research. 1 Nov 2011;**39**(20):e140-e140

[65] Adiconis X, Borges-Rivera D, Satija R, DeLuca DS, Busby MA, Berlin AM. et al. Comparative analysis of RNA sequencing methods for degraded or low-input samples. Nature Methods. 19 May 2013;**10**(7):623-629

[66] Knierim E, Lucke B, Schwarz JM, Schuelke M, Seelow D. Systematic comparison of three methods for fragmentation of long-range PCR products for next generation sequencing. Gilbert MTP, editor. PLoS One. 2011 30 Nov;**6**(11):e28240

[67] Hansen KD, Brenner SE, Dudoit S. Biases in Illumina transcriptome sequencing caused by random hexamer priming. Nucleic Acids Research. 1 Jul 2010;**38**(12):e131-e131

[68] van Gurp TP, McIntyre LM, Verhoeven KJF. Consistent errors in first strand cDNA due to random hexamer mispriming. Gibas C, editor. PLoS One. 30 Dec 2013;**8**(12):e85583

[69] Gubler U, Hoffman BJ. A simple and very efficient method for generating cDNA libraries. Gene. Nov 1983;**25**(2-3):263-269

[70] Zhu YY, Machleder EM, Chenchik A, Li R, Siebert PD. Reverse transcriptase template switching: A SMART approach for full-length cDNA library construction. Biotechniques. Apr 2001;**30**(4):892-897

[71] RNA-seq data analysis bioinformatic tools. Available from: https://omictools.com/rna-seq-category [Accessed: 3 February 2017]

[72] Afgan E, Baker D, van den Beek M, Blankenberg D, Bouvier D, Čech M. et al. The Galaxy platform for accessible, reproducible and collaborative biomedical analyses: 2016 update. Nucleic Acids Research. 8 Jul 2016;**44**(W1):W3-10

[73] Illumina BaseSpace. Available from: https://basespace.illumina.com [Accessed: 3 February 2017]

[74] Geneious. Available from: http://www.geneious.com [Accessed: 3 February 2017]

[75] FASTQ description. Available from: https://en.wikipedia.org/wiki/FASTQ_format [Accessed: 3 February 2017]

[76] Picard. Available from: http://broadinstitute.github.io/picard [Accessed: 3 February 2017]

[77] BamUtil. Available from: http://genome.sph.umich.edu/wiki/BamUtil [Accessed: 3 February 2017]

[78] Barnett DW, Garrison EK, Quinlan AR, Stromberg MP, Marth GT. BamTools: A C++ API and toolkit for analyzing and managing BAM files. Bioinformatics. 15 Jun 2011;**27**(12): 1691-1692

[79] Andrews S. FastQC: A quality control tool for high throughput sequence data. 2010. Available from: http://www.bioinformatics.babraham.ac.uk/projects/fastqc [Accessed: 3 February 2017]

[80] Schmieder R, Edwards R. Quality control and preprocessing of metagenomic datasets. Bioinformatics. 15 Mar 2011;**27**(6):863-864

[81] Del Fabbro C, Scalabrin S, Morgante M, Giorgi FM. An extensive evaluation of read trimming effects on illumina NGS data analysis. Seo J-S, editor. PLoS One. 23 Dec 2013;**8**(12):e85024

[82] Martin M. Cutadapt removes adapter sequences from high-throughput sequencing reads. EMBnet.journal. 2 May 2011;**17**(1):10

[83] FASTX-toolkit. Available from: http://hannonlab.cshl.edu/fastx_toolkit/index.html [Accessed: 3 February 2017]

[84] Bolger AM, Lohse M, Usadel B. Trimmomatic: a flexible trimmer for Illumina sequence data. Bioinformatics. 1 Aug 2014;**30**(15):2114-2120

[85] Williams CR, Baccarella A, Parrish JZ, Kim CC. Trimming of sequence reads alters RNA-Seq gene expression estimates. BMC Bioinformatics. 25 Dec 2016;**17**(1):103

[86] MacManes MD. On the optimal trimming of high-throughput mRNA sequence data. Frontiers in Genetics. 31 Jan 2014;**5**:13

[87] Tattini L, D'Aurizio R, Magi A. Detection of genomic structural variants from next-generation sequencing data. Frontiers in Bioengineering and Biotechnology. 25 Jun 2015;**3**:92

[88] Magoc T, Salzberg SL. FLASH: fast length adjustment of short reads to improve genome assemblies. Bioinformatics. 1 Nov 2011;**27**(21):2957-2963

[89] Zhang J, Kobert K, Flouri T, Stamatakis A. PEAR: A fast and accurate Illumina Paired-End reAd mergeR. Bioinformatics. 1 Mar 2014;**30**(5):614-620

[90] Le H-S, Schulz MH, McCauley BM, Hinman VF, Bar-Joseph Z. Probabilistic error correction for RNA sequencing. Nucleic Acids Research. 1 May 2013;**41**(10):e109-e109

[91] Song L, Florea L. Rcorrector: Efficient and accurate error correction for Illumina RNA-seq reads. Gigascience. 19 Dec 2015;**4**(1):48

[92] Altschul SF, Gish W, Miller W, Myers EW, Lipman DJ. Basic local alignment search tool. Journal of Molecular Biology. Oct 1990;**215**(3):403-410

[93] Fonseca NA, Rung J, Brazma A, Marioni JC. Tools for mapping high-throughput sequencing data. Bioinformatics. 1 Dec 2012;**28**(24):3169-3177

[94] Homer N, Merriman B, Nelson SF. BFAST: An alignment tool for large scale genome resequencing. Creighton C, editor. PLoS One. 11 Nov 2009;**4**(11):e7767

[95] Wu TD, Nacu S. Fast and SNP-tolerant detection of complex variants and splicing in short reads. Bioinformatics. 1 Apr 2010;**26**(7):873-881

[96] Li H, Ruan J, Durbin R. Mapping short DNA sequencing reads and calling variants using mapping quality scores. Genome Research. 1 Nov 2008;**18**(11):1851-1881

[97] Lee W-P, Stromberg MP, Ward A, Stewart C, Garrison EP, Marth GT. MOSAIK: A hash-based algorithm for accurate next-generation sequencing short-read mapping. Hsiao CK, editor. PLoS One. 5 Mar 2014;**9**(3):e90581

[98] Novoalign. Available from: http://www.novocraft.com [Accessed: 3 February 2017]

[99] Smith AD, Xuan Z, Zhang MQ. Using quality scores and longer reads improves accuracy of Solexa read mapping. BMC Bioinformatics. 2008;**9**(1):128

[100] Rumble SM, Lacroute P, Dalca A V., Fiume M, Sidow A, Brudno M. SHRiMP: Accurate mapping of short color-space reads. Wasserman WW, editor. PLoS Computational Biology. 22 May 2009;**5**(5):e1000386

[101] Langmead B, Salzberg SL. Fast gapped-read alignment with Bowtie 2. Nature Methods. 4 Mar 2012;**9**(4):357-359

[102] Kim D, Pertea G, Trapnell C, Pimentel H, Kelley R, Salzberg SL. TopHat2: Accurate alignment of transcriptomes in the presence of insertions, deletions and gene fusions. Genome Biology. 2013;**14**(4):R36

[103] Kim D, Langmead B, Salzberg SL. HISAT: A fast spliced aligner with low memory requirements. Nature Methods. 9 Mar 2015;**12**(4):357-360

[104] Li H, Durbin R. Fast and accurate short read alignment with Burrows-Wheeler transform. Bioinformatics. 15 Jul 2009;**25**(14):1754-1760

[105] Huang S, Zhang J, Li R, Zhang W, He Z, Lam T-W, et al. SOAPsplice: Genome-wide ab initio detection of splice junctions from RNA-Seq data. Frontiers in Genetics. 7 Jul 2011;**2**:46

[106] Dobin A, Davis CA, Schlesinger F, Drenkow J, Zaleski C, Jha S, et al. STAR: ultrafast universal RNA-seq aligner. Bioinformatics. 1 Jan 2013;**29**(1):15-21

[107] Chen LY, Wei K-C, Huang AC-Y, Wang K, Huang C-Y, Yi D, et al. RNASEQR—A streamlined and accurate RNA-seq sequence analysis program. Nucleic Acids Researc. 1 Mar 2012;**40**(6):e42-e42

[108] Lindner R, Friedel CC. A comprehensive evaluation of alignment algorithms in the context of RNA-Seq. Salzberg SL, editor. PLoS One. 26 Dec 2012;**7**(12):e52403

[109] Engström PG, Steijger T, Sipos B, Grant GR, Kahles A, Alioto T. et al. Systematic evaluation of spliced alignment programs for RNA-seq data. Nature Methods. 3 Nov 2013;**10**(12):1185-1191

[110] Li H, Handsaker B, Wysoker A, Fennell T, Ruan J, Homer N. et al. The sequence alignment/Map format and SAMtools. Bioinformatics. 15 Aug 2009;**25**(16):2078-2079

[111] Okonechnikov K, Conesa A, García-Alcalde F. Qualimap 2: Advanced multi-sample quality control for high-throughput sequencing data. Bioinformatics. 1 Oct 2015;btv566

[112] BAMstats. Available from: http://bamstats.sourceforge.net/ [Accessed: 3 February 2017]

[113] Lassmann T, Hayashizaki Y, Daub CO. SAMStat: Monitoring biases in next generation sequencing data. Bioinformatics. 1 Jan 2011;**27**(1):130-131

[114] Pan Q, Shai O, Lee LJ, Frey BJ, Blencowe BJ. Deep surveying of alternative splicing complexity in the human transcriptome by high-throughput sequencing. Nature Genetics. 2 Dec 2008;**40**(12):1413-1415

[115] Trapnell C, Williams BA, Pertea G, Mortazavi A, Kwan G, van Baren MJ. et al. Transcript assembly and quantification by RNA-Seq reveals unannotated transcripts and isoform switching during cell differentiation. Nature Biotechnology. 2 May 2010;**28**(5):511-515

[116] Guttman M, Garber M, Levin JZ, Donaghey J, Robinson J, Adiconis X. et al. Ab initio reconstruction of cell type–specific transcriptomes in mouse reveals the conserved multi-exonic structure of lincRNAs. Nature Biotechnology. 2 May 2010;**28**(5):503-510

[117] Pertea M, Pertea GM, Antonescu CM, Chang T-C, Mendell JT, Salzberg SL. StringTie enables improved reconstruction of a transcriptome from RNA-seq reads. Nature Biotechnology. 18 Feb 2015;**33**(3):290-295

[118] Florea LD, Salzberg SL. Genome-guided transcriptome assembly in the age of next-generation sequencing. IEEE/ACM Transactions on Computational Biology and Bioinformatics. 10(5):1234-1240

[119] Martin J, Bruno VM, Fang Z, Meng X, Blow M, Zhang T. et al. Rnnotator: An automated de novo transcriptome assembly pipeline from stranded RNA-Seq reads. BMC Genomics. 2010;**11**(1):663

[120] Robertson G, Schein J, Chiu R, Corbett R, Field M, Jackman SD. et al. De novo assembly and analysis of RNA-seq data. Nature Methods. 10 Nov 2010;**7**(11):909-912

[121] Martin JA, Wang Z. Next-generation transcriptome assembly. Nature Reviews Genetics. 7 Sep 2011;**12**(10):671-682

[122] Brown CT, Howe A, Zhang Q, Pyrkosz AB, Brom TH. A reference-free algorithm for computational normalization of shotgun sequencing data. 21 Mar 2012. arXiv:1203.4802v2 [q-bio.GN]. 1-18

[123] Grabherr MG, Haas BJ, Yassour M, Levin JZ, Thompson DA, Amit I. et al. Full-length transcriptome assembly from RNA-Seq data without a reference genome. Nature Biotechnology. 15 May 2011;**29**(7):644-652

[124] Schulz MH, Zerbino DR, Vingron M, Birney E. Oases: Robust de novo RNA-seq assembly across the dynamic range of expression levels. Bioinformatics. 15 Apr 2012;**28**(8): 1086-1092

[125] Jain P, Krishnan NM, Panda B. Augmenting transcriptome assembly by combining de novo and genome-guided tools. PeerJ. 15 Aug 2013;**1**:e133

[126] Li B, Fillmore N, Bai Y, Collins M, Thomson JA, Stewart R. et al. Evaluation of de novo transcriptome assemblies from RNA-Seq data. Genome Biology. 21 Dec 2014;**15**(12):553

[127] Smith-Unna R, Boursnell C, Patro R, Hibberd JM, Kelly S. TransRate: reference-free quality assessment of de novo transcriptome assemblies. Genome Research. 26 Aug 2016;(**8**): 1134-1144

[128] Simão FA, Waterhouse RM, Ioannidis P, Kriventseva E V, Zdobnov EM. BUSCO: Assessing genome assembly and annotation completeness with single-copy orthologs. Bioinformatics. 1 Oct 2015;**31**(19):3210-3212

[129] Thorvaldsdottir H, Robinson JT, Mesirov JP. Integrative Genomics Viewer (IGV): High-performance genomics data visualization and exploration. Briefings in Bioinformatics. 1 Mar 2013;**14**(2):178-192

[130] Milne I, Stephen G, Bayer M, Cock PJA, Pritchard L, Cardle L. et al. Using tablet for visual exploration of second-generation sequencing data. Briefings in Bioinformatics. Mar 2013;**14**(2):193-202

[131] Schmid-Burgk JL, Hornung V. BrowserGenome.org: web-based RNA-seq data analysis and visualization. Nature Methods. 29 Oct 2015;**12**(11):1001-1001

[132] Kuhn RM, Haussler D, Kent WJ. The UCSC genome browser and associated tools. Briefings in Bioinformatics. Mar 2013;**14**(2):144-161

[133] Wagner GP, Kin K, Lynch VJ. Measurement of mRNA abundance using RNA-seq data: RPKM measure is inconsistent among samples. Theory in Biosciences. 8 Dec 2012;**131** (4):281-285

[134] Liao Y, Smyth GK, Shi W. Feature counts: an efficient general purpose program for assigning sequence reads to genomic features. Bioinformatics. 1 Apr 2014;**30**(7):923-930

[135] Anders S, Pyl PT, Huber W. HTSeq--a Python framework to work with high-throughput sequencing data. Bioinformatics. 15 Jan 2015;**31**(2):166-169

[136] Tarazona S, Furió-Tarí P, Turrà D, Pietro A Di, Nueda MJ, Ferrer A. et al. Data quality aware analysis of differential expression in RNA-seq with NOISeq R/Bioc package. Nucleic Acids Research. 16 Jul 2015;gkv711

[137] Anders S, Huber W. Differential expression analysis for sequence count data. Genome Biology. 2010;**11**(10):R106

[138] Love MI, Huber W, Anders S. Moderated estimation of fold change and dispersion for RNA-seq data with DESeq2. Genome Biology. 5 Dec 2014;**15**(12):550

[139] Robinson MD, McCarthy DJ, Smyth GK. edgeR: A bioconductor package for differential expression analysis of digital gene expression data. Bioinformatics. 1 Jan 2010;**26**(1): 139-140

[140] Dillies M-A, Rau A, Aubert J, Hennequet-Antier C, Jeanmougin M, Servant N, et al. A comprehensive evaluation of normalization methods for Illumina high-throughput RNA sequencing data analysis. Briefings in Bioinformatics. 1 Nov 2013;**14**(6):671-683

[141] Li B, Dewey CN. RSEM: Accurate transcript quantification from RNA-Seq data with or without a reference genome. BMC Bioinformatics. 2011;**12**(1):323

[142] Trapnell C, Hendrickson DG, Sauvageau M, Goff L, Rinn JL, Pachter L. Differential analysis of gene regulation at transcript resolution with RNA-seq. Nature Biotechnology. 9 Dec 2012;**31**(1):46-53

[143] Glaus P, Honkela A, Rattray M. Identifying differentially expressed transcripts from RNA-seq data with biological variation. Bioinformatics. 1 Jul 2012;**28**(13):1721-1728

[144] Frazee AC, Pertea G, Jaffe AE, Langmead B, Salzberg SL, Leek JT. Ballgown bridges the gap between transcriptome assembly and expression analysis. Nature Biotechnology. 6 Mar 2015;**33**(3):243-236

[145] Bray NL, Pimentel H, Melsted P, Pachter L. Near-optimal probabilistic RNA-seq quantification. Nature Biotechnology. 4 Apr 2016;**34**(5):525-527

[146] Patro R, Duggal G, Love MI, Irizarry RA, Kingsford C. Salmon provides fast and bias-aware quantification of transcript expression. Nature Methods. Apr 2017;**14**(4):417-419

[147] Griffith M, Griffith OL, Mwenifumbo J, Goya R, Morrissy AS, Morin RD. et al. Alternative expression analysis by RNA sequencing. Nature Methods. 12 Oct 2010;**7**(10):843-847

[148] Wu AR, Neff NF, Kalisky T, Dalerba P, Treutlein B, Rothenberg ME. et al. Quantitative assessment of single-cell RNA-sequencing methods. Nature Methods. 20 Oct 2013; **11**(1):41-46

[149] Boley N, Stoiber MH, Booth BW, Wan KH, Hoskins RA, Bickel PJ. et al. Genome-guided transcript assembly by integrative analysis of RNA sequence data. Nature Biotechnology. 16 Mar 2014;**32**(4):341-346

[150] Altschul SF, Madden TL, Schäffer AA, Zhang J, Zhang Z, Miller W. et al. Gapped BLAST and PSI-BLAST: A new generation of protein database search programs. Nucleic Acids Research. 1 Sep 1997;**25**(17):3389-3402

[151] Camacho C, Coulouris G, Avagyan V, Ma N, Papadopoulos J, Bealer K. et al. BLAST+: Architecture and applications. BMC Bioinformatics. 2009;**10**(1):421

[152] Buchfink B, Xie C, Huson DH. Fast and sensitive protein alignment using DIAMOND. Nature Methods. 17 Nov 2014;**12**(1):59-60

[153] Zdobnov EM, Apweiler R. InterProScan—An integration platform for the signature-recognition methods in InterPro. Bioinformatics. Sep 2001;**17**(9):847-848

[154] Lowe TM, Eddy SR. tRNAscan-SE: A program for improved detection of transfer RNA genes in genomic sequence. Nucleic Acids Research. 1 Mar 1997;**25**(5):955-964

[155] Lagesen K, Hallin P, Rodland EA, Staerfeldt H-H, Rognes T, Ussery DW. RNAmmer: Consistent and rapid annotation of ribosomal RNA genes. Nucleic Acids Research. 16 Apr 2007;**35**(9):3100-3108

[156] Conesa A, Götz S, García-Gómez JM, Terol J, Talón M, Robles M. Blast2GO: A universal tool for annotation, visualization and analysis in functional genomics research. Bioinformatics. 15 Sep 2005;**21**(18):3674-3676

[157] Musacchia F, Basu S, Petrosino G, Salvemini M, Sanges R. Annocript: A flexible pipeline for the annotation of transcriptomes able to identify putative long noncoding RNAs. Bioinformatics. 1 Jul 2015;**31**(13):2199-2201

[158] Van Bel M, Proost S, Van Neste C, Deforce D, Van de Peer Y, Vandepoele K. TRAPID: An efficient online tool for the functional and comparative analysis of de novo RNA-Seq transcriptomes. Genome Biology. 2013;**14**(12):R134

[159] Trinotate. Available from: https://trinotate.github.io/ [Accessed: 3 February 2017]

[160] Subramanian A, Tamayo P, Mootha VK, Mukherjee S, Ebert BL, Gillette MA. et al. Gene set enrichment analysis: A knowledge-based approach for interpreting genome-wide expression profiles. Proceedings of the National Academy of Sciences. 25 Oct 2005;**102**(43):15545-15550

[161] Black DL. Mechanisms of alternative pre-messenger RNA splicing. Annual Review of Biochemistry. Jun 2003;**72**(1):291-336

[162] Matlin AJ, Clark F, Smith CWJ. Understanding alternative splicing: Towards a cellular code. Nature Reviews Molecular Cell Biology. May 2005;**6**(5):386-398

[163] Roy BM, Haupt LR. Griffiths L. Review: Alternative Splicing (AS) of genes as an approach for generating protein complexity. Current Genomics. 1 Apr 2013;**14**(3):182-194

[164] Wu TD, Reeder J, Lawrence M, Becker G, Brauer MJ. GMAP and GSNAP for genomic sequence alignment: Enhancements to speed, accuracy, and functionality. 2016;**1418**:283-334

[165] Wang K, Singh D, Zeng Z, Coleman SJ, Huang Y, Savich GL. et al. MapSplice: Accurate mapping of RNA-seq reads for splice junction discovery. Nucleic Acids Research. 1 Oct 2010;**38**(18):e178-e178

[166] Anders S, Reyes A, Huber W. Detecting differential usage of exons from RNA-seq data. Genome Research. 1 Oct 2012;**22**(10):2008-2017

[167] Shen S, Park JW, Lu Z, Lin L, Henry MD, Wu YN. et al. rMATS: Robust and flexible detection of differential alternative splicing from replicate RNA-Seq data. Proceedings of the National Academy of Sciences. 23 Dec 2014;**111**(51):E5593-E5601

[168] Vitting-Seerup K, Porse B, Sandelin A, Waage J. SpliceR: An R package for classification of alternative splicing and prediction of coding potential from RNA-seq data. BMC Bioinformatics. 2014;**15**(1):81

[169] Katz Y, Wang ET, Airoldi EM, Burge CB. Analysis and design of RNA sequencing experiments for identifying isoform regulation. Nature Methods. 7 Nov 2010;**7**(12):1009-1015

[170] Hu Y, Huang Y, Du Y, Orellana CF, Singh D, Johnson AR. et al. DiffSplice: The genome-wide detection of differential splicing events with RNA-seq. Nucleic Acids Research. 1 Jan 2013;**41**(2):e39-e39

[171] Mertens F, Johansson B, Fioretos T, Mitelman F. The emerging complexity of gene fusions in cancer. Nature Reviews Cancer. 22 May 2015;**15**(6):371-381

[172] Capdeville R, Buchdunger E, Zimmermann J, Matter A. Glivec (STI571, imatinib), a rationally developed, targeted anticancer drug. Nature Reviews Drug Discovery. Jul 2002; **1**(7):493-502

[173] Liu S, Tsai W-H, Ding Y, Chen R, Fang Z, Huo Z. et al. Comprehensive evaluation of fusion transcript detection algorithms and a meta-caller to combine top performing methods in paired-end RNA-seq data. Nucleic Acids Research. 18 Mar 2016;**44**(5):e47-e47

[174] Bashir A, Volik S, Collins C, Bafna V, Raphael BJ. Evaluation of Paired-End Sequencing strategies for detection of genome rearrangements in cancer. Ouzounis CA, editor. PLOS Computational Biology. 25 Apr 2008;**4**(4):e1000051

[175] Jia W, Qiu K, He M, Song P, Zhou Q, Zhou F. et al. SOAPfuse: An algorithm for identifying fusion transcripts from paired-end RNA-Seq data. Genome Biology. 2013;**14**(2):R12

[176] Nicorici D, Satalan M, Edgren H, Kangaspeska S, Murumagi A, Kallioniemi O, et al. FusionCatcher—A tool for finding somatic fusion genes in paired-end RNA-sequencing data. bioRxiv. 19 Nov 2014. 1:11

[177] Davidson NM, Majewski IJ, Oshlack A. JAFFA: High sensitivity transcriptome-focused fusion gene detection. Genome Medicine. 11 Dec 2015;**7**(1):43

[178] Carrara M, Beccuti M, Lazzarato F, Cavallo F, Cordero F, Donatelli S. et al. State-of-the-Art Fusion-Finder algorithms sensitivity and specificity. BioMed Research International. 2013;**2013**:1-6

[179] Lai EC. Micro RNAs are complementary to 3′ UTR sequence motifs that mediate negative post-transcriptional regulation. Nature Genetics. 18 Apr 2002;**30**(4):363-364

[180] Iorio M V, Croce CM. MicroRNA dysregulation in cancer: diagnostics, monitoring and therapeutics. A comprehensive review. EMBO Molecular Medicin. Mar 2012;**4**(3):143-159

[181] Tam S, Tsao M-S, McPherson JD. Optimization of miRNA-seq data preprocessing. Briefings in Bioinformatics. 1 Nov 2015;**16**(6):950-963

[182] Langmead B, Trapnell C, Pop M, Salzberg SL. Ultrafast and memory-efficient alignment of short DNA sequences to the human genome. Genome Biology. 2009;**10**(3):R25

[183] Friedman RC, Farh KK-H, Burge CB, Bartel DP. Most mammalian mRNAs are conserved targets of microRNAs. Genome Research. Jan19 2009;(1):92-105

[184] Friedländer MR, Mackowiak SD, Li N, Chen W, Rajewsky N. miRDeep2 accurately identifies known and hundreds of novel microRNA genes in seven animal clades. Nucleic Acids Research. Jan 2012;**40**(1):37-52

[185] Mathelier A, Carbone A. MIReNA: Finding microRNAs with high accuracy and no learning at genome scale and from deep sequencing data. Bioinformatics. Sep 15 2010;**26**(18):2226-2234

[186] Hackenberg M, Rodriguez-Ezpeleta N, Aransay AM. miRanalyzer: An update on the detection and analysis of microRNAs in high-throughput sequencing experiments. Nucleic Acids Research. 1 Jul 2011;**39**(Suppl):W132-W138

[187] Garmire LX, Subramaniam S. Evaluation of normalization methods in mammalian microRNA-Seq data. RNA. Jun 2012;**18**(6):1279-1288

[188] Ritchie ME, Phipson B, Wu D, Hu Y, Law CW, Shi W. et al. Limma powers differential expression analyses for RNA-sequencing and microarray studies. Nucleic Acids Research. 20 Apr 2015;**43**(7):e47

[189] Griffiths-Jones S, Grocock RJ, van Dongen S, Bateman A, Enright AJ. miRBase: MicroRNA sequences, targets and gene nomenclature. Nucleic Acids Research. 1 Jan 2006;**34**(Database issue):D140-D144

[190] Klein RJ. Complement factor H polymorphism in age-related macular degeneration. Science (80-). 15 Apr 2005;**308**(5720):385-389

[191] Westra H-J, Peters MJ, Esko T, Yaghootkar H, Schurmann C, Kettunen J. et al. Systematic identification of trans eQTLs as putative drivers of known disease associations. Nature Genetics. 8 Sep 2013;**45**(10):1238-1243

[192] Albert FW, Kruglyak L. The role of regulatory variation in complex traits and disease. Nature Reviews Genetics. Apr 2015;**16**(4):197-212

[193] Fehrmann RSN, Jansen RC, Veldink JH, Westra H-J, Arends D, Bonder MJ. et al. Trans-eQTLs reveal that independent genetic variants associated with a complex phenotype converge on intermediate genes, with a major role for the HLA. PLoS Genetics. Aug 2011;**7**(8):e1002197

[194] Nicolae DL, Gamazon E, Zhang W, Duan S, Dolan ME, Cox NJ. Trait-associated SNPs are more likely to be eQTLs: Annotation to enhance discovery from GWAS. PLoS Genetics. 1 Apr 2010;**6**(4):e1000888

[195] Pickrell JK, Marioni JC, Pai AA, Degner JF, Engelhardt BE, Nkadori E. et al. Understanding mechanisms underlying human gene expression variation with RNA sequencing. Nature. 1 Apr 2010;**464**(7289):768-772

[196] Dubois PCA, Trynka G, Franke L, Hunt KA, Romanos J, Curtotti A. et al. Multiple common variants for celiac disease influencing immune gene expression. Nature Genetics. Apr 2010;**42**(4):295-302

[197] Musunuru K, Strong A, Frank-Kamenetsky M, Lee NE, Ahfeldt T, Sachs K V. et al. From noncoding variant to phenotype via SORT1 at the 1p13 cholesterol locus. Nature. 5Aug 2010;**466**(7307):714-749

[198] Castel SE, Levy-Moonshine A, Mohammadi P, Banks E, Lappalainen T. Tools and best practices for data processing in allelic expression analysis. Genome Biology. 17 Sep 2015;**16**:195

[199] Stevenson KR, Coolon JD, Wittkopp PJ. Sources of bias in measures of allele-specific expression derived from RNA-seq data aligned to a single reference genome. BMC Genomics. 2013;**14**(1):536

[200] McKenna A, Hanna M, Banks E, Sivachenko A, Cibulskis K, Kernytsky A. et al. The genome analysis toolkit: A map reduce framework for analyzing next-generation DNA sequencing data. Genome Research. Sep 2010;**20**(9):1297-1303

[201] GTEx Consortium. The Genotype-Tissue Expression (GTEx) project. Nature Genetics. Jun 2013;**45**(6):580-585

Chapter 2

Practical Data Processing Approach for RNA Sequencing of Microorganisms

Toshitaka Kumagai and Masayuki Machida

Additional information is available at the end of the chapter

http://dx.doi.org/10.5772/intechopen.69157

Abstract

The rapid evolvement of sequencing technology has generated huge amounts of DNA/RNA sequences, even with the continuous performance acceleration. Due to the wide variety of basic studies and applications derived from the huge number of species and the microorganism diversity, the targets to be sequenced are also expanding. The huge amounts of data generated by recently developed high-throughput sequencers have required highly efficient data analysis algorithms using recently developed high-performance computers. We have developed a highly accurate and cost-effective mapping strategy that includes the exclusion of unreliable base calls and correction of the reference sequence through provisional mapping of RNA sequencing reads. The use of mapping software tools, such as HISAT and STAR, precisely aligned RNA-Seq reads to the genome of a filamentous fungus considering exon-intron boundaries. The accuracy of the expression analysis through the refinement of gene models was achieved by the results of mapped RNA-Seq reads in combination with ab initio gene finding tools using generalized hidden Markov models (GHMMs). Visualization of the mapping results greatly helps evaluate and improve the entire analysis in terms of both wet experiment and data processing. We believe that at least a portion of our approach is useful and applicable to the analysis of any microorganism.

Keywords: RNA sequencing, computational analysis, microorganisms, gene modeling, alternative splicing

1. Introduction

RNA sequencing (RNA-Seq) is currently one of the most powerful methods for the comprehensive analysis of the transcriptional expression of the entire genes of a particular organism. Due to recent extreme improvements in sequencing technology in terms of throughput and cost, large amounts of data have been accumulated, and the amount of data is increasing in

an accelerating manner. Multiplexing by so-called bar coding facilitates the flexible utilization of the high output capacity of sequencers for large numbers of samples without a significant increase in the overall sequencing cost. This technical improvement greatly contributes to the application of RNA-Seq to various microorganisms.

The purposes of using RNA-Seq are basically divided into two categories. One of these objectives is counting the number of tags to analyze the intensity of gene expression, and the other is determining the transcript sequences for various purposes, such as annotating the genome of non-model organisms and analyzing splice variants.

In a typical RNA-Seq expression analysis, once sequence reads, which are generally 10^7–10^9 reads with a length of 50–300 bases, are accumulated, they are mapped to the reference sequence, namely, a genome sequence corresponding to the organism that the RNA is prepared from Refs. [1–3]. The mapping can be achieved using a sequence similarity search between the reads and the reference sequence with a general purpose computer. Although this procedure is highly suitable for current high-throughput computing (HTC) accelerated by parallel processing, the amount of sequence reads is too large to analyze the sequence similarity in a conventional manner, even using current high-throughput computers, due to the balance of costs between sequencing and data analysis. This issue is the most important when a large number of samples are obtained in a short period of time at low cost, which is often the case in research and development using microorganisms.

The DNA sequencers developed even with the most recent technologies cannot avoid errors in sequence reads. The RNA quality might be reduced by difficult sample preparation due to a small number of samples (cells) and low RNA extraction efficiency from cells grown under particular cultivation conditions. This effect might increase the sequence errors and reduce the amount of data obtained, further complicating the mapping. Although sample preparation might often be improved by finding better conditions and/or better methods for RNA preparation, optimization generally requires time and money. Thus, a bioinformatics method with higher accuracy, higher efficiency, and lower cost is desired based on the balance of time and cost between wet experiments and computational analyses. Accuracy is the most important factor, which increases the motivation to improve the sample and computational analysis qualities, but the necessary quality of sequence reads is often unknown.

The sequencers currently available include those manufactured by Illumina [1], Life Technologies [2], Pacific Bioscience [4], and Oxford [5], and these have different specifications in terms of the number of reads, read length, accuracy, and cost. The choice of platform depends on the purpose of the experiment. A search for genes that cause phenotypic differences under different culture conditions might require a search for differentially expressed genes (DEGs) with high sensitivity among the conditions, and a sequencing platform that yields a higher number of reads rather than longer read lengths should be selected. In contrast, revealing the complete transcribed sequence of a gene of a higher eukaryote that has various isoforms would require a platform that outputs long sequences.

In addition to the various characteristics and output data formats, because sequencing technologies and their performance are continuously under development, it is also necessary to maintain current knowledge of the progress of the methods and software used for analysis. The important issue in such a fast-paced world is to not treat methods and software as complete "black boxes" but to understand the type of information included in a file of a certain format and the statistical nature of the data being processed.

Nearly 10,000 complete microorganism genomes have been published to date according to GOLD [6], and the number is increasing in an accelerating manner. Therefore, a genome sequence used as a reference for a particular species of interest might be found in the database. However, the strain to be analyzed is often not exactly the same. Sequence variations between strains cause serious problems in mapping, similar to the problem due to sequencing errors, as described above. Even if the reference and the experimental sample are from the same strain, the sequences might have variations due to multiple rounds of cultivation and/or long-term storage without appropriate freezing conditions during the distribution process.

The quality of a reference sequence in terms of nucleotide assignment accuracy, length of contigs or scaffolds, assembling reliability (artificial assembling rearrangement), and gene modeling reliability also affects the reliability of RNA-Seq results. Nucleotide assignment errors cause issues similar to sequencing errors and the variation (mutation) problems described above. Low-quality reference sequences might cause problems when calculating the expression of each gene. One of the advantages of gene expression analysis by RNA-Seq is to obtain precise information regarding the location of the transcripts, e.g., an intron-exon boundary, without preparation of probes considering various possibilities in the case of DNA microarray. This advantage is highly advantageous for the expression analysis of microorganisms for which no genomic information has been accumulated.

Although sequencing topics derived from sequencing platforms (chemistry, base calling method, hardware, etc.) and assembling are not addressed in this chapter, gene modeling, which defines CDSs (from coding DNA sequences), will be discussed because (i) RNA-Seq includes information that is important for correcting gene models and (ii) the calculation of expression levels from RNA-Seq depends on the gene model.

2. Factors affecting accuracy and efficiency

2.1. Quality control of sequence reads

If a reference sequence is available, a computational RNA-Seq analysis typically consists of mapping to the corresponding reference sequence and successive processes. The processes of removing unreliable reads and trimming unreliable segments of the reads are often applied without much consideration. Excluding bases with a lower quality score from the RNA-Seq reads improves the average quality score of the reads, which clearly improves the quality of the reads from the left to the right panel, as shown in **Figure 1A**. The upper panel of **Figure 1B**

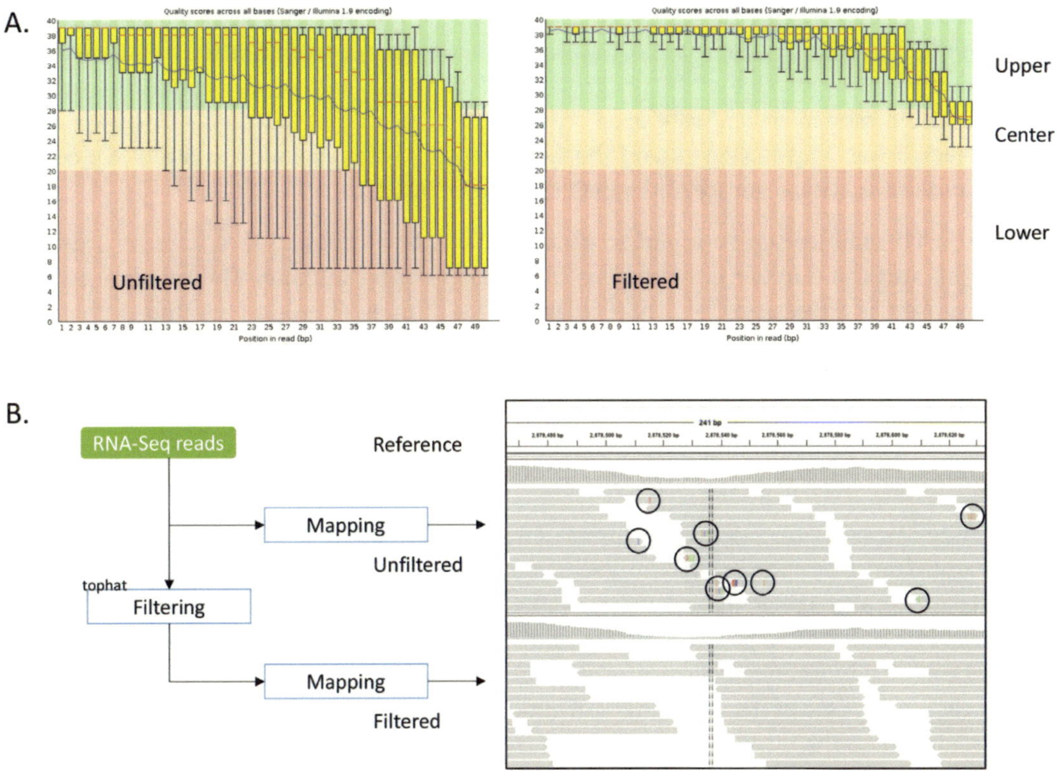

Figure 1. (A) Filtering of reads using quality values. The *Escherichia coli* genome was sequenced using a SOLiD 5500xl sequencer with a 50-bp read length and generated 5,869,272 reads. Quality score distribution of unfiltered (left) and filtered (right) reads visualized by FastQC (see **Table 1** for reference). The average quality values for each sequence position are indicated by a thin curved line. The right panel was obtained by the application of bases with a quality value ≥ 20 for more than or equal to 95%. "N" is less than or equal to 1. The number of reads after filtering was reduced to 2,697,082. For each position, a Box-Whisker-type plot, in which the central red line, yellow box, upper and lower whiskers, and blue line represent the median value, interquartile range (25–75%), 10 and 90% points, and mean quality, respectively. The *Y*-axis on the graph shows the quality scores. A higher score reflects better base call. The background of the graph divides the Y-axis into high (Upper), moderate (Center), and poor (Lower) quality calls. (B) Effect of filtering sequence reads. The sequence reads obtained before and after filtering, as indicated in A, were mapped to the reference genome and visualized. Mismatches are indicated by black circles.

shows a mapping result using unfiltered reads with the quality shown in the left panel of **Figure 1A**, indicating the presence of a significant number of bases mismatched to the reference sequence. However, using the reads in the right panel in **Figure 1A**, the mismatches are significantly decreased, as shown in the lower panel of **Figure 1B**. The filtering process requires only a relatively small calculation time but is thought to significantly improve reliability, which solves various problems derived from mismatches between reads and the reference.

Williams et al. showed that in RNA-Seq experiments, read trimming prior to mapping might have a substantial effect on the estimation of the gene expression level [7]. Therefore, if trimming is applied, extreme care should be taken, and other measures, such as length filtering, should be considered in the preprocessing pipeline to minimize the introduction of unwanted

Name	Category	Brief description[1]	Ref.	Link
FastQC	Quality control for raw reads	Providing a QC report to spot problems which originate either in the sequencer or in the starting library material.		https://www.bioinformatics.babraham.ac.uk/projects/fastqc/
Sickle	Reads trimming	Detection and trimming low quality region from all reads using sliding window.		https://github.com/najoshi/sickle
Cut adapt	Reads trimming	Searching for and removing adapters in all reads.		http://cutadapt.readthedocs.io/en/stable/index.html
BWA	Mapping	Mapping reads against a large reference genome sequence.		http://bio-bwa.sourceforge.net/
TopHat2	Mapping	A splice junction mapper for RNA-Seq reads.	[12]	https://ccb.jhu.edu/software/tophat/index.shtml
HISAT2	Mapping	A spliced alignment program, a successor to TopHat2.	[13]	http://www.ccb.jhu.edu/software/hisat/index.shtml
STAR	Mapping	Spliced transcripts alignment to a reference.	[14]	https://github.com/alexdobin/STAR
Cufflinks	Transcripto me assembly, etc.[2]	Assembling of transcripts, estimation of their abundances, and testing for differential expression and regulation in RNA-Seq samples.	[30]	http://cole-trapnell-lab.github.io/cufflinks/
Kallisto	Quantificati on of gene expression	Quantification of abundances of transcripts from RNA-Seq data based on the novel idea of pseudo-alignment for rapidly determining the compatibility of reads with targets, without the need for alignment.	[16]	https://pachterlab.github.io/kallisto/
Salmon	Quantificati on of gene expression	Quantification of the expression of transcripts using RNA-seq data using new algorithms (quasi-mapping) to provide accurate expression estimates with high throughput and little memory.	[17]	https://combine-lab.github.io/salmon/
VarScan2	Variant call	A mutation caller for targeted, exome, and whole-genome resequencing data.	[11]	http://dkoboldt.github.io/varscan/
AUGUSTUS	Gene finding	Prediction of genes in eukaryotic genomic sequences using extrinsic information as hints on the gene structure.	[18]	http://bioinf.uni-greifswald.de/augustus/
BRAKER1	Gene finding	A pipeline for unsupervised RNA-Seq-based genome annotation.	[19]	http://exon. gatech.edu/braker1.html
CodingQuarry	Gene finding	A self-training gene predicting tool dedicated to fungal genome working with assembled, aligned RNA-seq transcripts.	[20]	https://sourceforge.net/projects/codingquarry/
Tablet	Genome viewer	A graphical viewer for next generation sequence assemblies and alignments.	[36]	https://ics.hutton.ac.uk/tablet/

Name	Category	Brief description[1]	Ref.	Link
Artemis	Genome viewer	A genome browser and annotation tool that allows visualization of sequence features, next generation data.	[37]	http://www.sanger.ac.uk/science/tools/artemis
IGV	Genome viewer	Interactive exploration of genomic datasets supporting various data types, including array-based and next-generation sequence data, and genomic annotations.	[38, 39]	http://software.broadinstitute.org/software/igv/
CLC Genomics Workbench	Integrated solutions	Integrated package of software tools for genomic analysis and visualization supporting various data types, including array-based and next-generation sequence data, and genomic annotations.		https://www.qiagenbioinformatics.com/products/clc-genomics-workbench
Genome Traveler	Integrated solutions	Integrated package of software tools for genomic analysis and visualization supporting various data types, including array-based and next-generation sequence data, and genomic annotations.		http://www.insilicobiology.jp/index.php?option=com_content&view=article&id= 107&Itemid=73&lang=en

[1]Functions related to the topics in this chapter are briefly summarized. Reading the references and/or accessing the web sites is required for details and other functions especially for the integrated package of software.

[2]Transcriptome assembly, quantification of gene expression and testing differential expression genes.

Table 1. Overview of software tools for transcriptome analysis.

bias. In our follow-up examination of the reads obtained using an Illumina MiSeq platform, we concluded that for relatively long sequencing reads, such as 100 or 150 bases, with low sequence errors, aggressive trimming of sequencing reads is generally no longer necessary for estimating the gene expression level. In the following section, we propose correction of the reference sequence using RNA-Seq reads in cases in which the genome sequence of the same strain used in the RNA-Seq experiment is not available to avoid mismatches between the RNA-Seq reads and the reference. The removal and trimming of unreliable sequences are necessary for this purpose.

2.2. Pipelines and peripheral tools

Figure 2A shows a typical pipeline for analyzing gene expression based on RNA-Seq reads. The pipeline effectively works for microorganisms, genome sequences, and gene models, which are reliable due to significant correction and curation by the efforts of a large number of researchers. Typical examples of such microorganism are *Escherichia coli, Bacillus subtilis, Saccharomyces cerevisiae, Schizosaccharomyces pombe, Neurospora crassa,* and *Aspergillus nidulans,* which are known as model organisms. Among microorganisms, filamentous fungi generally have the largest genome sizes and introns in most existing genes and are thus thought to require a pipeline with the highest performance and various functions for the analyses. Furthermore, filamentous fungi are potential producers of various

http://dx.doi.org/10.5772/intechopen.69157

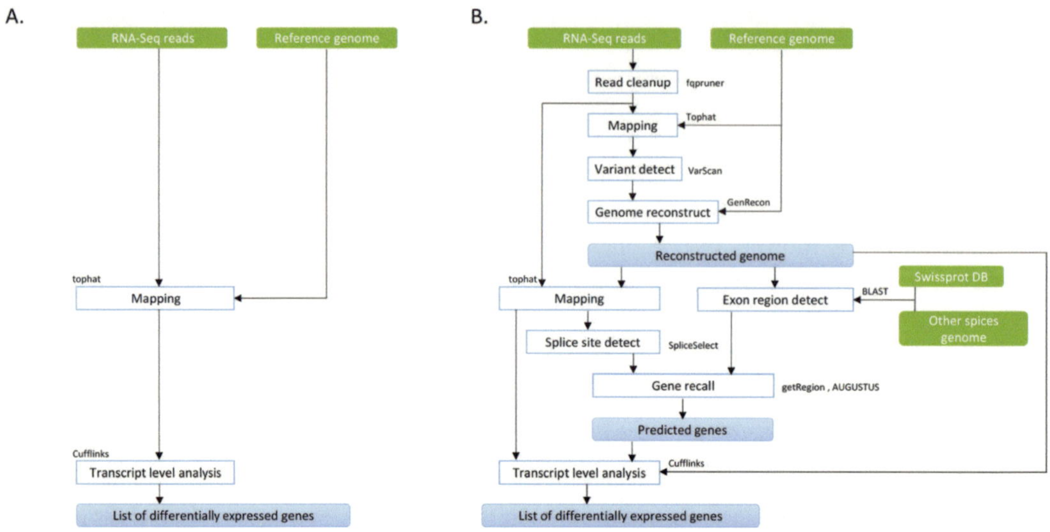

Figure 2. Example of the RNA-Seq analysis pipeline. (A) Typical simple pipeline. First, RNA-Seq reads are mapped to a reference sequence using a mapping tool such as TopHat. Next, tools such as Cufflinks count the number of reads mapped to each genomic feature and extract differentially expressed genes (DEGs). (B) Proposed pipeline for microorganisms whose reference sequence and gene models are not extensively corrected or curated. Fqpruner, GenRecon, SpliceSelect, and getRegion in the figure are in-house scripts. Fqpruner is a program written in C++ to trim the 3′-end of low-quality reads and has almost the same function as the combination of sickle (see **Table 1** for reference) and Cutadapt [10]. GenRecon is a Perl script that outputs a consensus sequence based on output by the variant detect tool, VarScan [11]. SpliceSelect is a Perl script that integrates splice site positions from multiple TopHat output files. GetRegion is a Perl script that receives the BLAST results and outputs genomic regions to execute AUGUSTUS for the prediction of genes from genomic loci involving homologous genes with known amino acid sequences.

secondary metabolites, which are economically important and have a large number of highly diverse secondary metabolism-related genes. Thus, the genomes of filamentous fungi and actinomycetes remain attractive targets in this field. To effectively and accurately analyze RNA-Seq reads from filamentous fungi without publicly available genomic information, we have developed several tools and introduced into the pipeline, as shown in **Figure 2B**.

RNA-Seq reads can be analyzed without their corresponding genome sequence as a reference through the de novo assembly of the reads. Long-read technologies, such as PacBio RS II (Pacific Bioscience) and MinION (Oxford Nanopore Technologies), should lead to better results than sequencers that generate short reads using this approach. However, we do not include the de novo assembly of RNA-Seq reads in this chapter because sequencing the genome of a microorganism using next-generation sequencers, such as Illumina technology, is relatively inexpensive in terms of cost and time. For example, we have used the improved pipeline for the analysis of the genome sequences obtained from a short-read sequencer, SOLiD 500xl, in combination with the de novo assembly pipeline that the manufacturer developed for mate-paired sequences [8] with successive automatic annotation. Illumina and Life Technologies platforms, such as HiSeq/MiSeq/NextSeq and Ion Torrent/Ion PGM, respectively, might also generate a reference genome sequence that is adequate for this purpose in an easy and cost-effective manner. Based on the assumption that the genome sequence is

available as a reference for the microorganism, the strategy of mapping the transcriptome is not included in this chapter.

The sequencing platforms described above are widely used, and bioinformatics tools have been extensively developed for each platform. The characteristics of the errors depend on the sequencing platform, such as those manufactured by Illumina, Life Technologies, and Pacific Bioscience. The number of reads, read length, and data format also varies by platform. Furthermore, more than one platform, such as a combination of Illumina and Pacific Bioscience or Life Technologies and Illumina [9], might be used, which also requires a specific methodology for obtaining reasonable results.

2.3. Basic mapping problems

The mapping of RNA-Seq reads to the reference genome has been a serious problem in RNA-Seq analysis due to the extremely large data size (e.g., more than 500 Gb are obtained from a single run of HiSeq 2500) and sequence errors in both the RNA-Seq reads themselves and the reference. Most of the mapping tools search the nucleotide sequences with a similarity greater than a certain threshold value in the reference sequence for each RNA-Seq read. Multiple mapping algorithms are widely used to accurately identify the most homologous positions on the reference sequence. However, a shorter read length than the repetitive elements in the reference sequence and sequencing errors complicates the problem.

A typical RNA-Seq experiment consists of the sequencing of both ends of a cDNA fragment to generate two reads (a read pair) separated by a sequence of variable length. The accurate alignment of these read pairs is essential to the downstream analysis of an RNA-Seq experiment, but RNA-Seq read alignment is challenging due to the noncontiguous nature of mRNA transcripts resulting from the existence of introns in eukaryotic genes. Recently developed mapping tools, such as TopHat [12], STAR [13], and HISAT [14], perform spliced alignment by considering an exon-intron boundary for the RNA-Seq reads. Software programs that support splice alignment use different strategies from several perspectives [15]. The method of determining the position on the reference sequence where a read is mapped can be roughly classified into two groups: exon first and seed and extend.

Exon-first methods, such as TopHat, utilize a two-step process. First, they map reads to the reference sequence without allowing large gaps. Subsequently, the unmapped reads are divided into short segments, and each is independently aligned to the reference sequence. The discontinued region on the genome where contiguous segments are mapped is treated as a candidate of two connected exons obtained by splice alignment. The exon-first approach is the most effective in cases in which a majority of the reads can be mapped without gaps. If retrotransposed genes or pseudogenes originating from transcripts with multiple exons are present in the genome sequence, software that employs the exon-first approach might preferentially map the reads to the retrotransposed region. In seed-and-extend methods, such as STAR, reads are divided into short seeds (k-mers), the positions where they are present in the genome are searched, and alignments are built and extended using this information.

Seed-and-extend methods are generally considered more sensitive but slower than exon-first methods. However, with great efforts, excellent software programs using seed-and-extend or hybrid methods have been developed in recent years. Substantial effort has been spared, and software using the seed-and-extend method has become sufficiently fast. In a typical expression analysis of microorganisms using RNA-Seq, the computational processing time required for mapping reads to the reference genome sequence is no longer a major problem.

For transcript quantification, software such as Kallisto [16] and Salmon [17], which use newer algorithms that do not require the pre-mapping of reads to a reference sequence, has become increasingly faster. A very large-scale expression analysis with RNA-Seq could be performed using this type of software.

2.4. Mapping problems caused by mutation

Our analysis of RNA-Seq data from *S. cerevisiae* encountered another type of problem, which derived from the accumulation of mutations in the genome. Widely distributed strains, such as *S. cerevisiae* BY4741 and W303, can undergo a large number of mutations possibly during the distribution process due to relatively long-term storage without freezing and multiple rounds of inoculation and successive cultivation. The mutation frequency can be decreased by careful handling, such as decreasing the number of inoculation processes and avoiding stressful conditions. However, the introduction of mutations cannot be completely prevented due to spontaneous mutation, which is a natural characteristic of all organisms. The basic procedure for resolving this problem is to sequence the genome of the strain for which RNA-Seq is performed. However, because the sequencing strategy, including sample preparation, for genome sequencing is different from that used for RNA-Seq and because of the cost- and time-saving requirements, RNA-Seq data sometime have to be analyzed using the reference sequence deposited in a public database. To overcome this problem without losing reliability, we have addressed the correction of the reference sequence using RNA-Seq reads based on two methods: (1) RNA-Seq reads are mapped to the reference sequence using the spliced mapper mentioned in the previous section, and the reference sequence is corrected using the consensus of the mapped reads. (2) The de novo transcriptome assembly of RNA-Seq reads is aligned to the reference genome. The former method was almost completely automatable and worked well for small variations, such as single-base substitution. With the latter method, it was necessary to process a number of isoform candidates at the same loci of the reference genome outputted by the transcriptome assembler, which required time and effort to tune the various parameters and threshold values. Unless the genome has undergone a complicated structural change from the reference sequence, the former method is sufficient. After correcting the reference sequence, the reads were again mapped to the corrected reference sequence. This strategy worked fairly well.

2.5. Gene finding using RNA-Seq

Typical examples of the gene modeling problem are found by analyzing filamentous fungi. Industrially important fungi are often isolated due to their production of useful secondary

metabolites. Because their genomes are generally unknown, sequencing and successive gene modeling are indispensable but are performed by a limited number of researchers with a limited amount of knowledge. In such cases, RNA-Seq reads can be used to correct gene models prior to expression analysis to obtain accurate expression levels.

Several researchers have attempted to improve the accuracy of predicting protein-coding genes, and these attempts have included the use of RNA-Seq. AUGUSTUS is a gene prediction program that uses a generalized hidden Markov model (GHMM) [18], which is widely used for eukaryote genome sequencing projects. AUGUSTUS can incorporate hints of the gene structure from extrinsic sources. After RNA-Seq reads are mapped to the genome, spliced mapped reads can be used as valuable information for gene finding.

In recent years, gene prediction software using RNA-Seq for both model training and gene prediction with the trained model has been developed and has demonstrated high accuracy for gene structure prediction [19, 20]. The training of conventional gene finding depends on the gene models in the genomes of species other than the target one. However, the gene models of the species already deposited in public databases have not always been experimentally confirmed but are the results of predictions based on the results of other genomes. Thus, the use of the results of RNA-Seq read mapping, which provides direct information of the CDSs of the target species, in combination with recent gene finding algorithms, enables significant improvement in gene modeling.

We used an internally developed pipeline that performs training with RNA-Seq read mapping and ab initio gene prediction (**Figure 2B**). In this pipeline, exon-intron boundary information is predicted using mapped RNA-Seq, and coding sequence candidates is obtained by homology searches between the genome sequence and protein sequence databases, such as the Swiss-Prot database. Subsequently, AUGUSTUS was trained using these pieces of information, and all of the genes in the genome were predicted. This pipeline worked well for gene prediction of non-model organisms and has been used for the genome analysis of various filamentous fungi. The improvements in the predicted gene structures are thought to contribute to more accurate RNA-Seq expression quantification as transcript references.

In the case of bacteria, which do not have poly-A tails, the degradation of ribosomal RNA is required for the extraction of mRNA. Because the degradation will not be complete, the ribosomal RNA sequences have to be removed after sequencing by searching the consensus sequence in the reads. Another problem is that bacterial genes are sometimes overlapped on the genome and might be transcribed even in different orientations. This can be problematic for identifying CDSs based on the RNA-Seq mapping results. To solve this problem, strand-specific RNA-Seq has the advantage of obtaining useful information for gene modeling. However, because bacterial mRNA does not have poly-A tails, as described above, preparation of a strand-specific library is more difficult than the preparation of eukaryotic mRNA. A strand-specific library for bacteria can be prepared basically by two methods [21]: (i) adapter ligation to the first strand synthesized in the cDNA preparation [22] and (ii) chemical modification of RNA or the second strand of the cDNA [23–25].

2.6. Quantification of gene expression and identification of differentially expressed genes

Expression analysis with RNA-Seq typically begins by counting the number of reads mapped to reference transcript sequences. We can resolve the various mapping problems mentioned above and perform mapping to the genome with accurately predicted gene structures or assembled transcript sequences using transcriptome assembly software.

Microarrays are widely used for the quantification of the abundance of mRNAs corresponding to genes. In microarray experiments, the gene expression level is measured as a continuous value, intensity. RNA-Seq differs from microarrays in that it addresses nonnegative discrete values, i.e., the number of reads mapped to the gene, in order to measure the expression of a gene. Analytical methods for microarray data that assume a Gaussian distribution, such as linear discriminant analysis, might not perform as well for RNA-Seq data with a discrete distribution.

Let us consider the problem of quantifying gene expression levels using discrete RNA-Seq data and a related problem, namely, the identification of differentially expressed genes (DEGs) between conditions. In RNA-Seq experiments, transcribed mRNA is fragmented into a certain length, cDNA is subsequently synthesized, and sequencing is performed. Thus, the total number of observed reads for a transcript is proportional to the number of expressed mRNAs for the transcript multiplied by the length of the transcript. To compensate for this bias, it is a common practice to divide the number of mapped reads by the transcript length. RPKM (Reads Per Kilobase transcript per Million mapped reads) is the most commonly used method for length and sample size normalization.

Unfortunately, this correction is not sufficient to test whether gene expression differs between conditions. Oshlack and Wakefield showed that the power of a *t*-test of the count data, regardless of whether it is divided by the length of the transcript, is proportional to the square root of the length of the transcript [26]. Therefore, for a given expression level, the test becomes more significant for longer transcripts.

Many methods have been developed for assessing differential expression from RNA-Seq data. Count data, such as the counts of mapped fragments of RNA-Seq data, are often modeled as a Poisson distribution. The Poisson distribution has equal mean and variance values, and DEGs can be identified by conducting a likelihood ratio test between conditions. Real RNA-Seq data often exhibits overdispersion. The count data measured via RNA-Seq often has a variance that is larger than the mean due to various biases and errors as well as length bias. A negative binomial distribution is widely used for modeling such cases. Several RNA-Seq data analysis software packages incorporating these models have been developed. Soneson and Delorenzi evaluated eleven software packages that implemented various methods to model count data for differential expression analyses of RNA-Seq data [27]. When designing experiments to analyze differential expressions using RNA-Seq, it is necessary to carefully consider the type of method used for DEG extraction and the amount of biological replications that are needed. Three replicates often give reproducible results in successive independent experiments in

terms of the assignment of a gene(s) with the expression of interest, although a single experiment often fails to yield reproducible results.

The comparison of the transcriptome for each condition often shows a large number of DEGs. Therefore, outlining the changes in the expression profile by extracting features common to genes whose expression intensity has changed is a common approach. Gene set enrichment analysis (GSEA) is a popular method for condensing information from gene expression profiles into a summary of pathways or functional groups. GSEA was developed for microarray data and can also be used for RNA-Seq data. However, most RNA-Seq data obtained so far have only small replicates, which enforces application of the gene-permuting GSEA method (or preranked GSEA), resulting in a great number of false positives due to the inter-gene correlation in each gene set. Yoon et al. demonstrated that the incorporation of the absolute gene statistic in one-tailed GSEA considerably improves the false-positive control and the overall discriminatory ability of the gene-permuting GSEA methods for RNA-Seq data [28].

2.7. Alternative splicing

As shown recently, RNA-Seq also enables the detection of alternative slicing from various fungi and higher organisms, such as mammals and plants. Alternative splicing from RNA-Seq can also be performed using bioinformatics software, such as GESS (graph-based exon-skipping scanner) [29] and Cufflinks [30]. Both tools can detect isoforms of transcripts based on mapping information generated by TopHat using a graph-based method. The former outputs all isoforms detected in the GTS format and requires MISO [31] to calculate the RPKM values for each isoform, whereas the latter is able to calculate the values. These tools are widely used for the analysis of higher organisms, such as mammals and plants, but not fungi.

Splicing variants have been found in various fungi, including *Aspergillus oryzae* [32], *Magnaporthe grisea* [33], *Cryptococcus neoformans* [34], and *Trichoderma longibrachiatum* [35], by deep RNA-Seq despite their significantly lower frequency compared with that found in higher organisms. Alternative splicing might affect the calculation of the FPKM (Fragments Per Kilobase of exon per Million fragments mapped)/RPKM values; however, because of the relatively low frequency (less than 10% of the entire genes on a genome) and abundance of "intron retention" [35], the results might not be significant without specific measures. Isoforms might also be detected through an inaccurate mapping of RNA-Seq reads resulting from base call errors and incorrect exon-intron boundaries. Thus, the calculation of RPKM values for the entire CDSs could be performed, particularly for the initial analysis.

2.8. Visualization and evaluation of the analysis

Visualization of RNA-Seq results is useful and strongly recommended during the analysis process for a rapid evaluation of the reliability of the analysis. Typical views of the results, including mapping, models, and nucleotide sequences, are shown in **Figure 3B** using Genome Traveler/in silico Molecular Cloning (GT/IMC) available from in silico biology, Inc. Various software tools, such as Tablet [36], Artemis [37], Integrative Genome Viewer (IGV) [38, 39], and CLC Genomics Workbench, were developed by the James Hutton Institute, Sanger Institute, Broad Institute, and CLC Bio, respectively. Some of these tools are operating system

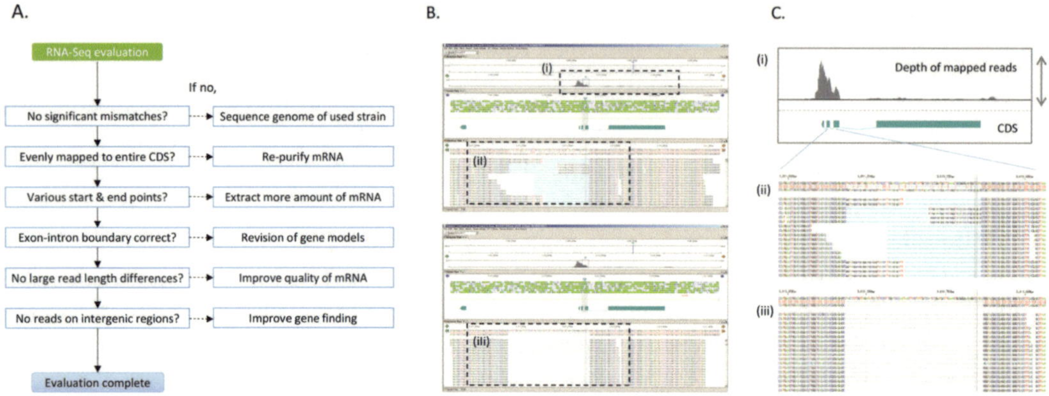

Figure 3. Visualization of the results. The RNA-Seq reads of *Aspergillus flavus* NRRL3357 (NCBI BioProject Accession: PRJNA299060) were mapped to the corresponding reference genome sequence with annotations (http://genome.jgi.doe.gov/pages/dynamicOrganismDownload.jsf?organism=Aspfl1) analyzed by the Joint Genome Institute (JGI) [41]. Genome Traveler (GT) from in silico biology is used to visualize the read mapping, gene models, and nucleotide sequences in a single window. (A) Schematic diagram of RNA-Seq analysis evaluation. (B) Mapping result using BWA (upper) and HISAT (lower). Each panel shows the depth of the RNA-Seq reads (top panel), a gene model (middle panel), and the nucleotide sequences of the mapped reads (bottom panel). The top of the middle panel shows termination codons in six frames with vertical lines and relatively long ORFs with solid rectangles. The bottom of the middle panel shows the predicted exons. The width of the bottom panel corresponds to the region indicated by brackets with triangles in the top and middle panels. (C) Magnified version of the regions indicated by the dotted rectangle in (B).

specific, but the others are executable on multiple platforms, e.g., by using Java. Because recent sequencing platforms output huge amounts of data, the operating system should be 64 bits with a memory size of at least 16 Gbytes. Differently from de novo assembly for genome sequencing, mapping requires less memory and lower CPU performance. Introduction of a small-scale server equipped with eight CPUs and 32 Gbytes of memory might help reduce the required time with a relatively low cost. The sequencing quality can also be validated by the read lengths and their variation, particularly when the reads are trimmed based on the quality.

Figure 3A presents a schematic diagram of how RNA-Seq analysis is achieved in combination with visual evaluation. The read mapping and alignment are displayed as shown in **Figure 3B and C**. When the reads have sufficient quality for the subsequent analyses, they are aligned without a significant number of mismatches. The read lengths aligned to the reference might sometimes have large differences in length, even after using a platform of fixed read length, such as Illumina and SOLiD. This effect occurs due to the low-quality values of the nucleotides at the end of a read sequence, which are removed by a trimming process, as discussed above. High-quality reads have nearly the maximum or indicated read length of the sequencing platform used. It is important that each read does not have the same starting and ending positions on the reference to confirm that excess PCR amplification, which often occurs when the RNA quality is low, was not applied.

Another important indicator of experimental quality is the depth of reads inside CDSs. High AT or GC proportions, such as 70% and greater, in a particular region might cause a lower depth of coverage depending on the sequencing platform due to insufficient amplification during emulsion PCR. The depth of the reads should be roughly the same throughout the entire CDS.

Deeper coverage at the 3′ end than at the 5′ end indicates low mRNA quality, probably due to partial degradation, when poly-A-tailed RNA capture is applied in the preparation process.

In the case of fungi, introns might not be clearly displayed by a simple mapping approach without considering the exon-intron boundary because of the short intron length (typically in the range of 5–100 nt), even when using short reads of 50 bp. The predicted CDS at the center of **Figure 3B** and **C** shows two short exons close to the 5′-end. Mapping by BWA [40], which does not consider the intron-exon boundary, aligned some reads to the intron, introducing mismatches (the upper panel of **Figure 3B** and **C—(ii)**). By referring to the mismatches between the reference and the consensus of the mapped reads, the location of the intron can be assumed to be the region where gray asterisks instead of red vertical bars are clustered at the top of the bottom panel. In contrast, read mapping using HISAT2 (the lower panel of **Figure 3B** and **C—(iii)**) and STAR (data not shown), both of which consider the intron-exon boundary, fairly accurately mapped the reads connecting two adjacent exons, introducing an intron between the exons.

The above CDS has another long intron-predicted upstream of the two short introns mentioned above, although this third intron might be too long for a gene from a filamentous fungus. Furthermore, the depth of reads for the first exon is much lower than those for the second and third exons (**Figure 3C—(i)**). Considering the precipitous change in depths between the first and second exons and the almost even distribution of the depth in the first exon despite its large size, the large difference in depth is not thought to result from partial mRNA degradation. Consequently, it is believed that the first exon should be separated from the other exons, resulting in two CDSs. In agreement with this consideration, RNA-Seq reads are also mapped to the region of the long intron with a depth similar to that of the first exon (the upstream part of the two CDSs after division) after a short intron is detected by HISAT2 (data not shown).

2.9. Perspective

Recently developed long-read sequencers, such as PacBio RS II, PacBio Sequel, and Oxford Nanopore MinION, promise to deliver more complete genome assemblies with fewer gaps. Higher error rates, low yields per cost, and stringent DNA requirements might be concerns. Short-read sequencers have an advantage for measuring transcriptional expression due to the production of a greater number of reads. In contrast, long-read sequencers have the potential to accurately analyze the structure of transcripts, including the linkage between multiple splicing variations [42]. The selection and combination of appropriate bioinformatics tools as well as sequencing platforms should be a key issue depending on the purpose of the analysis.

Acknowledgements

This work was supported by the commission for the Development of Artificial Gene Synthesis Technology for Creating Innovative Biomaterial from the Ministry of Economy, Trade and Industry (METI), Japan. This work was also supported by the project focused on developing key technology of discovering and manufacturing drug for the next-generation treatment and

diagnosis from the Ministry of Economy, Trade and Industry (METI) and the Japan Agency for Medical Research and Development (AMED). We thank the American Journal Experts 479 for proofing the manuscript.

Author details

Toshitaka Kumagai and Masayuki Machida*

*Address all correspondence to: m.machida@aist.go.jp

Fermlab Inc., National Institute of Advanced Industrial Science and Technology (AIST), Tokyo, Japan

References

[1] Bentley DR, Balasubramanian S, Swerdlow HP, Smith GP, Milton J, Brown CG, et al. Accurate whole human genome sequencing using reversible terminator chemistry. Nature. 2008;**456**(7218):53-59

[2] Perkel J. Making contact with sequencing's fourth generation. Biotechniques. 2011;**50** (2):93-95

[3] Cloonan N, Forrest AR, Kolle G, Gardiner BB, Faulkner GJ, Brown MK, et al. Stem cell transcriptome profiling via massive-scale mRNA sequencing. Nature Methods. 2008;**5**(7):613-619

[4] Eid J, Fehr A, Gray J, Luong K, Lyle J, Otto G, et al. Real-time DNA sequencing from single polymerase molecules. Science. 2009;**323**(5910):133-138

[5] Jain M, Olsen HE, Paten B, Akeson M. The Oxford Nanopore MinION: Delivery of nanopore sequencing to the genomics community. Genome Biology. 2016;**17**(1):239

[6] Mukherjee S, Stamatis D, Bertsch J, Ovchinnikova G, Verezemska O, Isbandi M, et al. Genomes OnLine Database (GOLD) v.6: Data updates and feature enhancements. Nucleic Acids Research. 2017;**45**(D1):D446-D456

[7] Williams CR, Baccarella A, Parrish JZ, Kim CC. Trimming of sequence reads alters RNA-Seq gene expression estimates. BMC Bioinformatics 2016;**17**:103

[8] Umemura M, Koyama Y, Takeda I, Hagiwara H, Ikegami T, Koike H, et al. Fine de novo sequencing of a fungal genome using only SOLiD short read data: Verification on *Aspergillus oryzae* RIB40. PLoS One. 2013;**8**(5):e63673

[9] Ikegami T, Inatsugi T, Kojima I, Umemura M, Hagiwara H, Machida M, et al. Hybrid de novo genome assembly using MiSeq and SOLiD short read data. PLoS One. 2015;**10**(4):e0126289

[10] Martin M. Cutadapt removes adapter sequences from high-throughput sequencing reads. EMBnet.journal. 2011;**17**(1):10-12

[11] Koboldt DC, Zhang Q, Larson DE, Shen D, McLellan MD, Lin L, et al. VarScan 2: Somatic mutation and copy number alteration discovery in cancer by exome sequencing. Genome Research. 2012;**22**(3):568-576

[12] Kim D, Pertea G, Trapnell C, Pimentel H, Kelley R, Salzberg SL. TopHat2: Accurate alignment of transcriptomes in the presence of insertions, deletions and gene fusions. Genome Biology. 2013;**14**(4):R36

[13] Dobin A, Davis CA, Schlesinger F, Drenkow J, Zaleski C, Jha S, et al. STAR: Ultrafast universal RNA-seq aligner. Bioinformatics. 2013;**29**(1):15-21

[14] Kim D, Langmead B, Salzberg SL. HISAT: A fast spliced aligner with low memory requirements. Nature Methods. 2015;**12**(4):357-360

[15] Garber M, Grabherr MG, Guttman M, Trapnell C. Computational methods for transcriptome annotation and quantification using RNA-seq. Nature Methods. 2011;**8**(6):469-477

[16] Bray NL, Pimentel H, Melsted P, Pachter L. Near-optimal probabilistic RNA-seq quantification. Nature Biotechnology. 2016;**34**(5):525-527

[17] Patro R, Duggal G, Love MI, Irizarry RA, Kingsford C. Salmon provides fast and bias-aware quantification of transcript expression. Nature Methods. 2017;**14**:417-419

[18] Stanke M, Schoffmann O, Morgenstern B, Waack S. Gene prediction in eukaryotes with a generalized hidden Markov model that uses hints from external sources. BMC Bioinformatics. 2006;**7**:62

[19] Hoff KJ, Lange S, Lomsadze A, Borodovsky M, Stanke M. BRAKER1: Unsupervised RNA-Seq-Based Genome Annotation with GeneMark-ET and AUGUSTUS. Bioinformatics. 2016;**32**(5):767-769

[20] Testa AC, Hane JK, Ellwood SR, Oliver RP. CodingQuarry: Highly accurate hidden Markov model gene prediction in fungal genomes using RNA-seq transcripts. BMC Genomics 2015;**16**:170

[21] Mills JD, Kawahara Y, Janitz M. Strand-specific RNA-Seq provides greater resolution of transcriptome profiling. Current Genomics. 2013;**14**(3):173-181

[22] Croucher NJ, Fookes MC, Perkins TT, Turner DJ, Marguerat SB, Keane T, et al. A simple method for directional transcriptome sequencing using Illumina technology. Nucleic Acids Research. 2009;**37**(22):e148

[23] Levin JZ, Yassour M, Adiconis X, Nusbaum C, Thompson DA, Friedman N, et al. Comprehensive comparative analysis of strand-specific RNA sequencing methods. Nature Methods. 2010;**7**(9):709-715

[24] He Y, Vogelstein B, Velculescu VE, Papadopoulos N, Kinzler KW. The antisense transcriptomes of human cells. Science. 2008;**322**(5909):1855-1857

[25] Borodina T, Adjaye J, Sultan M. A strand-specific library preparation protocol for RNA sequencing. Methods in Enzymology. 2011;**500**:79-98

[26] Oshlack A, Wakefield MJ. Transcript length bias in RNA-seq data confounds systems biology. Biology Direct. 2009;**4**:14

[27] Soneson C, Delorenzi M. A comparison of methods for differential expression analysis of RNA-seq data. BMC Bioinformatics. 2013;**14**:91

[28] Yoon S, Kim SY, Nam D. Improving gene-set enrichment analysis of RNA-Seq data with small replicates. PLoS One. 2016;**11**(11):e0165919

[29] Ye Z, Chen Z, Lan X, Hara S, Sunkel B, Huang TH, et al. Computational analysis reveals a correlation of exon-skipping events with splicing, transcription and epigenetic factors. Nucleic Acids Research. 2014;**42**(5):2856-2869

[30] Roberts A, Pimentel H, Trapnell C, Pachter L. Identification of novel transcripts in annotated genomes using RNA-Seq. Bioinformatics. 2011;**27**(17):2325-2329

[31] Katz Y, Wang ET, Airoldi EM, Burge CB. Analysis and design of RNA sequencing experiments for identifying isoform regulation. Nature Methods. 2010;**7**(12):1009-1015

[32] Wang B, Guo G, Wang C, Lin Y, Wang X, Zhao M, et al. Survey of the transcriptome of *Aspergillus oryzae* via massively parallel mRNA sequencing. Nucleic Acids Research. 2010;**38**(15):5075-5087

[33] Ebbole DJ, Jin Y, Thon M, Pan H, Bhattarai E, Thomas T, et al. Gene discovery and gene expression in the rice blast fungus, *Magnaporthe grisea*: Analysis of expressed sequence tags. Molecular Plant-Microbe Interactions. 2004;**17**(12):1337-1347

[34] Loftus BJ, Fung E, Roncaglia P, Rowley D, Amedeo P, Bruno D, et al. The genome of the basidiomycetous yeast and human pathogen *Cryptococcus neoformans*. Science. 2005;**307**(5713):1321-1324

[35] Xie BB, Li D, Shi WL, Qin QL, Wang XW, Rong JC, et al. Deep RNA sequencing reveals a high frequency of alternative splicing events in the fungus *Trichoderma longibrachiatum*. BMC Genomics 2015;**16**:54

[36] Milne I, Stephen G, Bayer M, Cock PJ, Pritchard L, Cardle L, et al. Using Tablet for visual exploration of second-generation sequencing data. Briefings in Bioinformatics. 2013;**14**(2):193-202

[37] Rutherford K, Parkhill J, Crook J, Horsnell T, Rice P, Rajandream MA, et al. Artemis: Sequence visualization and annotation. Bioinformatics. 2000;**16**(10):944-945

[38] Thorvaldsdottir H, Robinson JT, Mesirov JP. Integrative Genomics Viewer (IGV): High-performance genomics data visualization and exploration. Briefings in Bioinformatics. 2013;**14**(2):178-192

[39] Robinson JT, Thorvaldsdottir H, Winckler W, Guttman M, Lander ES, Getz G, et al. Integrative genomics viewer. Nature Biotechnology. 2011;**29**(1):24-26

[40] Li H, Durbin R. Fast and accurate long-read alignment with Burrows-Wheeler transform. Bioinformatics. 2010;**26**(5):589-595

[41] Nordberg H, Cantor M, Dusheyko S, Hua S, Poliakov A, Shabalov I, et al. The genome portal of the Department of Energy Joint Genome Institute: 2014 updates. Nucleic Acids Research. 2014;**42**(Database issue):D26-D31

[42] Tilgner H, Grubert F, Sharon D, Snyder MP. Defining a personal, allele-specific, and single-molecule long-read transcriptome. Proceedings of the National Academy of Sciences of the United States of America. 2014;**111**(27):9869-9874

Chapter 3

Transcriptome Analysis for Non-Model Organism: Current Status and Best-Practices

Vahap Eldem, Gokmen Zararsiz, Tunahan Taşçi,
Izzet Parug Duru, Yakup Bakir and Melike Erkan

Additional information is available at the end of the chapter

http://dx.doi.org/10.5772/intechopen.68983

Abstract

Since transcriptome analysis provides genome-wide sequence and gene expression information, transcript reconstruction using RNA-Seq sequence reads has become popular during recent years. For non-model organism, as distinct from the reference genome-based mapping, sequence reads are processed via *de novo* transcriptome assembly approaches to produce large numbers of contigs corresponding to coding or non-coding, but expressed, part of genome. In spite of immense potential of RNA-Seq–based methods, particularly in recovering full-length transcripts and spliced isoforms from short-reads, the accurate results can be only obtained by the procedures to be taken in a step-by-step manner. In this chapter, we aim to provide an overview of the state-of-the-art methods including (i) quality check and pre-processing of raw reads, (ii) the pros and cons of *de novo* transcriptome assemblers, (iii) generating non-redundant transcript data, (iv) current quality assessment tools for *de novo* transcriptome assemblies, (v) approaches for transcript abundance and differential expression estimations and finally (vi) further mining of transcriptomic data for particular biological questions. Our intention is to provide an overview and practical guidance for choosing the appropriate approaches to best meet the needs of researchers in this area and also outline the strategies to improve on-going projects.

Keywords: whole transcriptome, *de novo* assembly, genome-wide expression, non-model organism

1. Introduction

The on-going advances in sequencing technologies and a drastic drop in the cost of sequencing allow us to obtain genome-wide genetic information for virtually all kingdoms of life.

Particularly, making large-scale DNA sequencing more affordable and accessible for small-scale laboratories has greatly promoted genomic research studies on non-model organisms genetically linked to a specific biological question of interest [1, 2]. Despite huge effort, *de novo* sequencing of an entire genome is not an easy task, even now, and this also makes 'RNA sequencing (hereafter, RNA-Seq)-based transcriptomic analysis' appealing for non-model organisms that are generally described as having no or limited genomic resources and transcriptomic datasets as well as molecular tools [3–6]. In the field of '-omics' disciplines, RNA-Seq is among high-throughput experimental methods and widely used for identifying all functional elements in the genome. In other words, RNA-Seq data are directly derived from functional genomic elements, mostly protein-coding genes. Therefore, analysing the expressed part of genome by RNA-Seq gives substantial information about the genome-wide transcriptome structure, profile and dynamics for non-model organism at genome-wide scale. Currently, large-scale sequencing efforts such as 'Fish-T1K (Transcriptomes of 1000 fishes)', '1KITE (1K insect transcriptome evolution)' and '1KP (1000 Plants Project)' have been initiated to serve as valuable source of transcriptome composition and dynamics. In spite of immense potential of RNA-Seq–based methods, particularly in recovering full-length transcripts and spliced isoforms from short-reads, the accurate results can be only obtained by the procedures to be taken in a step-by-step manner.

Compelling evidence show that a number of factors *de novo* transcript construction procedure were reported, such as error-prone and biased (e.g. GC%) nature of sequencing technologies, limitations of assembler algorithm and multi k-mer approaches [7–9], read length [10], coverage depth of reads [11], pre-processing options of raw reads [12, 13] and transcript complexity of organism (e.g. sequence variations at terminal regions, alternative splicing, antisense transcription, overlapping genes) [14]. Therefore, the state-of-the-art advancements in methodologies

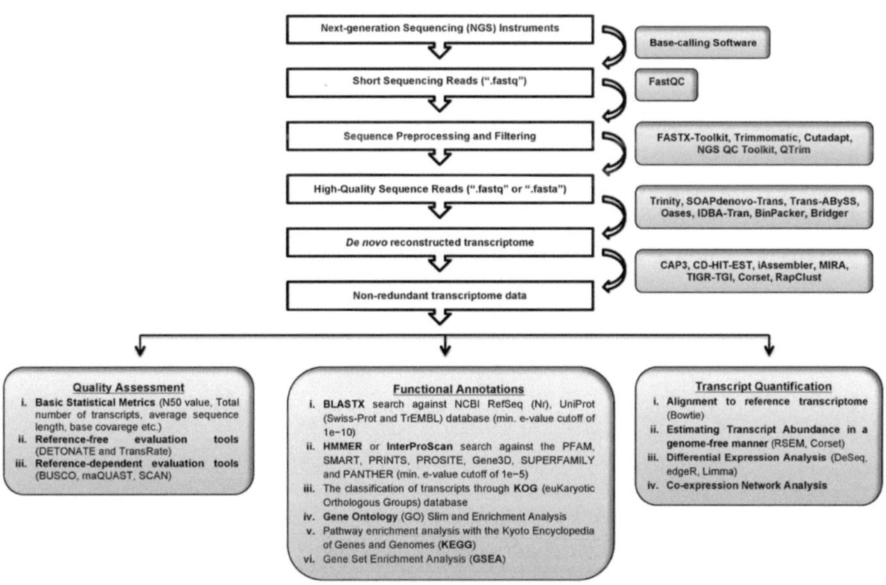

Figure 1. An overview of *de novo* transcriptome analysis pipelines from assembly to quality checking and pre-processing to assembly and transcript quantification.

and applications for transcriptome assembly should be meticulously considered while planning a project. As no consensus procedure exists, researchers mainly in the field of ecology and evolution use many different approaches and tools from sequence pre-processing to functional annotations (**Figure 1**). In this context, establishing a guideline that facilitates and standardizes the transcriptome assembly and post-assembly analysis provides a good starting point.

2. *De novo* transcriptome assembly methods and mining transcriptome data for non-model organism

2.1. Quality check and pre-processing of raw reads

Following sequencing reaction and initial processing, next-generation sequencing instruments generate raw image files that are automatically processed via instrument base calling software to output a massive quantity of raw sequence data in ".fastq" format. The ".fastq" is a text format containing both sequence read and base calling information encoded in ASCII characters. The read quality at each base or quality score can be obtained by converting the ASCII characters into Phred score (Q) indicating the probability of an erroneous base call. Compelling evidences show that a minimum threshold of Phred score for assembly and alignment is 20 (equivalent to 99% probability of being correct) for each base in raw read. Despite remarkable progress in sequencing chemistry and base detection approaches, the instruments can still produce incomplete, erroneous and ambiguous reads. Therefore, a pre-processing step (quality checking and read filtering) is considered an essential prerequisite prior to *de novo* transcriptome assembly because erroneous and ambiguous bases can often lead to fragmented and misassembled transcripts.

Quality checking and visualization of raw reads (in fastq) start with the FastQC tool (a standalone Java program available at http://www.bioinformatics.babraham.ac.uk/projects/fastqc/). FastQC generates a HTML output containing a number of graphical illustrations providing the number and length of raw reads and duplication rate, but two main component of the FastQC tool: (i) *per base sequence content* and (ii) *per base sequence quality* are particularly useful in guiding pre-processing step. The most popular pre-processing tools are FASTX-Toolkit [15], Trimmomatic [16], Cutadapt [17], NGS QC Toolkit [18] and Qtrim [19], and regardless of the tools used, common pre-processing steps include: (i) removing adapter sequences, (ii) discarding the low quality reads ($Q \leq 20$) and ambiguous nucleotides (Ns), (iii) removing the short-read length sequences (length below 50 base pair (bp)) and (iv) trimming low quality bases at the both ends of reads (generally first 10 bp) (**Figure 1**) [20]. After pre-processing, resulting high-quality reads are ready for downstream analysis; *de novo* transcriptome assembly.

2.2. A brief glance at *de novo* transcript assemblers

Currently, the length of sequence reads from NGS instruments (e.g. sequencing by synthesis from Illumina HiSeq Models) is ranged from 150 to 250 base pairs (bp) and, following quality checking and filtering step, the high-quality sequence reads have to be *de novo* assembled for

transcript reconstruction. The sequence read length is shown to be one of the key parameters in determining *de novo* assembly strategy. While the overlap-layout consensus (OLC) approach has been used for the assembly of long reads generated from the third-generation sequencing instruments such as PacBio Sequel or Oxford Nanopore, *de Bruijn* graph approach has been used in both *de novo* genome and transcriptome assembly because this computationally effective algorithm can process billions of short reads to reconstruct the transcriptome as complete as possible. In the *de Bruijn* methods, the graphs are constructed from short reads and then paths in this graph are used to generate contigs. In graph construction, a given read is broken into k-mer seeds (nodes) and edges are added between consecutive k-mers (in manner; the suffix of length k−1 of one node is the prefix of length k−1 of the other) and then, these k-mers are arranged into a *de Bruijn* graph structure (**Figure 2**). Contigs are obtained by inversely transforming the optimal path in the *de Bruijn* graph into sequences [21]. However, *de Bruijn* graph-based strategy between *de novo* genome and transcriptome assembly is slightly modified because of the following reasons: (i) while the DNA sequencing depth is expected to be uniform across the genome (except in repetitive regions), the sequencing depth of transcripts can vary considerably, (ii) Genome assembly graph is considered as linear (theoretically one graph for each chromosome), but due to alternative splicing, transcriptome assembly is more complex than genome and requires a graph to represent the multiple alternative transcripts per locus [1, 21]. By considering these challenges, several *de novo* assembly tools such as Trinity [1], SOAPdenovo-Trans [22], Trans-AbySS [23], Oases [24], IDBA-Tran [25], BinPacker [26] and Bridger [27] have been developed so far (Box 1). Most of these tools, which are initially developed for *de novo* genome assembly (except for Trinity) use *de Bruijn* graph-based assembly strategy and have their own pros and cons in transcript reconstruction.

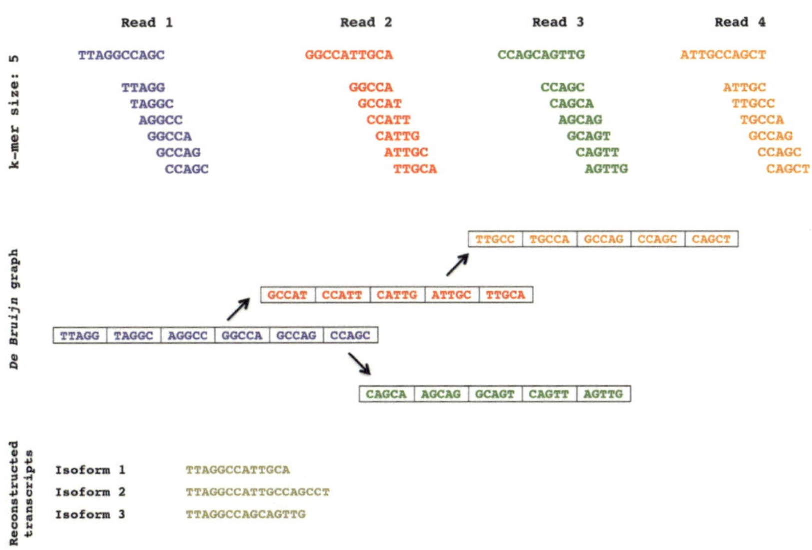

Figure 2. The *de Bruijn* graph approach is instrumental for reference-free transcriptome assembly and *de Bruijn* graphs are built from the short reads. These short reads are split into short k-mers (here, k-mer length, 5) and then k-mers are connected by overlapping prefix and suffix (k−1)-mers. When the *de Bruijn* graph is built from reads, the optimal paths are obtained in the graphs and reconstructed transcripts (or contigs) are recovered by inversely transforming the optimal path in the *de Bruijn* graph.

The quality of assemblies in terms of transcript number and length generated by such assemblers is highly influenced by k-mer length or hash length. Schulz et al. [24] reported that although assemblies generated using short k-mer have the risk of introducing misassemblies, rare transcripts can only be retrieved by selecting short k-mers while longer k-values perform best on high expression genes. In order to identify the full spectrum of transcript abundance and isoforms, *de novo* assemblers utilize an iterative multi-kmer approach from 21 to 71, except for Trinity whose k-mer length is fixed to 25. Due to its apparent importance, an informed k-mer selection tool, KREATION, has been recently developed using fit-based algorithm, limiting the number of k-mer values without significant loss in assembly quality but with saving in assembly time [28]. KREATION first clusters the assemblies generated from single k-mer to determine *"extended clusters"* showing the assembly quality and then, a heuristic model is applied to predict the optimal stopping threshold for a multi k-mer assembly study.

Box 1. A general overview of *de novo* transcriptome assembly tools from short-reads.

Trinity

Trinity's main difference from other transcriptome assembly programs is that it is directly manufactured for *de novo* RNA assembly. It uses the parallel calculation method to create alternate spliced isoforms and transcripts with *de Bruijn* method [1]. Trinity has three functional modules; *Inchworm*, *Chrysalis* and *Butterfly* of which work in succession and perform different tasks [29]. *Inchworm* uses greedy extension model based on k-mer overlap and reports full-length transcripts for a dominant isoform. Then, *Chrysalis* clusters overlapping contigs and constructs *de Bruijn* graphs. Finally, *Butterfly* process these graphs in parallel and reconstructs full-length transcripts for each isoform. In addition to reconstruct accurate transcripts from RNA-Seq data, Trinity exhibit superior performance in recovering isoforms. Trinity requires extensive computational resources and running time, but it performs best in terms of assembly quality such as N50 value, fewer chimeras and transcript coverage.

SOAPdenovo-Trans

SOAPdenovo-Trans is *de Bruijn* graph-based assembler, which derived from its genome assembler version SOAPdenovo2 [22]. In SOAPdenovo-Trans algorithm, two module error-removal and heuristic graph traversal methods are borrowed from Trinity and Oases, respectively. The algorithm has two main steps: (i) contig assembly and (ii) transcript assembly. Contigs are generated using SOAPdenovo after globally and locally error removal. SOAPdenovo-Trans uses both single-end reads and paired-end reads which mapped back onto the contigs to build scaffolds and then it applies a strict transitive reduction method to simplify the scaffolding graphs, and provide more accurate results. SOAPdenovo-Trans uses less memory and shortest running time than other assembler programs. Although SOAPdenovo-Trans performed best in base coverage, the minimum, first quartile, median, mean and third quartile length of transcripts obtained from SOAPdenovo-Trans is shorter than that in BinPacker, Bridger, IDBA-Tran and Trinity.

Trans-AbySS

Trans-abyss is a method and pipeline for the collection and analysis of short transcriptomic data. Abyss assembly process consists of single-ended and double-ended stages. The single-ended stage is also based on the *de Bruijn* graph structure; when parameter k is given, it is transformed into tiled k-mer represented as read nodes and (k-1) bases are superimposed as directed edges. Allelic differences, minor changes in the sequence and repetitive random base invocation errors lead to 'bubbles' throughout the graph. Once these errors have been removed in the k-mer space, the single-ended contigs defined by the 'walk' clear across the graph. In the matched tier phase, the pairs aligned in the single-ended contigs define the empirical distribution of the distances of the pairs. Single-ended readings of different contigs to the co-aligned pairs and empirical distribution then intercontig distance and combined to form contigs are paired end contigs that can be combined [23]. Trans-AbySS reaches the end by creating direct sequenced readings with Bruijn graphics, removing possible errors from the middle and solving each connected Bruijn graph for each connected component. Compared to other assembler programs the lowest percentage of chimera is seen in Trans-AbySS [30]. Comparative studies showed that with Trinity, Trans-ABySS performed best in gene coverage and number of recovered full-length transcripts [31].

Oases

Oases is a RNA transcriptome assembler that contains many developmental constructs. Combines multiple k-mers and topological analysis methods. In addition, it uses the dynamic error correction feature developed for RNA-Seq data. Assembly process of Oases takes place by creating independent assemblies, which vary according to the length of the k-mers, and then assembling them all together in one assembly. In each assembly, readings are used to generate *de Bruijn*, and then faults are simplified, organized into a scaffold, divided into loci and eventually analysed. Then dynamic correction is performed and Oases creates contigs sets of clusters called loci. Since it is more likely to be unique, long contigs treated first when the scaffold is constructed and faults that may arise from alternative splices are eliminated. Oases provide a robust pipeline from RNA-Seq readings to generate full-length assemblies of transcripts. Especially designed for dealing with RNA-Seq condition, unequal coverage and alternative spliced situations [24]. Oases-Velvet produced the highest number of chimeric transcripts at different k-mer sizes and it has the highest RAM (i.e. random access memory) usage among all assemblers.

IDBA-Tran

IDBA-Tran uses a different approach. Firstly, it produces small *de Bruijn* graphs and enlarges the graph with larger k values. Subsequently, transcripts are found on a large Bruijn graph,

where the same genetic transcripts usually form a single component [25]. IDBA-Tran modulates the products of the k-mers of the same composition with a very normal distribution, which depends on the expression levels of the corresponding isoforms. IDBA-Tran obtains a large number of small components, each representing a single gene. For each small component, IDBA-Tran retrieves the isoform sequences with matched-ended reads by looking for compound pathways. Based on more than one normal distribution and contig length, IDBA-Tran calculates a local threshold to determine whether a k-mer or contigs in error. Using the probabilities and depths that connect the two components together, taking into account the length of the path, the graphics that make up the IDBA-Tran components detect and remove faulty paths. For this reason, IDBA-Tran produces more contigs for low-expressed transcripts and performs better than Oases and Trinity [25].

BinPacker

BinPacker reshapes the problems and generates full-length transcripts by following the aggregated graph line generated by various techniques used in Bridger. Some advantages of BinPacker: (i) BinPacker allows the use of user-defined k-mer values for best performance and (ii) BinPacker uses a strict mathematical model. This allows the BinPacker to achieve a lower false positive rate at the same sensitivity level. (iii) BinPacker makes full use of the step depth applied to graphics, so that the assembly results are more accurate. BinPacker combines transcripts on every merging graph it creates [26]. BinPacker is more unsuccessful than other programs on chimeric data [31].

Bridger

Using a multi-k strategy to achieve high sensitivity leads to more false positives. However, identifying the optimal set of paths that represent the potential isoform can significantly reduce false positive estimates. Bridger's basic idea is to build a bridge between two popular assemblers, Cufflinks (reference-based assembler) and Trinity (*de novo* assembler). Bridger uses a rigorous mathematical model called the minimum path envelope to search for the lowest path set (transcript) supported by RNA-Seq readings. Bridger runs very fast and requires less memory space and CPU (i.e. Central Processing Unit) time than other methods and generates splicing graphics for all genes [27].

2.3. Generating non-redundant transcript data

As described in the previous section in detail, a reference transcriptome for non-model organism can be built using various types of *de novo* transcriptome assemblers. All these assemblers are successful to some extent in recovering expressed transcripts; however, constructing full-length transcripts from short reads remains a daunting and complicated task. Therefore, to obtain more accurate data, researchers performed several studies to optimize a number of

key parameters affecting assembly results such as optimal sequencing depth [11], the read length [10], multi k-mer approaches [7–9], the quality score and error correction of sequence reads [12, 13]. However, transcriptome software themselves follow a multi-stage procedure to avoid introducing misassemble, chimeric assembly and transcript artefacts and to obtain all spliced isoforms from the same gene. For instance, the Inchworm module of Trinity assembles short-reads using greedy extension based on k-mer overlap and reports full-length transcripts for a dominant isoform. Then, the final module, Butterfly, processes the individual graphs in parallel and reconstructs full-length transcripts for each isoform after Chrysalis clusters overlapping contigs, and constructs de Bruijn graphs. Despite all these efforts, *de novo* assembly of short-reads, regardless of software used, results in hundreds of thousands of contigs, a set of contiguous transcript sequences. Without any further analysis such as clustering or post-assembling, the final set of contigs includes (i) partial transcripts and rudimentary isoforms (splice variants), (ii) redundant transcripts (different lengths of the same transcripts, mostly fragments) and (iii) chimeric (fusion) and misassembled sequences [3].

Creating non-redundant transcript dataset with various bioinformatics approaches is a first step after *de novo* transcript assembly. Because, eliminating redundant transcripts and retaining one representative of each transcript isoform (generally, correct and longest in each transcript cluster) are particularly important for downstream applications such as the analysis of transcript structure, gene expression, phylogenomics and identification of SNP variants [8, 30, 32]. To date, several clustering algorithm and post-assembly implementations were developed and used in a significant number of articles for the purpose of creating a non-redundant consensus dataset. The most popular tools used to reduce redundancy in the assembled dataset are CAP3 [33], CD-HIT-EST [34], iAssembler [35], MIRA [36] and TIGR-TGI Clustering tool [37] as well as Corset [32], if performing a differential gene expression analysis. In addition to these tools, some assemblers such as Oases and Trans-ABySS have their own "merging tools" to generate a consensus transcript set when applied multiple k-mer approaches.

So far, all studies using *de novo* transcriptome assembly procedure have included either post-assembly or clustering analysis. Among the assembly-based approaches, CAP3 [33] is one of the first large-scale EST-based assembly tool, which filters for redundant information by detecting overlaps between the contigs and generate the consensus sequence for each transcript. As an overlap-layout-consensus (OLC)-based assembly pipeline, TIGR gene indices clustering tool (TGICL) [37] was developed for producing larger and more complete consensus sequences. In this pipeline, a final set of contigs is first clustered based on pairwise sequence similarity and then each cluster is assembled so that consensus sequences (or non-redundant unigenes) are generated. Yet these methods are successful in removing redundancy, the methods have failed to satisfy the needs of generating a contig per transcripts. It was suggested that there are two type problems, which might be responsible for such failure. The problems frequently observed during assembly are (i) the misassembly of spliced transcripts or paralogs and (ii) contigs derived from the same transcript fail to be assembled together. The iAssembler [35] specially developed to overcome these problems encountered and it consists of seven modules grouped into three functional phases: general controller (input, output and assembly parameters), assembler and error corrector phases. The iAssembler utilizes the approaches of

CAP3 and MIRA assemblers for initial assembly of transcripts, and subsequently, the pairwise alignment information of overlapped transcripts is obtained using Megablast to assemble them into one contig if those transcripts fail to be assembled by either MIRA or CAP3. The assembly process finishes after correcting the above-mentioned errors via error corrector phases, which is the main contribution of iAssembler. A comparison showed that iAssembler has a superior performance over CAP3, MIRA and TGICL in terms of generating much less assembly errors in assembling [35].

Another widely used approach to reduce redundancy in contig assembly is clustering sequences. In this regard, by far the most popular tool is CD-HIT-EST [34]. The CD-HIT-EST is generally used to remove the shorter redundant transcripts and duplicate contigs in large-scale transcriptome datasets. Compared to assembly-based approaches, the CD-HIT-EST is dramatically faster in practice due to its novel parallelization strategy. Corset [32] as a state- of-the-art approach was proposed for hierarchically clustering contigs using information about shared reads. The performance evaluation showed that Corset outperformed CD-HIT-EST in recall (i.e. true positives/(true positives + false negatives)) for genes with no fragmentation and the authors suggested that CD-HIT-EST is not the most effective contig clustering tool while Corset gives a convenient method to cluster contigs [32]. More recently, a clustering tool, RapClust [38] has been developed for *de novo* transcriptome clustering based on the relationships exposed by multi-mapping sequencing fragments and it generates clusters of comparable or better quality than current clustering approaches and does so substantially faster. Although accumulating evidences have indicated that the sequence identity threshold should be set above 90% in both assembly and clustering approaches, a detailed comparison analysis is required for those approaches in terms of accuracy and capability for removing redundant sequences.

2.4. Quality assessment tools for *de novo* transcriptome assemblies

Quality assessment of *de novo* assembled transcripts using reference-free or evidence-based tools seems to be a prerequisite for meaningful interpretation of downstream analysis such as discovery of novel transcripts and correct identification of differentially expressed genes. From a practical point of view, the quality assessment of assembled transcriptome sequences can be handled in three different ways: (i) basic statistical metrics, (ii) reference-free evaluation tools and (iii) reference-dependent or sequence homology-based approaches. Generally, calculating basic statistical metrics is considered as first step in the evaluation of assembled transcriptome. These metrics include total number of transcripts, total base coverage, transcript coverage, N50 value, the presence of chimeric transcripts, longest transcript length, average length of transcripts, etc. These metrics are simple and useful to obtain information about the transcript numbers and coverage at a first glance, but provides no information about accuracy or reliability of transcripts. For instance, N50 value is a median length of a set of contigs (assembled transcripts), but it measures the continuity of contigs but not their accuracy. Recently, reference-free evaluation tools were developed for the accuracy and completeness of *de novo* transcriptome assemblies (see Box 2, i.e. RSEM-EVAL and TransRate). These approaches only process high-quality sequence reads and assembled transcriptome

based on their strong background models and producing scores indicating assembly quality. As for sequence homology-based quality metric, it is seen as standard evaluation criteria for transcriptome assemblies. In this approach, each contig in the assembled transcriptome set was aligned against a reference database (rnaQUAST) or publicly available databases using BLAST, BLAT or SCAN methods (Box 2). Besides, now it is well known that the genome of all living organisms from bacteria to mammals contains evolutionary conserved and phylogenetic clades characteristic of single-copy orthologous gene sets. Therefore, it is considered as an indicator of quality and completeness of transcriptome assembly (see BUSCO in Box 2).

Box 2. A general overview and framework of *de novo* transcriptome assembly evaluation tools.

DETONATE

Li et al. [39] proposed a software package called DETONATE (DE novo TranscriptOme rNa-seq Assembly with or without the Truth Evaluation) which is a methodology for assessing and ranking of *de novo* transcriptome assemblies obtained from various assemblers. DETONATE software is consisted of two parts: RSEM-EVAL and REF-EVAL. As a reference-free evaluation method, RSEM-EVAL is considering as main contribution of the software and uses a probabilistic model that requires only an assembly and the RNA-Seq reads to compute the joint probability. RSEM-EVAL provides a score obtained from calculation of three components; maximum likelihood (ML) estimate, an assembly prior and a Bayesian information criterion (BIC) penalty, reflecting whether resulting contigs are supported by RNA-Seq reads or not. Then, RSEM-EVAL ranks these scores in descending order (from highest to lowest) and highest-scoring assembly is considered as ground truth, in other words, most reliable and compact assembly.

rnaQUAST

Bushmanova et al. [40] developed a quality evaluation tool for transcriptome assemblies. The tool, rnaQUAST, basically maps assembled transcripts to reference genome using BLAT [41] or GMAP [42] and comparing resulting alignments to gene database for measuring quality metrics. In addition to the basic descriptors for contig continuity such as total length, average length of assembled transcripts, longest transcripts and N50 value, the principal contribution of rnaQUAST is arised from the alignments of transcripts to isoforms' positions and analyses them to estimate how well the isoforms are covered by the assembly. For *de novo* quality assessment, rnaQUAST takes advantage of other tools like BUSCO.

BUSCO

In an evolutionary context, Simao et al. [43] presented a software package, BUSCO (Benchmarking Universal Single-Copy Orthologs) for assessment of transcriptome assembly and completeness.

For that purpose, BUSCO scans transcriptome assembly for the presence of near-universal single-copy orthologous gene-sets generated from OrthoDB database of orthologs (http://www.orthodb.org). Covering a high proportion of single-copy orthologous gene-sets indicates completeness of assembled transcripts. BUSCO sets are generated for six major phylogenetic clades; 3023 genes for vertebrates, 675 for arthropods, 843 for metazoans, 1438 for fungi and 429 for eukaryotes. Accumulating evidence showed that above 90% covering of single-copy orthologous gene-sets indicates a good completeness of transcriptome assembly.

TransRate

Despite relative success in generating *de novo* transcriptome assemblies from short-reads, due to wide range of multiple and flexible parameters of *de novo* assembly methods, this methods can generate different assemblies, even if same data were used. These assemblies include chimeras, structural errors, incomplete assembly (e.g. hybrid assembly of gene families, spurious insertions in contigs) and base errors. To overcome frequently occurring problems and filtering, optimization as well as comparison of assemblies, Smith-Unna et al. [44] developed a reference-free transcriptome assembly evaluation tool for the accuracy and completeness of *de novo* transcriptome assemblies using only input reads and assembled contigs. TransRate first aligns the input reads to final assembly, processes those alignments, and calculates contig scores using the full set of processed read alignments. Following these processes, TransRate classifies contigs into two classes; well assembled and poorly assembled, by learning a score cut-off from the data that maximizes the overall assembly score. TransRate gives two types of reference-free statistics; TransRate contig score and assembly score which are calculated by considering these errors. Therefore, TransRate is seen as a diagnostic quality score tool while RSEM-EVAL, another reference-free transcriptome assembly evaluation tool.

SCAN

Comparing assembled transcripts against a reference nucleotide or proteome is a routine task for annotating transcripts. By utilizing this information, Misner et al. [45] described an analytical R package called SCAN (sequence comparative analysis using networks) which generates gene-similarity networks illustrating sequence similarities between transcript assemblies and reference data. The SCAN differs from other software such as BLAST [46] or BLAT [41] in that it provides a robust statistical support in a biological context.

2.5. Current approaches for transcript quantification from RNA-Seq

Following to the assembly procedures, next step is to map the reads to a reference genome or transcriptome, quantify the transcript abundances and detect the differentially expressed transcripts among interested biological conditions. In this section, we give a brief overview of algorithms used is each analysis procedure (**Figure 3**).

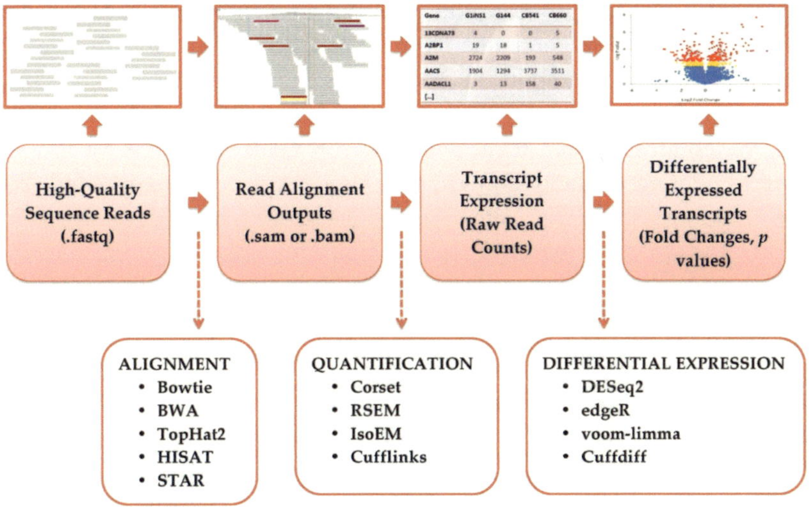

Figure 3. Schematic representation of transcript quantification from alignment to differential expression analysis.

Alignment is an important step in RNA-Seq analysis, which refers to the mapping of the reads to a reference genome or transcriptome, if it is available. Aligners can be classified as spliced and unspliced aligners. Unspliced aligners, e.g. Burrows-Wheeler alignment tool (BWA) and Bowtie, align the reads to the transcriptome by using Burrows-Wheeler or seed methods. These aligners do not properly control intron-sized gaps since they are not designed for spliced alignments. For accurate and fast alignment of the sequence reads over exon/intron boundaries, spliced aligners are proposed which use either exon-first or seed-extended methods [47]. While mapping reads using splice-aware aligners such as HISAT [48], TopHat2 [49] and STAR [50] are generally preferred for genome alignment, the software that is particularly developed for differential gene expression analysis for *de novo* assembled transcriptome uses Bowtie alignment program with '—best' option [32, 51]. Alignment process can be complicated due to several factors: sequencing errors, polymorphisms, imperfect annotation, intron-sized gaps, intron signal, alternative splicing and pathological splicing. Moreover, alignment results directly affect the results of downstream analysis, e.g. transcript quantification, differential expression, gene ontology and pathway analysis [52].

After mapping, the next step is the quantification of each transcript for each sample. It has been reported that the number of reads aligned to the reference genome is linearly related to the abundance of transcripts. Large number of transcript quantification algorithms is available in the literature. rSeq models the sequence reads assumed to follow Poisson distribution with parameters related to the transcript abundances [53]. RSEM is a widely used approach that uses expectation-maximization (EM) algorithm to compute the maximum-likelihood estimates of θ parameters, where θ_i is the probability of a fragment derived from ith transcript. Gibbs sampling is used as well to estimate the posterior means and confidence intervals of transcript abundances. RSEM does not require reference genome or transcriptome files from the users. RSEM conducts a quality score data within the scope of its statistical model or uses a position-dependent error model based on the FASTQ or FASTA input data

types, respectively [51, 54]. Scripture uses the gapped alignments of the reads across splice junctions and the annotated transcripts and produces transcript expressions as RPKM (read per kilobase per million mapped reads) values [55]. Cufflinks assume the sequence reads are sampled independently with uniform probability along transcripts and proportional to the abundances among transcripts. A Bayesian method is used in parameter estimation [56]. IsoEM method exploits information from the distribution of insert sizes and estimates the isoform abundances using an EM algorithm [57]. MMSeq estimates haplotype, isoform and gene-specific expression using a Poisson-based model and EM algorithm. The priors of transcript abundances are assumed to follow a Gamma distribution [58]. BitSeq models the posterior probabilities sequence reads with Markov chains and estimates the transcript expressions using a Bayesian approach [59]. eXpress has a similar methodology to cufflinks. However, it can determine the transcript abundances real-time, and can model indels and errors [60]. CEM identifies the RNA-Seq biases, i.e. positional, sequencing and mapping biases, with quasi-multinomial distribution model and estimates the isoform abundances with component elimination EM approach [61]. Sailfish is an alignment-free approach that is based on indexing and counting k-mers of sequence reads. EM method is used in maximum-likelihood estimation of the transcript abundances. Sailfish is reported as the fastest quantification method as compared to other methods [62]. TIGAR2 models the insertion, deletion and substitution errors in a probabilistic framework, given the gapped alignment of reads to the reference genome. TIGAR2 uses a generative model, including alignment state, nucleotides, the read length distribution and read qualities at first and second positions, to estimate the transcript isoform expressions [63].

Kanitz et al. [64] benchmarked these methods on both simulated and an experimental datasets. The performances are found to be very similar for all algorithms. Teng et al. [65] described several evaluation metrics and compared 7 quantification algorithms and reported that Flux Capacitor and eXpress underperformed, while RSEM outperformed other methods. We believe that RSEMs accuracy may result from its ability to properly handling short transcripts, poly (A) tails and the reads that map to multiple genes. Moreover, this method does not require a reference genome, which is stated to be challenging mostly for eukaryotic species, whose RNA transcripts are spliced and polyadenylated [51]. Beyond these methods, Corset has shown to be another powerful method, which clusters the transcripts into genes and calculates the counts for each gene in a single step [32].

After mapping, per transcript read counts can be used as a relative measure of transcript abundance. In a perfect world, transcript abundance of steady-state mRNA should be directly proportional to the number of reads: a transcript from gene A with twice the cellular concentration of transcript B should have twice as many reads. This relationship should hold across a large range of expression levels spanning several orders of magnitude. Generated transcript abundances can be input to various analysis pipelines. In most cases, the objective is to identify the differentially expressed transcripts between given biological conditions. A key data assumption here is that the data should not contain any technical biases, which may arise from sequence composition, transcript length, sequence depth, sampling bias in library preparation, presence of majority fragments, etc. To enable comparison of genes across samples, these technical biases should be identified and corrected before starting

differential expression analysis. Total count (TC), upper quartile (UQ) and median methods are quantile-based methods, which divide transcript read counts by total number of reads, 3rd quartile and median, respectively. The disadvantage of these methods is that the greater counts can dominate the lower counts in downstream analysis, e.g. differential expression analysis. Reads per kilobase per million mapped reads (RPKM) adjusts read counts both for sequence depth and gene length. RPKM produces unbiased estimates of number of reads; however, this affects the variance. Trimmed mean of M values (TMM) and DESeq2 median ratio approaches are considered as effective library size approaches. These methods assume that a majority of transcripts is not differentially expressed and thus minimize the effect of majority sequences. TMM trims the data based on the log-fold-changes and absolute intensities, then computes the weighted average of genewise log-fold-changes using delta method [66]. DESeq2 median ratio approach generates a pseudo reference sample, which is the geometric mean across samples. Size factors are obtained from the counts and the pseudo reference sample across all genes [67]. An important problem in differential expression analysis is to statistically model the obtained RNA-Seq counts. The preceding studies applied microarray-based methods to log-transformed counts [68, 69]. Some of the studies preferred modelling these data using Poisson distribution [61, 70]. Poisson distribution has a single parameter that represents both mean and variance. Nagalakshmi et al. [71] stated that the presence of biological replicates leads the variance exceeds the mean. This problem is referred to as overdispersion, which led to the development of novel approaches using negative binomial (NB) distribution. DESeq2 and edgeR are the two popular and NB-based approaches to model RNA-Seq data. Both approaches are based on the estimation of mean and variance relationship based on NB distribution. DESeq2 conducts local regression, while edgeR uses a single proportionality constant in this estimation [72, 73]. More recently, Law et al. [74] proposed the voom method, which estimates the mean and variance relationship from log-counts at observational level. Voom provides both gene expression estimates and the corresponding precision weights for downstream analysis. Integration of this method with limma (linear models for microarray and RNA-Seq data) method provided the best control of type-I error, best power and lowest false discovery rate. Wang and Gribskov [31] points out that there may be differences on the differential expression results, between reference genome-based and *de novo* transcriptome assembly approaches. Incomplete and incorrect reference annotation, exon level expression differences and fragmentation of low coverage transcripts are pointed as the reasons of these differences. The authors suggest to perform both approaches even the reference genome is present.

2.6. Transcriptomics tells more: focusing on specific annotation tools and guidelines

The general analysis framework of *de novo* assembled transcripts has three phases: (i) generating non-redundant transcripts and quality assessment, (ii) basic sequence annotations including homology-based sequence annotations (BlastX), gene ontology (GO Slim and Enrichment), pathway analysis (KEGG Enrichment) and (iii) transcript quantifications (**Figure 1**). Although annotation process (beyond the scope of this chapter) provides significant information regarding cellular component, molecular functions and biological process in which transcripts involved, more information can be obtained if transcriptomic data can be further analysed and

interpreted in line with the study objectives and research questions. For instance, in evolutionary perspective, transcriptome data can be used for detecting positively selected or fast evolving genes (PSG, FEG) and are increasingly used in genome-wide phylogenetic studies [75–77] following the steps: orthologs gene detection (particularly single copy genes), multiple sequence alignment of coding regions with PRANK and GUIDANCE pipeline (PRANK algorithm is based on an exhaustive search of the best pairwise solution; the guidance assigning a confidence score for each residue, column and sequence in a multi-alignment from Prank [78], so Guidance [79] can be used for weighting, filtering or masking unreliably aligned positions in sequence alignments before positive selection using the branch-site dN/dS test). Following a multiple sequence alignment, the phylogeny is inferred by Phyml [80] based on proteins residues translated from multi-alignments of single copy orthologous. Then, multiple sequence alignment is used to detect positive selection using the branch-site model with the CodeML program of the PAML [81].

In the context of genome-wide sequence polymorphism within species, mining *de novo* constructed transcripts by appropriate variant calling tools may help us to elucidate the nucleotide-level organismal differences. Among the genetic markers, single nucleotide polymorphisms (SNPs) are the most frequent DNA variation across genome and these genetic markers are widely used for characterising genetic diversity and population structure at genome level, construction of linkage and QTL mapping and association mapping due to their high density/frequency and low mutation rate over generations. In non-model organism, lack of genome sequence information, the standard approach for identification of SNPs or insertion-deletion (InDels) starts by mapping high-quality reads against a reference transcript set constructed *de novo* and detect variations. Briefly, the high-quality reads were aligned against reference transcript set using unspliced aligners such as Burrows-Wheeler alignment tool (BWA) [82] or Bowtie2 [83] and then mapped file '.bam' is obtained for variant calling. After sorting aligned reads and removing duplicates and merging '.bam' alignment results, GATK2 (genome analysis tool kit) [84] is used to perform SNP calling. GATK2 software first filters, realigns and recalibrates reads using its standard filter and data pre-processing methods. The resulting analysis ready reads are parsed to detect SNPs using GATK-UnifiedGenotyper tool with parameters of "-stand_call_conf 30" and "-stand_emit_conf 10". Following this step, SNP calls are hard-filtered using GATK-VariantFiltration tool with parameters of "quality by depth > 5", "unfiltered read depth ≥ 10" and "read mapping quality ≥ 40" to obtain reliable and accurate SNPs [85–87].

The eukaryotic genome harbours a large number of non-coding RNAs, which include small and long non-coding RNAs (lncRNAs). LncRNAs are RNA molecules that are longer than 200 nucleotides in length and do not contain protein-encoding sequences. Recent studies have shown that although human genome contains about 19,000 protein-encoding genes (approximately 2% of the genome) [88], 58,684 high-quality lncRNAs have been identified in the genome using a large-scale transcriptome analysis [89]. Accumulating evidence showed that the protein-coding genes are accounted for only 50% of final assembled transcriptome data. Mining final non-redundant transcriptome data via long non-coding RNA identification tools such as PLEK [90], lncRScan-SVM [91], FEELnc [92] or measuring protein coding potential of transcripts using various tools such as coding potential calculator (CPC) [93], coding potential

assessment tool (CPAT) [94], coding-non-coding index (CNCI) [95] provides us more information about the transcriptome landscape of non-model organism.

Acknowledgements

All authors contributed to the editing of the manuscript and the content is solely the responsibility of the authors. This work was partly supported by the Istanbul University Scientific Research Project (Project No. 46473 and 29506) and also partly supported by Marmara University Research Fund (Grant Number: FEN-A-100616-0275).

Author details

Vahap Eldem[1*], Gokmen Zararsiz[2], Tunahan Taşçi[3], Izzet Parug Duru[4], Yakup Bakir[5] and Melike Erkan[1]

*Address all correspondence to: vahap.eldem@istanbul.edu.tr

1 Department of Biology, Faculty of Sciences, Istanbul University, Istanbul, Turkey

2 Department of Medical Statistics, Faculty of Medicine, Erciyes University, Kayseri, Turkey

3 Department of Medical Imaging Techniques, Vocational School of Health Services, Istanbul Bilgi University, Istanbul, Turkey

4 Department of Physics, Faculty of Science and Art, Marmara University, Istanbul, Turkey

5 Department of Biology, Faculty of Science and Art, Marmara University, Istanbul, Turkey

References

[1] Grabherr MG, Haas BJ, Yassour M, Levin JZ, Thompson DA, Amit I, et al. Full-length transcriptome assembly from RNA-Seq data without a reference genome. Nature Biotechnology. 2011;**29**(7):644-652. DOI: 10.1038/nbt.1883

[2] Ekblom R, Galindo J. Applications of next generation sequencing in molecular ecology of non-model organisms. Heredity. 2011;**107**(1):1-15. DOI: 10.1038/hdy.2010.152

[3] Cahais V, Gayral P, Tsagkogeorga G, Melo-Ferreira J, Ballenghien M, Weinert L, et al. Reference-free transcriptome assembly in non-model animals from next-generation sequencing data. Molecular Ecology Resources. 2012;**12**(5):834-845. DOI: 10.1111/j.1755-0998.2012.03148.x

[4] Todd EV, Black MA, Gemmell NJ. The power and promise of RNA-seq in ecology and evolution. Molecular Ecology. 2016;**25**(6):1224-1241. DOI: 10.1111/mec.13526

[5] da Fonseca RR, Albrechtsen A, Themudo GE, Ramos-Madrigal J, Sibbesen JA, Maretty L, et al. Next-generation biology: Sequencing and data analysis approaches for non-model organisms. Marine Genomics. 2016;**30**:3-13. DOI: 10.1016/j.margen.2016.04.012

[6] Honaas LA, Wafula EK, Wickett NJ, Der JP, Zhang Y, Edger PP, et al. Selecting superior de novo transcriptome assemblies: Lessons learned by leveraging the best plant fenome. PloS one. 2016;**11**(1):e0146062. DOI: 10.1371/journal.pone.0146062

[7] Surget-Groba Y, Montoya-Burgos JI. Optimization of de novo transcriptome assembly from next-generation sequencing data. Genome Research. 2010;**20**(10):1432-1440. DOI: 10.1101/gr.103846.109

[8] Zhao QY, Wang Y, Kong YM, Luo D, Li X, Hao P. Optimizing de novo transcriptome assembly from short-read RNA-Seq data: A comparative study. BMC Bioinformatics. 2011;**12**(Suppl 14):S2. DOI: 10.1186/1471-2105-12-S14-S2

[9] Haznedaroglu BZ, Reeves D, Rismani-Yazdi H, Peccia J. Optimization of de novo transcriptome assembly from high-throughput short read sequencing data improves functional annotation for non-model organisms. BMC Bioinformatics. 2012;**13**:170. DOI: 10.1186/1471-2105-13-170

[10] Chang Z, Wang Z, Li G. The impacts of read length and transcriptome complexity for de novo assembly: A simulation study. PloS one. 2014;**9**(4):e94825. DOI: 10.1371/journal.pone.0094825

[11] Francis WR, Christianson LM, Kiko R, Powers ML, Shaner NC, Haddock SH. A comparison across non-model animals suggests an optimal sequencing depth for de novo transcriptome assembly. BMC Genomics. 2013;**14**:167. DOI: 10.1186/1471-2164-14-167

[12] Macmanes MD, Eisen MB. Improving transcriptome assembly through error correction of high-throughput sequence reads. PeerJ. 2013;**1**:e113. DOI: 10.7717/peerj.113

[13] Mbandi SK, Hesse U, Rees DJ, Christoffels A. A glance at quality score: Implication for de novo transcriptome reconstruction of Illumina reads. Frontiers in Genetics. 2014;**5**:17. DOI: 10.1186/s12859-015-0492-5

[14] Wang B, Tseng E, Regulski M, Clark TA, Hon T, Jiao Y, et al. Unveiling the complexity of the maize transcriptome by single-molecule long-read sequencing. Nature Communications. 2016;**7**:11708. DOI: 10.1038/ncomms11708

[15] Gordon A, Hannon GJ. FastX-Toolkit. FASTQ/A Short-reads Preprocessing Tools [Internet]. 2010. Available from: http://hannonlab.cshl.edu/fastx_toolkit/ [Accessed: 01-01-2017]

[16] Bolger AM, Lohse M, Usadel B. Trimmomatic: A flexible trimmer for Illumina sequence data. Bioinformatics. 2014;**30**(15):2114-2120. DOI: 10.1093/bioinformatics/btu170

[17] Martin M. Cutadapt removes adapter sequences from high-throughput sequencing reads.[Internet]. 2011 [Accessed: 01-01-2017]

[18] Patel RK, Jain M. NGS QC Toolkit: A toolkit for quality control of next generation sequencing data. PloS one. 2012;**7**(2):e30619. DOI: 10.1371/journal.pone.0030619

[19] Shrestha RK, Lubinsky B, Bansode VB, Moinz MB, McCormack GP, Travers SA. QTrim: A novel tool for the quality trimming of sequence reads generated using the Roche/454 sequencing platform. BMC Bioinformatics. 2014;**15**:33. DOI: 10.1186/1471-2105-15-33

[20] Eldem V, Zararsiz G, Erkan M, Bakir Y. De novo assembly and comprehensive characterization of the skeletal muscle transcriptomes of the European anchovy (*Engraulis encrasicolus*). Marine Genomics. 2015;**20**:7-9. DOI: 10.1016/j.margen.2015.01.001

[21] Martin JA, Wang Z. Next-generation transcriptome assembly. Nature Reviews Genetics. 2011;**12**(10):671-682. DOI: 10.1038/nrg3068

[22] Xie Y, Wu G, Tang J, Luo R, Patterson J, Liu S, et al. SOAPdenovo-Trans: De novo transcriptome assembly with short RNA-Seq reads. Bioinformatics. 2014;**30**(12):1660-1666. DOI: 10.1093/bioinformatics/btu077

[23] Robertson G, Schein J, Chiu R, Corbett R, Field M, Jackman SD, et al. De novo assembly and analysis of RNA-seq data. Nature Methods. 2010;**7**(11):909-912. DOI: 10.1038/nmeth.1517

[24] Schulz MH, Zerbino DR, Vingron M, Birney E. Oases: Robust de novo RNA-seq assembly across the dynamic range of expression levels. Bioinformatics. 2012;**28**(8):1086-1092. DOI: 10.1093/bioinformatics/bts094

[25] Peng Y, Leung HC, Yiu SM, Lv MJ, Zhu XG, Chin FY. IDBA-tran: A more robust de novo de Bruijn graph assembler for transcriptomes with uneven expression levels. Bioinformatics. 2013;**29**(13):i326-i334. DOI:10.1093/bioinformatics/btt219

[26] Liu J, Li G, Chang Z, Yu T, Liu B, McMullen R, et al. BinPacker: Packing-Based de novo transcriptome assembly from RNA-seq data. PLOS Computational Biology. 2016;**12**(2):e1004772. DOI: 10.1371/journal.pcbi.1004772

[27] Chang Z, Li G, Liu J, Zhang Y, Ashby C, Liu D, et al. Bridger: A new framework for de novo transcriptome assembly using RNA-seq data. Genome Biology. 2015;**16**:30. DOI: 10.1186/s13059-015-0596-2

[28] Durai DA, Schulz MH. Informed kmer selection for de novo transcriptome assembly. Bioinformatics. 2016;**32**(11):1670-1677. DOI: 10.1093/bioinformatics/btw217

[29] Haas BJ, Papanicolaou A, Yassour M, Grabherr M, Blood PD, Bowden J, et al. De novo transcript sequence reconstruction from RNA-seq using the Trinity platform for reference generation and analysis. Nature Protocols. 2013;**8**(8):1494-1512. DOI: 10.1038/nprot.2013.084

[30] Yang Y, Smith SA. Optimizing de novo assembly of short-read RNA-seq data for phylogenomics. BMC Genomics. 2013;**14**:328. DOI: 10.1186/1471-2164-14-328

[31] Wang S, Gribskov M. Comprehensive evaluation of de novo transcriptome assembly programs and their effects on differential gene expression analysis. Bioinformatics. 2017; **33**(3):327-333. DOI: 10.1093/bioinformatics/btw625

[32] Davidson NM, Oshlack A. Corset: Enabling differential gene expression analysis for de novo assembled transcriptomes. Genome Biology. 2014;**15**(7):410. DOI: 10.1186/s13059-014-0410-6

[33] Huang X, Madan A. CAP3: A DNA sequence assembly program. Genome Research. 1999;**9**(9):868-877

[34] Fu L, Niu B, Zhu Z, Wu S, Li W. CD-HIT: Accelerated for clustering the next-generation sequencing data. Bioinformatics. 2012;**28**(23):3150-3152. DOI: 10.1093/bioinformatics/bts565

[35] Zheng Y, Zhao L, Gao J, Fei Z. iAssembler: A package for de novo assembly of Roche-454/Sanger transcriptome sequences. BMC Bioinformatics. 2011;**12**:453. DOI: 10.1186/1471-2105-12-453

[36] Chevreux B, Pfisterer T, Drescher B, Driesel AJ, Muller WE, Wetter T, et al. Using the miraEST assembler for reliable and automated mRNA transcript assembly and SNP detection in sequenced ESTs. Genome Research. 2004;**14**(6):1147-1159. DOI:10.1101/gr.1917404

[37] Pertea G, Huang X, Liang F, Antonescu V, Sultana R, Karamycheva S, et al. TIGR gene indices clustering tools (TGICL): A software system for fast clustering of large EST datasets. Bioinformatics. 2003;**19**(5):651-652

[38] Srivastava A, Sarkar H, Malik L, Patro R. Accurate, fast and lightweight clustering of de novo transcriptomes using fragment equivalence classes. arXiv preprint arXix. 2016:1604.03250

[39] Li B, Fillmore N, Bai Y, Collins M, Thomson JA, Stewart R, et al. Evaluation of de novo transcriptome assemblies from RNA-Seq data. Genome Biology. 2014;**15**(12):553. DOI: 10.1186/s13059-014-0553-5

[40] Bushmanova E, Antipov D, Lapidus A, Suvorov V, Prjibelski AD. rnaQUAST: A quality assessment tool for de novo transcriptome assemblies. Bioinformatics. 2016;**32**(14):2210-2212. DOI:10.1093/bioinformatics/btw218

[41] Kent WJ. BLAT--the BLAST-like alignment tool. Genome Research. 2002;**12**(4):656-664. DOI: 10.1101/gr.229202

[42] Wu TD, Watanabe CK. GMAP: A genomic mapping and alignment program for mRNA and EST sequences. Bioinformatics. 2005;**21**(9):1859-1875. DOI: 10.1093/bioinformatics/bti310

[43] Simao FA, Waterhouse RM, Ioannidis P, Kriventseva EV, Zdobnov EM. BUSCO: Assessing genome assembly and annotation completeness with single-copy orthologs. Bioinformatics. 2015;**31**(19):3210-3212. DOI: 10.1093/bioinformatics/btv351

[44] Smith-Unna R, Boursnell C, Patro R, Hibberd JM, Kelly S. TransRate: Reference-free quality assessment of de novo transcriptome assemblies. Genome Research. 2016;**26**(8):1134-1144. DOI: 10.1101/gr.196469.115

[45] Misner I, Bicep C, Lopez P, Halary S, Bapteste E, Lane CE. Sequence comparative analysis using networks: Software for evaluating de novo transcript assembly from next-generation sequencing. Molecular Biology and Evolution. 2013;**30**(8):1975-1986. DOI: 10.1093/molbev/mst087

[46] Altschul SF, Madden TL, Schaffer AA, Zhang J, Zhang Z, Miller W, et al. Gapped BLAST and PSI-BLAST: A new generation of protein database search programs. Nucleic Acids Research. 1997;**25**(17):3389-3402

[47] Heras Saldana S, Al-Mamun HA, Ferdosi MH, Khansefid M, Gondro C. RNA sequencing applied to livestock production. In: Kadarmideen HN, editor. Systems Biology in Animal Production and Health. 1st ed. Switzerland: Springer; 2016. pp. 63-94. DOI: 10.1007/978331943335.ch4

[48] Kim D, Langmead B, Salzberg SL. HISAT: A fast spliced aligner with low memory requirements. Nature Methods. 2015;**12**(4):357-360. DOI: 10.1038/nmeth.3317

[49] Kim D, Pertea G, Trapnell C, Pimentel H, Kelley R, Salzberg SL. TopHat2: Accurate alignment of transcriptomes in the presence of insertions, deletions and gene fusions. Genome Biology. 2013;**14**(4):R36. DOI: 10.1186/gb-2013-14-4-r36

[50] Dobin A, Davis CA, Schlesinger F, Drenkow J, Zaleski C, Jha S, et al. STAR: Ultrafast universal RNA-seq aligner. Bioinformatics. 2013;**29**(1):15-21. DOI: 10.1093/bioinformatics/bts635

[51] Li B, Dewey CN. RSEM: Accurate transcript quantification from RNA-Seq data with or without a reference genome. BMC Bioinformatics. 2011;**12**:323. DOI: 10.1186/1471-2105-12-323

[52] Baruzzo G, Hayer KE, Kim EJ, Di Camillo B, FitzGerald GA, Grant GR. Simulation-based comprehensive benchmarking of RNA-seq aligners. Nature Methods. 2017;**14**(2):135-139. DOI: 10.1038/nmeth.4106

[53] Jiang H, Wong WH. Statistical inferences for isoform expression in RNA-Seq. Bioinformatics. 2009;**25**(8):1026-1032. DOI: 10.1093/bioinformatics/btp113

[54] Li B, Ruotti V, Stewart RM, Thomson JA, Dewey CN. RNA-Seq gene expression estimation with read mapping uncertainty. Bioinformatics. 2010;**26**(4):493-500. DOI: 10.1093/bioinformatics/btp692

[55] Guttman M, Garber M, Levin JZ, Donaghey J, Robinson J, Adiconis X, et al. Ab initio reconstruction of cell type-specific transcriptomes in mouse reveals the conserved multi-exonic structure of lincRNAs. Nature Biotechnology. 2010;**28**(5):503-510. DOI: 10.1038/nbt.1633

[56] Trapnell C, Williams BA, Pertea G, Mortazavi A, Kwan G, van Baren MJ, et al. Transcript assembly and quantification by RNA-Seq reveals unannotated transcripts and isoform switching during cell differentiation. Nature Biotechnology. 2010;**28**(5):511-515. DOI: 10.1038/nbt.1621

[57] Nicolae M, Mangul S, Mandoiu, II, Zelikovsky A. Estimation of alternative splicing isoform frequencies from RNA-Seq data. Algorithms for Molecular Biology. 2011;**6**(1):9. DOI: 10.1186/1748-7188-6-9

[58] Turro E, Su SY, Goncalves A, Coin LJ, Richardson S, Lewin A. Haplotype and isoform specific expression estimation using multi-mapping RNA-seq reads. Genome Biology. 2011;**12**(2):R13. DOI: 10.1186/gb-2011-12-2-r13

[59] Glaus P, Honkela A, Rattray M. Identifying differentially expressed transcripts from RNA-seq data with biological variation. Bioinformatics. 2012;**28**(13):1721-1728. DOI: 10.1093/bioinformatics/bts260

[60] Roberts A, Pachter L. Streaming fragment assignment for real-time analysis of sequencing experiments. Nature Methods. 2013;**10**(1):71-73. DOI: 10.1038/nmeth.2251

[61] Li W, Jiang T. Transcriptome assembly and isoform expression level estimation from biased RNA-Seq reads. Bioinformatics. 2012;**28**(22):2914-2921. DOI: 10.1093/bioinformatics/bts559

[62] Patro R, Mount SM, Kingsford C. Sailfish enables alignment-free isoform quantification from RNA-seq reads using lightweight algorithms. Nature Biotechnology. 2014;**32**(5):462-464. DOI: 10.1038/nbt.2862

[63] Nariai N, Kojima K, Mimori T, Sato Y, Kawai Y, Yamaguchi-Kabata Y, et al. TIGAR2: Sensitive and accurate estimation of transcript isoform expression with longer RNA-Seq reads. BMC Genomics. 2014;**15**(Suppl 10):S5. DOI: 10.1186/1471-2164-15-S10-S5

[64] Kanitz A, Gypas F, Gruber AJ, Gruber AR, Martin G, Zavolan M. Comparative assessment of methods for the computational inference of transcript isoform abundance from RNA-seq data. Genome Biology. 2015;**16**:150. DOI: 10.1186/s13059-015-0702-5

[65] Teng M, Love MI, Davis CA, Djebali S, Dobin A, Graveley BR, et al. A benchmark for RNA-seq quantification pipelines. Genome Biology. 2016;**17**:74. DOI: 10.1186/s13059-016-0940-1

[66] Robinson MD, Oshlack A. A scaling normalization method for differential expression analysis of RNA-seq data. Genome Biology. 2010;**11**(3):R25. DOI: 10.1186/gb-2010-11-3-r25

[67] Anders S, Huber W. Differential expression analysis for sequence count data. Genome Biology. 2010;**11**(10):R106. DOI: 10.1186/gb-2010-11-10-r106

[68] Parikh A, Miranda ER, Katoh-Kurasawa M, Fuller D, Rot G, Zagar L, et al. Conserved developmental transcriptomes in evolutionarily divergent species. Genome Biology. 2010;**11**(3):R35. DOI: 10.1186/gb-2010-11-3-r35

[69] Perkins TT, Kingsley RA, Fookes MC, Gardner PP, James KD, Yu L, et al. A strand-specific RNA-Seq analysis of the transcriptome of the typhoid bacillus Salmonella typhi. PLoS Genetics. 2009;**5**(7):e1000569. DOI: 10.1371/journal.pgen.1000569

[70] Wang L, Feng Z, Wang X, Wang X, Zhang X. DEGseq: An R package for identifying differentially expressed genes from RNA-seq data. Bioinformatics. 2010;**26**(1):136-138. DOI: 10.1093/bioinformatics/btp612

[71] Nagalakshmi U, Wang Z, Waern K, Shou C, Raha D, Gerstein M, et al. The transcriptional landscape of the yeast genome defined by RNA sequencing. Science. 2008;**320**(5881): 1344-1349. DOI: 10.1126/science.1158441

[72] Love MI, Huber W, Anders S. Moderated estimation of fold change and dispersion for RNA-seq data with DESeq2. Genome Biology. 2014;**15**(12):550. DOI: 10.1186/s13059-014-0550-8

[73] Robinson MD, McCarthy DJ, Smyth GK. edgeR: A Bioconductor package for differential expression analysis of digital gene expression data. Bioinformatics. 2010;**26**(1):139-140. DOI: 10.1093/bioinformatics/btp616

[74] Law CW, Chen Y, Shi W, Smyth GK. Voom: Precision weights unlock linear model analysis tools for RNA-seq read counts. Genome Biology. 2014;**15**(2):R29. DOI: 10.1186/gb-2014-15-2-r29

[75] Yang Y, Wang L, Han J, Tang X, Ma M, Wang K, et al. Comparative transcriptomic analysis revealed adaptation mechanism of Phrynocephalus erythrurus, the highest altitude Lizard living in the Qinghai-Tibet Plateau. BMC Evolutionary Biology. 2015;**15**:101. DOI: 10.1186/s12862-015-0371-8

[76] Yang L, Wang Y, Zhang Z, He S. Comprehensive transcriptome analysis reveals accelerated genic evolution in a Tibet fish, *Gymnodiptychus pachycheilus*. Genome Biology and Evolution. 2014;**7**(1):251-261. DOI: 10.1093/gbe/evu279

[77] Shao Y, Wang LJ, Zhong L, Hong ML, Chen HM, Murphy RW, et al. Transcriptomes reveal the genetic mechanisms underlying ionic regulatory adaptations to salt in the crab-eating frog. Scientific Reports. 2015;**5**:17551. DOI: 10.1038/srep17551

[78] Loytynoja A, Goldman N. webPRANK: A phylogeny-aware multiple sequence aligner with interactive alignment browser. BMC Bioinformatics. 2010;**11**:579. DOI: 10.1186/1471-2105-11-579

[79] Penn O, Privman E, Ashkenazy H, Landan G, Graur D, Pupko T. GUIDANCE: A web server for assessing alignment confidence scores. Nucleic Acids Research. 2010;**38**(Web Server issue):W23-W28. DOI: 10.1093/nar/gkq443

[80] Guindon S, Dufayard JF, Lefort V, Anisimova M, Hordijk W, Gascuel O. New algorithms and methods to estimate maximum-likelihood phylogenies: Assessing the performance of PhyML 3.0. Systematic Biology. 2010;**59**(3):307-321. DOI: 10.1093/sysbio/syq010

[81] Yang Z. PAML 4: Phylogenetic analysis by maximum likelihood. Molecular Biology and Evolution. 2007;**24**(8):1586-1591. DOI: 10.1093/molbev/msm088

[82] Li H, Durbin R. Fast and accurate short read alignment with Burrows-Wheeler transform. Bioinformatics. 2009;**25**(14):1754-1760. DOI: 10.1093/bioinformatics/btp324

[83] Langmead B, Salzberg SL. Fast gapped-read alignment with Bowtie 2. Nature Methods. 2012;**9**(4):357-359. DOI: 10.1038/nmeth.1923

[84] McKenna A, Hanna M, Banks E, Sivachenko A, Cibulskis K, Kernytsky A, Garimella K, Altshuler D, Gabriel S, Daly M, DePristo MA. The genome analysis toolkit: A MapReduce framework for analyzing next-generation DNA sequencing data. Genome Research. 2010;**20**(9):1297-1303. DOI: 10.1101/gr.107524.110

[85] Lopez-Maestre H, Brinza L, Marchet C, Kielbassa J, Bastien S, Boutigny M, Monnin D, El Filali A, Carareto CM, Vieira C, Picard F, Kremer N, Vavre F, Sagot MF, Lacroix V. SNP calling from RNA-seq data without a reference genome: identification, quantification, differential analysis and impact on the protein sequence. Nucleic Acids Research. 2016;**44**(19). DOI: 10.1093/nar/gkw655

[86] Li Y, Zhou Z, Tian M, Tian Y, Dong Y, Li S, Liu W, He C. Exploring single nucleotide polymorphism (SNP), microsatellite (SSR) and differentially expressed genes in the jellyfish (*Rhopilema esculentum*) by transcriptome sequencing. Marine Genomics. 2017. DOI: 10.1016/j.margen.2017.01.007

[87] Humble E, Thorne MA, Forcada J, Hoffman JI. Transcriptomic SNP discovery for custom genotyping arrays: Impacts of sequence data, SNP calling method and genotyping technology on the probability of validation success. BMC Research Notes. 2016;**9**(1):418. DOI: 10.1186/s13104-016-2209-x

[88] Ezkurdia I, Juan D, Rodriguez JM, Frankish A, Diekhans M, Harrow J, et al. Multiple evidence strands suggest that there may be as few as 19,000 human protein-coding genes. Human Molecular Genetics. 2014;**23**(22):5866-5878. DOI: 10.1093/hmg/ddu309

[89] Iyer MK, Niknafs YS, Malik R, Singhal U, Sahu A, Hosono Y, et al. The landscape of long noncoding RNAs in the human transcriptome. Nature Genetics. 2015;**47**(3):199-208. DOI: 10.1038/ng.3192

[90] Li A, Zhang J, Zhou Z. PLEK: A tool for predicting long non-coding RNAs and messenger RNAs based on an improved k-mer scheme. BMC Bioinformatics. 2014;**15**:311. DOI: 10.1186/1471-2105-15-311

[91] Sun L, Liu H, Zhang L, Meng J. lncRScan-SVM: A tool for predicting long non-coding RNAs using support vector machine. PloS one. 2015;**10**(10):e0139654. DOI: 10.1371/journal.pone.0139654

[92] Wucher V, Legeai F, Hedan B, Rizk G, Lagoutte L, Leeb T, et al. FEELnc: A tool for long non-coding RNA annotation and its application to the dog transcriptome. Nucleic Acids Research. 2017. DOI: 10.1093/nar/gkw1306

[93] Kong L, Zhang Y, Ye ZQ, Liu XQ, Zhao SQ, Wei L, et al. CPC: Assess the protein-coding potential of transcripts using sequence features and support vector machine. Nucleic Acids Research. 2007;**35**(Web Server issue):W345-W349. DOI: 10.1093/nar/gkm391

[94] Wang L, Park HJ, Dasari S, Wang S, Kocher JP, Li W. CPAT: Coding-potential assessment tool using an alignment-free logistic regression model. Nucleic Acids Research. 2013;**41**(6):e74. DOI: 10.1093/nar/gkt006

[95] Sun L, Luo H, Bu D, Zhao G, Yu K, Zhang C, et al. Utilizing sequence intrinsic composition to classify protein-coding and long non-coding transcripts. Nucleic Acids Research. 2013;**41**(17):e166. DOI: 10.1093/nar/gkt646

Chapter 4

Models of RNA Interaction from Experimental Datasets: Framework of Resilience

William Seffens

Additional information is available at the end of the chapter

http://dx.doi.org/10.5772/intechopen.69452

Abstract

Resilience is a network property of systems responding under stress, which for biomedicine correlates to chronic or acute insults. Current need exists for models and algorithms to study whole transcriptome differences between tissues and disease states to understand resilience. Goal of this effort is to interpret cellular transcription in a dynamic system biology framework of RNA molecules forming an information structure with regulatory properties acting on individual transcripts. We develop and evaluate a bioinformatics framework based on information theory that utilizes RNA expression data to create a whole transcriptome model of interaction that could lead to the discovery of new biological control mechanisms. This addresses a fundamental question as to why transcription yields such a small fraction of protein products. We focus on a transformative concept that individual transcripts collectively form an "information cloud" of sequence words, which for some genes may have significant regulatory impact. Extending the concept of *cis*- and *trans*-regulation, we propose to search for RNAs that are modulated by interactions with the transcriptome cloud and calling such examples *nebula* regulation. This framework has implications as a paradigm change for RNA regulation and provides a deeper understanding of nucleotide sequence structure and -omic language meaning.

Keywords: transcriptome, RNA, diffusion, secondary structure, resilience, information theory

1. Introduction

The concept of resilience is receiving increasing attention in chronic stress-related disease conditions. Resilience has been shown in clinical studies to play a protective role in patients

with chronic disease conditions including osteoarthritis, breast and ovarian cancer, diabetes, and cardiovascular disease. The purpose of this study is to explore the relationships between RNA-RNA interactions and to devise a related measure of resilience from network properties of the whole transcriptome.

1.1. RNA physiology

At various levels, RNA is processed by alternate mechanisms [1], suggesting a biological framework that supports important system network features such as resilience. Trafficking of RNAs is essential for cellular function and homeostasis, but only recently it has become possible to visualize molecular events *in vivo*. Analysis of RNA motion within the cell nucleus has been particularly intriguing as they have revealed an unanticipated degree of dynamics within the organelle [2]. Single-molecule RNA imaging methods have revealed that the intranuclear and cytoplasmic trafficking occurs largely by energy-independent mechanisms and is driven by diffusion. RNA molecules undergo constrained diffusion, largely limited by the spatial constraint imposed by chromatin and chromatin-binding proteins if in the nucleus as demonstrated in numerous studies. In the cell, transcripts move by a stop-and-go mechanism, where free diffusion is interrupted by random association with cellular structures [3]. The ability and mode of motion of RNAs has implications for how they find nuclear targets on chromatin or cellular sub-compartments and how macromolecular complexes are assembled *in vivo*. Most importantly, the dynamic nature of RNAs is emerging as a means to control physiological cellular responses and pathways [4]. For example, unexpectedly complicated nuclear egress and nuclear import of small RNAs is more common than previously appreciated [5].

Much attention has been focused on noncoding RNAs and their physiological/pathological implications [6]. This focus in RNA research is ultimately directed toward understanding the regulation of protein-coding gene networks, but ncRNAs also form well-orchestrated regulatory interaction networks [7]. For example, computational prediction of miRNA target sites suggests a widespread network of miRNA-lncRNA interaction [8]. Others suggest the possibility of widespread interaction networks involving competitive endogenous RNAs (ceRNAs) where ncRNAs could modulate regulatory RNA by binding and titration of binding sites on protein coding messengers [9]. Cellular uptake and trafficking of RNA could be widespread [10]. As the number of experiments increases rapidly, and transcriptional units are better annotated, databases indexing RNA properties and function will become essential tools to understand physiologic processes in the transcriptome.

1.2. Biological-omic information theory

Much of bioinformaticians sequence analyses focuses on methodologies based on string alignment algorithms. However, such approaches fail to discover genomic aspects of systemic nature regarding dynamics or resilience. An alternative framework is based on alignment-free methods of genome analysis, where global properties of genomes are investigated [11]. A key concept of informational analysis is that of probability distributions. A genomic, or in our case transcriptomic, distribution associates to discrete values defined on transcripts, the number of

times these values occur in a given transcriptome. The general concept of discrete probability distribution, called information source, was the starting point of information theory developed by Shannon [12]. Links between information theory and biology emerged from Shannon's Ph. D. thesis, titled "An Algebra for Theoretical Genetics" (1940), where the notion of information entropy was introduced [13]. For example, distributions of codons have shown characteristic properties that are linked to biological meanings, such as secondary structure free energy [14]. Other approaches based on the recurrence of genomic elements and on correlation structures in DNA sequences use mutual information, which plays a central role in the mathematical analysis of message transmission. Dictionary-based methodologies analyze sequences through properties of collections of words. Dictionaries are concepts from formal language theory, probability, and information theory that provide new perspective which may uncover the physiology of internal transcriptome structures.

2. Methods

We formally define the transcriptome as an information structure, and then construct several simple models as examples. The most realistic model is used to examine real datasets of partitioned RNAs for validation of framework.

2.1. Transcriptome information theory structure

RNA sequence is abstractly represented as a string over the nucleotide alphabet $\mathfrak{R} = \{A, C, G, U\}$. This can be extended to modified nucleotides with an extended alphabet $\mathfrak{R} \cong \{A, C, G, U, N\}$, such that symbol N represents a modified nucleotide. W_k denotes a set of alphabet letters of length k, called k-mers and $\mathfrak{W}$ denotes the set of all possible nonempty strings over the alphabet $\mathfrak{R}$. Given a transcript string $S = s1, s2, \ldots$ to sn, of length n, $S[i, j]$ with $1 \le i \le j \le n$ is the substring of S from position i to position j (included). The length of S is $|S| = n$. Substrings of S of length k are called k-words or simply words of S. In the following, the entire transcriptome is denoted by W based on k-mer dictionaries and entropies, which are aimed at defining and computing informational indexes for representative sets of transcriptomes. We assume that the complexity of a transcriptome increases with its distance from randomness, as identified by suitable comparison between transcriptomes of the same length. This framework provides clues about the appropriate k length to consider for analysis of transcriptome properties.

2.2. Spatial transcriptome information cloud (STIC) model construction

We hypothesized that miRNA localization in cellular compartments is an emergent property from Brownian motion interactions of a cloud of RNA sequences and RNA-binding proteins that can be analyzed in W [15]. There k-mer words of miRNA functional size were added to a dictionary from sliding windows of transcript sequences S. A prediction from this cloud model is that anomalous diffusion can occur if random-walk transcripts interact with their surrounding scaffold as a stochastic semantic cloud, and if the cloud relaxation time is a longer time frame than transit [16]. We showed that RNAs with sequences similar to the whole transcriptome exhibit modified or enhanced transport compared to RNA sequences without

similar sequences [17]. Thus, RNAs were found to partition into different cellular compartments based on a semantic similarity of word compositions within W_k. We determine the frequency of all k-mers in the transcriptome as a matrix composed of RNA sequences and their word copy levels. For each transcript, we count the number of k-mer words in common within W_k or dictionary as a semantic similarity measure to the transcriptome, and we can also able to compare such counts to randomized W_k sequence words.

Model assumptions are: (1) RNA diffuses away from point of transcription creating a cloud of k-mer sequences. (2) All RNAs comprise the transcriptome, and each transcript is affected by local RNAs with effective interaction windows of some sequence word length k nucleotides (nt). We assume significant k-mer word size to be 3–22 nt, which is equal to the functional miRNA size at the high side, and down to below the size of the "core" sequence [18]. (3) The diffusion rate of individual RNAs depends on degree of (a) sequence similarity and (b) reverse complementarity of RNA words at that location in the STIC (**Figure 1**). (4) Cloud dictionaries (collection of transcriptome word sets in W_k) change as function of distance from transcriptome site and cell state. (5) The cloud affects anomalous RNA diffusion that can give rise to an emergent and patterned behavior in the cell [19].

We model the RNA sequence word content of the transcriptome cloud as a function of distance from transcription site at the chromosome. RNA molecule diffusion in nuclear compartments would lead to cytoplasmic and extracellular localization of RNA if the transcript half-life is greater than its transit time. Calculations at arbitrary transit distances could be determined

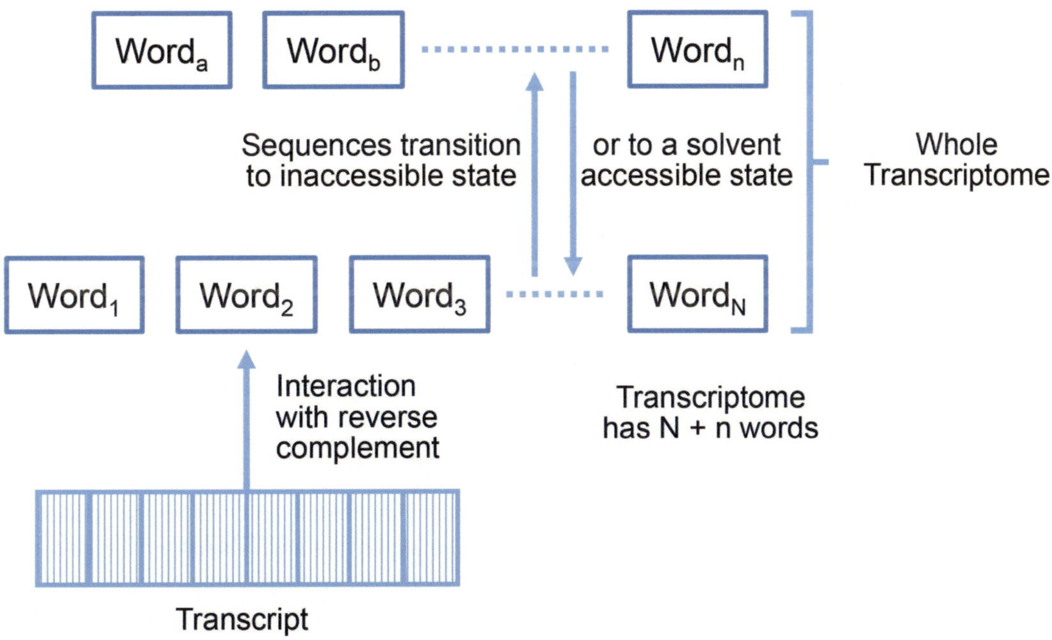

Figure 1. K-mer words classified as solvent-accessible or inaccessible. Note that in this framework, k-mer words are generated from a sliding window and not from a contiguous word segments as could be interpreted by the figures adjacent to word blocks. Transcriptome is a dictionary of $N + n$ words and their associated frequencies. Interaction of transcript with transcriptome affects diffusion from solvent-accessible bases (words). Transcript itself is a part of the transcriptome.

http://dx.doi.org/10.5772/intechopen.69452

from this model with a large set of partial differential equations modeling RNA mobility, but was described as computationally prohibitive [15] for any realistic sized transcriptome. Each sequence S would be dynamically modeled with a neighborhood sized number of RNA-RNA interactions. Instead, we pursue a thermodynamic approach based on the Fokker-Planck equation to quantify stochastic processes in liquid medium [20]. RNA interactions are assumed to function over sequence lengths encompassing small single-stranded and solvent-accessible regions.

Assuming smallest word in the cloud is 3 nt long, corresponding to the lower limit of size for a seed sequence in miRNA [18]. The upper limit for word size is set at 22 nt, corresponding to the size of a typical mature miRNA. Again, this is the same as the miRNA response elements (MRE) size in the simpler related ceRNA hypothesis by Salmena [9]. Instead, we determine the frequency of all words in the transcriptome as a matrix composed of RNA sequences and copy levels from RNA-seq datasets. For each transcript, count number of words in common with the cloud dictionary as a similarity measure to the transcriptome (tCount), and also count reverse complement words (rcCount) for RNA-RNA interactions. These raw counts can be multiplied by the frequencies of repetitive words in W to yield tWord = tCount * tFreq and rcWord = rcCount * rcFreq. As shown by Seffens [17], miRNAs with greater similarity to the transcriptome, i.e., greater tCount and tWord, are suggested to diffuse differentially based on spatial partitioning. In addition, greater intramolecular RNA-RNA interaction would be expected to hinder diffusion. This work proposes a general RNA sequence function that combines the influence of similarity with native (NAM) and reverse complementarity (RCM) measures as a cloud interaction function: $\mathfrak{C}$[W, NAM, RCM], such that cloud interactions increase with RCM, and decrease with NAM. Transcripts with low $\mathfrak{C}$ would have "ideal solution" diffusion coefficients and found in cytoplasmic compartment, and those with greater $\mathfrak{C}$ would be slowed by RNA-RNA interactions and hence enriched in nuclear or perinuclear compartments.

2.2.1. *Accessibility of an RNA sequence word*

For each component word of a transcript, determine whether it is expected to be in a single-stranded and solvent-accessible state (state "A"), or double-stranded or buried within the RNA molecule and is inaccessible (state "I"). For model calculations and preliminary studies (Model-1 W^1 discussed later), we assume all words are accessible in state "A," and the transcriptome is uniform within the cell (i.e., ignore distance r from transcription site). Construct a matrix $W_k(T, f_A, f_I, r)$ for each word size k, and populate the respective matrix with the component words of the transcriptome from RNA-seq reads such that S is the actual word sequence, f_A is the frequency or number of accessible words of that sequence, and f_I is the frequency or number of inaccessible words. Matrix W_k then contains information of all transcript sub-sequences and is a representation of the spatial transcriptome information cloud in some volume elements of the cell fraction. Let the diffusion coefficient for a transcript be described [24]as D_{RNA} [21]. Then the effect of interaction of that transcript with the cloud would yield

$$D_{RNA} = {D_{RNA}}^{ideal} - \mathfrak{C}\left[W_k(S, f_A, f_I, r), S\right] = {D_{RNA}}^{ideal} - \text{RCM} + \text{NAM} \qquad (1)$$

where $\mathfrak{C}$ is the cloud interaction term for molecule RNA exhibiting probabilities of RNA-RNA interactions as a function of the STIC represented by matrix W_k at some position r in the cell.

For RNA expression data from the whole cell, r is ignored. In experiments from purified nuclei, r ranges from 0 to the radius of the cell's nucleus, r_N. In experiments derived from the cytosol, r ranges from r_N to the cellular membrane radius r_C. Experimental data from extracellular vesicles will have $r > r_C$ and RNA half-life becomes important to consider as a factor. As a first approximation for the $\mathfrak{C}$ function, we assume that the deviation from ideal D_{RNA} scales as the number of reverse complement words (rcCount) in common with transcriptome W_k and is measured by difference to the number tCount of words in common with W_k, which normalizes for transcript size. We could also compare to ranCount, number of words in common with a randomized W_k. Putting together, we have

$$\mathfrak{C}[W_k, S] = \alpha \text{ rcCount}/4^k \tag{2}$$

to normalize number of words, or alternately,

$$\mathfrak{C}[W_k, S] = \alpha(\text{rcCount} * \text{rcFreq} - \text{tCount} * \text{tFreq}) = \text{RCM for } \alpha = 1.0 \tag{3}$$

where α is a scaling factor and is dimensionless. The reverse complement measure (RCM), which factors rcCount word frequencies by rcFreq, then subtracting the count of words in common with transcriptome (tCount) by the corresponding tFreq, is one of several possible measures for correlation to measured compartmentalization of individual transcripts from RNA-expression datasets. The content of $W_k(r)$ changes as a function of r due to changing concentrations of transcripts in the cell. Boundary condition on whole cell measurement from microarray or RNA-seq experiments would be

$$W_k = \int_0^{r_C} W_k(r)\, dr \tag{4}$$

assuming no export from the cell. If there are no reverse complement words in common between transcript S and W_k, then $\mathfrak{C}$ $[W_k, S]$ is zero and the diffusion of that molecule is ideal. As a first approximation for the $\mathfrak{C}$ function, we assume that the deviation from ideal D_{RNA} scales as the number (rcCount) of reverse complement words in common with W_k and is compared by a difference to the number tCount of words in common with W_k to normalize for transcript size. We could also compare to ranCount, number of words in common with a randomized W_k. Reverse complement measure (RCM) factors word frequencies to assess transcript-cloud interactions that correlate to measured compartmentalization of individual transcripts [17].

2.2.2. Words that are solvent-accessible

The above model treatment assumed that all RNA sequences are available for reverse complementarity interactions. RNAs except for miRNAs typically have regions that are solvent-inaccessible and/or double-stranded, preventing intramolecular interactions [22]. mRNAs have more secondary structures or intra-strand base pairing than expected by chance [23]. We have determined the secondary structure of all RefSeq transcripts to predict single-stranded regions using RNAfold [24], while others have used RNA structure predictors (RNAplfold in

Refs. [25, 26]) in a pooling predictor using machine learning [27]. Additionally, nucleotide solvent-accessibility in RNA structures could be estimated by the neural network method of Singh [22] using models of window size 3 nt, which could be expanded to 5–9 nt windows for k length. Alternatively, accessible surface area can be calculated by a publically available program NACCESS [28] to refine the STIC transcriptome words to those populated from single-stranded regions only, along with confidence measures. Solvent accessibility estimates for each transcript word partition the frequency entries in the transcriptome matrix $W_k(S, f_A, f_I, r)$ by reducing f_A in the amount that f_I increases. Shifts of f_A to f_I could be caused by RNA-binding factors (RNA or protein) that cover a word in the transcript or the word in the transcriptome, or indirectly by binding to some other region of the RNA causing a *cis*-type of structural alteration leading to solvent inaccessibility (**Figure 2**). Transcriptome cloud or *nebula* regulation is introduced here and is proposed to occur as an indirect result of some factor that changes f_A/f_I for some word that then alters a different interacting transcript's diffusion coefficient. Conversely, f_I to f_A shifts could be caused by the release of binding factors or conformational change leading to exposure of the particular word and to nearby target RNAs. Dictionaries with this dynamic accounting of the transcriptome are labeled T, instead of the simpler W word matrix.

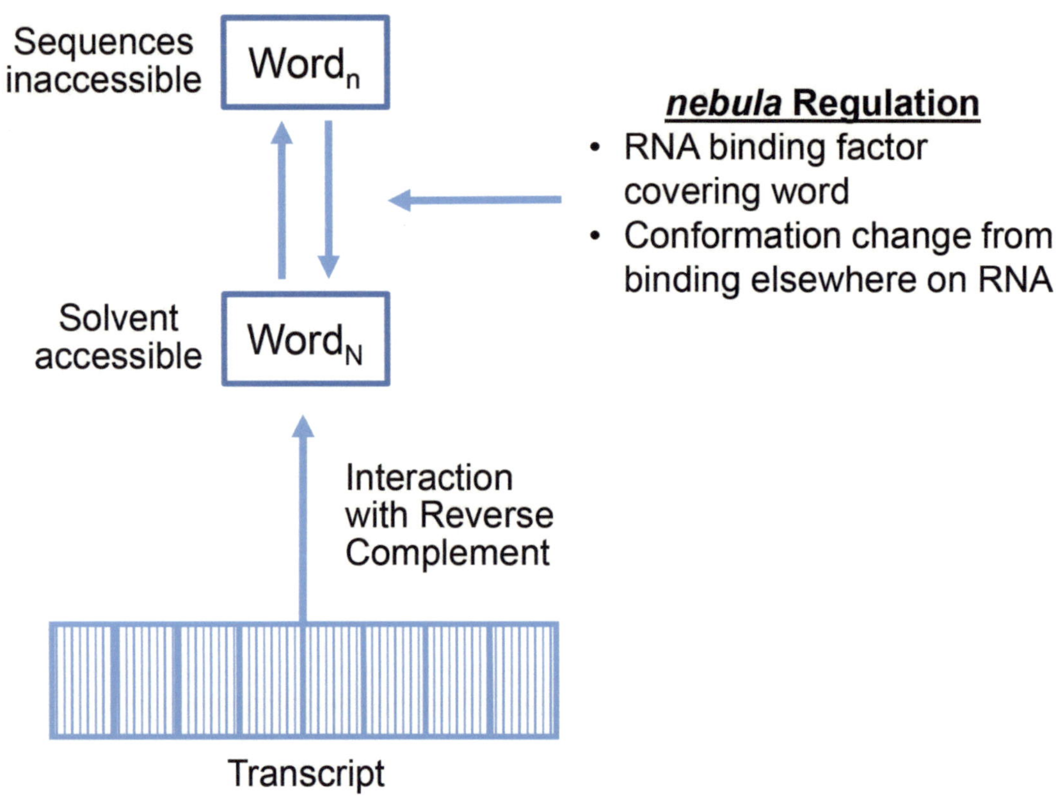

Figure 2. Words classified as solvent-accessible or -inaccessible in dynamic transitions. Interaction of RNA binding-proteins and other RNA affects balance of solvent-accessible words in transcriptome and transcript.

2.2.3. *Genome-wide profiling of* in vivo *RNA structure*

Recent transcriptome-wide RNA structure profiling through application of structure-probing enzymes or chemicals combined with high-throughput sequencing promises *in vivo* RNA structural information availability. Resultant datasets provide opportunity to investigate RNA structural information on global scale for STIC development. The analysis of high-throughput RNA structure profiling data requires considerable computational effort and currently dataset are not readily available. StructureFold processes and performs analysis of raw high-throughput RNA structure profiling data [29], incorporating wet-bench structural information from chemical probes and ribonucleases to restrain RNA structure prediction via RNAstructure and ViennaRNA package algorithms. StructureFold is deployed via the Galaxy platform. Alternatively, structure-seq is a recent quantitative and high-throughput method that provides genome-wide information on RNA structure with single-nucleotide resolution [30]. The methodology can perform both *in vitro* and *in vivo* RNA structure-function determinations, with insights to RNA regulation of gene expression and RNA processing. Implementation of structure-seq begins with chemical RNA structure probing under single-hit kinetics conditions. Modified RNA is then subjected to reverse transcription using random hexamer primers, then reverse transcription executed until it is blocked by chemically modified residues. Resultant cDNAs are amplified by adapter-based polymerase chain reaction (PCR) which are subjected to high-throughput sequencing, subsequently allowing retrieval of structural information on a genome-wide scale. A single structure-seq experiment can provide information on tens of thousands of RNA structures in a matter of weeks. Ding et al. [31] used RNAstructure calculated for each of thousands of mRNAs a positive predictive value (PPV), which they use to compare relative frequencies of base pairing *in vivo* constrained RNA structures to *in silico* predicted RNA structure. They found that most mRNAs do not fold *in vivo* as to *in silico*-predicted structures, as evident from a broad PPV distribution. Interestingly, mRNAs of cold and metal ion stress-response genes folded *in vivo* significantly different from their unconstrained *in silico* predictions. These stressors are known to affect RNA structure and thermo-stability like melting temperature T_m. Instead, genes involved with basic biological functions such as gene expression, protein maturation or processing, and peptide metabolic processes show little change in their *in vivo*-constrained and *in silico*-predicted RNA secondary structures. Ding speculated mRNAs related to cell maintenance and showing high PPV may have evolved to resist large conformational changes in order to maintain homeostasis, an idea suggesting RNA resilience. This bias may be detectable in our transcriptome model W. As genome-wide profiling of *in vivo* RNA structure datasets becomes easily available [32], the information can be incorporated into the STIC model by adding custom transform and load tools for each dataset.

2.3. Simplest models of transcriptomes

We consider simplest models of the transcriptome to examine some limits on the model parameters and functions. Component of a transcriptome are listed in **Table 1**.

2.3.1. *Transcriptome model 0 (W^0)*

Simplest model considers a spatially uniform transcriptome composed of ribosomes, tRNA, and a minor number of mRNAs. Here, the distribution of transcripts is assumed uniform and the transcriptome model lacks spatial elements. Further, consider a transcriptome where

Transcriptome construction		
Class	**Biotype**	**Network system function**
ncRNA	rRNA	Most abundant; constant character
ncRNA	tRNA	Most frequent; constant character
Protein coding	mRNA	Act as gene; bigger than coded protein
ncRNA	miRNA	Block some mRNA; smallest func. RNA
Processed transcripts	lncRNA	Block or regulate some other RNA
Transcriptome = $\Sigma\ W^{Biotype}$		

Notes: Sequence words summed into dictionary over all transcript types.

Table 1. Transcriptome construction from different RNA biotypes. Transcriptome model W^1 is a subset of 8 human rRNA and tRNA types.

ribosomes and tRNAs are all "A" for adenosine, and the mRNAs are also all "A." We can construct transcriptome model W^0 using transcript values found in **Table 1** from Seffens [17], with sizes n and respective abundances. The number of nonunique words (of size k) would be $n - k + 1$ for each transcript. Using sizes and respective abundance values in **Table 1** [17], gives 2.8×10^{10} words, composed of all "A"s. Assume mRNAs are 2 kb "A"s, then there are no reverse complement interactions, so RCM should be zero, while NAM would be maximal (RCM and NAM defined in Section 2.2). The diffusion coefficient for these mRNAs would be ideal since there are no base-pairing interactions within W^0 and transcript similarity to the transcriptome is maximal. Now assume the mRNAs are all "U"s, they now strongly interact with the majority of W^0. RCM becomes $2000 \times 2.8 \times 10^{10}$ or 5.6×10^{13} for each mRNA transcript (while NAM would be zero). This would be the expected maximal value for RCM with mRNAs of 2 kb size, yielding diffusion coefficients smaller than ideal values. These RNAs would exhibit larger intramolecular RNA-RNA interactions, and they do not look (NAM = 0) and behave ($D_{RNA} \ll D_{RNA}{}^{ideal}$) as the rest of the transcriptomes.

2.3.2. *Transcriptome model 0-R ($W^{0\text{-}R}$)*

Now assume that the transcriptome W^0 is composed of completely random sequences of *A, C, G, Us*-labeled $W^{0\text{-}R}$. How many of the 2.8×10^{10} words of length k composed of four different letters would be unique (not identical) in the model? Combination of all possible k-mer words would be $4^{22} = 1.76 \times 10^{13}$ since there are four possible nucleotide letters at each of the k positions. Since there are about 1000 times more possible combinations than there are $k = 22$ words, we could assume that all 22-mer words are unique. Smaller values of k will result in repeats or duplicate words increasing frequency values in W_k. These calculations give an expected value for RCM based on no biases in the sequences.

2.3.3. *Transcriptome model 1 (W^1)*

The next more realistic model is composed of eight real human RNA transcripts comprising a simple representation of the transcriptome in a cell (**Table 1** and in Ref. [17]). It is assembled

from four of the most prevalent human tRNAs with lengths of $n = 71$–73 nt, and four of the major subunits of the eukaryotic ribosome with sizes from $n = 121$ to 5034 nt, with the total number of nucleotides N being the sum of the nucleotides in each transcript, or $N = 7470$ nt. Then the frequency of words with length k that are contained in each transcript is a subset of the number of possible k-mer words which is $n - k + 1$. In Model-1 labeled as W^1, for each word length from $k = 3$ to 22, word count was calculated along with the sum of the frequencies of those words extracted from the simple eight RNA transcripts. The intermediate output from program TIC-generator (for transcriptome information cloud generator, described in Ref. [17]) listed all k-mer words contained in each transcript, together with their frequency of occurrence. These lists from the eight rRNA and tRNA transcripts were combined, and then duplicate words resolved to form dictionary W_k^1. With the total possible number of words of length $k = 4^k$, the fraction of all the words actually present in W_k^1 decreased for increasing word size [17]. It is interesting that the peak in unique and total duplicate (blue diamonds in Ref. [17]) words is maximal at the same size as the miRNA "seed" sequence as defined in Ref. [18].

2.3.4. *Randomized transcriptome of Model-1 ($W^{1\text{-}R}$)*

We ran TIC-generator with shuffled-sequence transcripts labeled Model 1-R. Base composition of Model-1 transcriptome is 1341 "A," 2320 "C," 2519 "G," and 1291 "T," or 18% "A," 31% "C," 34% "G," and 17% "T." Using a random letter generator, we assembled four random transcriptomes with the same transcript length for the eight sequences and equal Model-1 base composition. We examined mostly word lengths k of 7 and 8 in preliminary studies shown below.

2.4. Real model validation

As a validation of this transcriptome model framework, we utilized the simple transcriptome model version (simple model W^1) that used real highly expressed genes, and for comparison separately, randomized sequences of that transcriptome ($W^{1\text{-}R}$). This simple realistic model is composed of only eight real human RNA transcripts as a basic representation of the transcriptome in a cell. Experimental validation of the basic model transcriptome for k-mers considered various trial functions of semantic word similarity and reverse complementarity, which were calculated using published data sets. For example, trial functions evaluated include tWord for transcriptome words in common with target multiplied by respective word frequency in W_k. A total of seven RNA studies, with data sources grouped into high and low study parameter sets, were statistically analyzed by mean values and t-test calculated as two-tail t-test under two-sample equal variance assumption models (**Table 2**). Validation for the STIC model examined various functions of reverse complementarity using these published data sets. Here, we assume that appearance in exosomes or microparticles requires greater mobility and hence larger diffusion coefficients than cytoplasmic or nuclear RNAs [17]. Several functions tested include tWord for transcriptome words in common with target multiplied by word frequency in the transcriptome, rcWord (reverse complement k-mer words in common times frequency), RCM = rcWord – tWord, reverse complement count (RCC) measure = tCount – rcCount, Z-RCC as a z-score of RCC compared to four randomized transcriptomes Model 1-R, Z-RCM as the z-score of RCM, RCC-Ran which subtracts the value computed from 1-R and finally (RCC-Ran)/Len which

is normalized for sequence length. The first five studies examined miRNA, while the Chen [33] and Friedel [34] studies measured mRNAs. Description of data sources that were grouped into high and low study parameter sets, with mean values and t-tests calculated detailed in sections below.

2.4.1. Model 1 validation with miRNA from exosome datasets

The Villarroya-Beltri [35] work reports on microarray datasets of exosome and cellular fractions from activated and resting human T lymphocyte cultures. They differentially assessed whether RNAs are specifically enriched within exosomes by performing microarray analysis of activation-induced variations in mRNA and miRNA profiles from primary T lymphoblast and their secreted exosomes. Data found in their supplementary data and also data publicly available at gene expression omnibus as Gene Expression Omnibus (GEO) Series accession number GSE50972 were used for **Table 2**. They showed that for most cases, miRNAs modulated upon activation are differentially found in cells and exosomes for either upregulated or downregulated miRNAs. This suggests that mRNA and miRNA loading into exosomes is not a simple passive process. Specific miRNAs were more highly expressed in exosomes than found in the cells, and in most cases this difference is preserved under cellular resting or activated conditions. Similarly, most miRNAs that are preferentially found in cells than in exosomes also keep this tendency regardless of the activation state of the cell. As such, Villarroya-Beltri classified some miRNAs as specifically sorted into exosomes (labeled EXOmiRNAs), whereas others are specifically retained in cells (as CLmiRNAs). We calculated tCount and rcCount as a count (**Table 2** in Ref. [17]), and tWord and rcWord, the latter which factor the expression level of that word. Other measures compared counts and words to a randomized transcriptome (RAN). We used a word size $k = 7$ roughly equal to the miRNA seed sequence length [17]. Values of rcWord (mean 10.31) were lower than tWord (mean 12.45), and hence RCM and RCC were more negative for exosomes compared to cytoplasmic miRNAs. This supports the STIC model since exosome transcripts must diffuse further than cytoplasmic (CL) RNA, so avoid reverse complementarity. In summary, all trial measures calculated from this dataset showed significant support for the transcriptome model except for Z-RCM.

2.4.2. Model 1 validation with nuclear-enriched miRNAs

Park et al. [36] study compared microarray analysis of cytoplasmic and in this case nuclear fractions of hct116 colon cancer cells. They identified various miRNAs that exist in isolated nuclei from miRNA profiles correlated between cytoplasmic and nuclear fractions from multiple microarray analyses. Nuclear confinement of the mature form of miRNAs was validated by controlling reverse transcriptase RT-PCR conditions excluding the presence of precipitate forms of miRNA (e.g., as pri-miRNA or pre-miRNA). They found that elevated levels of representative miRNAs in purified nuclei support the idea that significant numbers of mature miRNAs survive not only in the cytoplasm but also in the nucleus. We sorted their data by N/C ratio and *partitioned these data into two groups: $N/C > 0.47$, which was nuclear-enriched (45 samples), and $N/C < 0.47$, which was preferentially found in the cytoplasm (33 samples). We found that tCount was 4.02 for nuclear-enriched, and 5.00 for cytoplasmic, with a t-test p-value of 0.116 between the groups; while tWord was 4.73 for nuclear and 10.58 for cytoplasmic

Source experiment	N	tWord	rcWord	RCM	RCC	Z-RCC	Z-RCM	RCC-Ran	(RCC-Ran)/Len
Villarroya-Beltri									
EXO-CL resting	75	4×10^{-7}**	2×10^{-5}**	0.08*	0.023**	0.029**	0.603	0.04**	0.038**
EXO-CL activated	67	4×10^{-7}**	1×10^{-5}**	0.206	0.008 **	0.033**	0.503	0.032**	0.028**
Park paper									
$N/C > 0.471$ nuclear	43	0.024**	0.021**	0.62	0.76	0.77	0.31	0.41	0.42
Huang paper									
Top-low rcmm	100	0.522	0.02**	0.002 **	0.042 **	0.83	0.16	0.078*	0.072*
Cheng paper									
Top-low	50	0.128	0.002 **	0.035 **	0.002 **	0.062*	0.25	0.132	nc
Guduric-Fuchs paper									
Ratio EV/cell top-low	10	0.093*	0.39	0.3	0.075*	0.046**	0.178	0.03**	nc
EV RPMM top-low	10	0.79	0.973	0.736	0.96	0.268	0.816	0.306	nc
Chen paper									
Perinuclear-cell	6	0.62	0.76	0.24	0.14	0.15	0.18	0.076*	0.095*
Friedel									
mRNA half-life	15	0.017**	0.025**	0.86	nc	nc	0.44	nc	nc

Notes: Double-asterisk cells have significance below 0.05, while single-asterisk cells have significance below 0.10 but above 0.05. Cells with "nc" were not calculated from randomized transcriptome.

Table 2. t-Tests of case studies with STIC model parameters.

miRNAs, with a significant t-test p-value of 0.023 between nuclear and cytoplasmic groups. We also found nuclear-enriched miRNAs have higher rcWord values compared to cytoplasmic miRNA (p-value = 0.021 in **Table 2**), suggesting those transcripts have greater potential to interact with other transcriptome RNAs and hence may have lower than expected diffusion coefficients. The other evaluated measures did not show significance between groups.

2.4.3. *Model 1 validation with additional RNA studies*

Huang et al. [37] study utilized RNA-seq with exosomes from human plasma. We found that the top 100 abundant miRNAs in exosomes had tCount (mean 4.80) and tWord (mean 6.72) measures compared to those lower 100 with low "rcmm" reads (mean 4.64 and 7.41, respectively). In support of the STIC model, exosome transcripts have more similarity to the simple model transcriptome. Exosome abundant miRNAs had negative RCM (mean −0.87) and RCC (mean −0.27) measures compared to those with low rcmm reads (mean 1.37 and 0.55, respectively). The most significant trial function was RCM (p-value = 0.002) followed by rcWord (p-value = 0.02) measure. From these data, we find similarity that exosome transcripts have less reverse complementarity to the simple Model-1 transcriptome. Again, these results are supported by Cheng et al. [38] study of exosomes in human blood. From 50 most abundant miRNAs in exosome samples labeled "Plasma UC Exo," we find mean tCount and tWord

values of 4.56 and 6.00 compared to 5.58 and 8.80, respectively, for low abundance transcripts. This set of exosome miRNAs had RCM and RCC values of −1.54 and 3.8 compared to 0.36 and 5.8 for low abundance transcripts, again supporting the STIC model. Several of the trial functions in **Table 2** were significant measures for data sets in that study.

Pursuing in-depth understanding of the mechanism supporting selective exportation of miRNAs to extracellular vesicles (EVs), Guduric-Fuchs [39] employed next generation sequencing to discriminate global expression patterns of small RNAs in HEK293T cells and the EVs that they released. Enrichment of overexpressed miRNA in EVs was measured by RT-qPCR in HEK293T cells, mesenchymal stem cells, macrophages, and immune cells. We sorted data from Guduric-Fuchs by EV/cell ratio, then compared the top 10 (exosome-enriched) and bottom (cytoplasmic enriched) miRNAs by evaluating the measures listed in **Table 2**. Only trial functions Z-RCC and RCC-RAN were significant from this dataset. Overall from using EV/cell in various measures examined across the studies, tWord and tCount (from Ref. [17]), along with their difference (tW–tC), have values that progress from lower for nuclear, higher for cytoplasmic, and highest for exosomal miRNAs. Therefore, we consider under transitivity, EXO > CL > NUC for these transcriptome measures of similarity. This supports the notion that miRNAs with sequence similarity to the overall transcriptome can random-walk furthest from their points of transcription if the secretion mechanism requires a great distance to travel. These conclusions on trial functions are most significant with the tCount measure, with a p-value close to zero for the Villarroya-Beltri study, and 0.016 for the Guduric-Fuchs study, while the Park study showed little difference (p-value = 0.122) for tCount between nuclear and cytoplasmic enrichment.

2.4.4. *Word count normalization from RNA-seq datasets*

Normalization is a crucial step in the analysis of RNA-seq data and has a strong impact on the detection of differentially expressed genes sought to validate the STIC model. Several normalization strategies have been proposed to correct for between-sample distributional differences in read counts, such as differences in total counts (i.e., sequencing depths), and within-sample gene-specific effects, such as gene length or GC-content effects [40]. Global-scaling normalization adjusts gene-level counts by a single factor per sample, such as the per-sample total read count, or reads per kilobase of exon model per million mapped reads (RPKM), or some housekeeping gene count. Statistical corrections by a quantile per-sample count distribution or other robust summaries obtained by relating each sample to a reference sample (e.g., trimmed mean of M values (TMM) and methods of Anders and Huber [41]). Although there have been efforts to systematically compare normalization methods [42], this important aspect of RNA-seq analysis is still not fully resolved. When data arise from complex experiments as in Section 2 above, involving cell fractionation, low-input RNA or different batches and read lengths, there may be more to correct for than differences in sequencing depth, referred to as unknown nuisance technical variation error. One methodology correction is the addition of spike-in controls within the normalization procedure [43]. Control designs have been successfully employed in microarray normalization, for miRNA and mRNA arrays [44]. Negative controls in the normalization procedure test the assumption that the majority of genes are not differentially expressed between study conditions. This assumption can be violated when a

global shift in expression occurs between conditions, such that control-based normalization may be necessary for technical variation, and a global mean read for global differences in RNA levels.

3. Spatial and temporal localization

We follow with a description of possible experimental data sets for populating transcriptome model in W. RNA-seq data sets would be the preferred source for fine structure of word contents, but microarray expression data could also be used for overall population of W.

3.1. Spatial localization by RNA imaging

The only method that provides insight into both the level and localization in single cells is *in situ* hybridization (ISH), which has increased considerably in importance in RNA research. ISH along with multiplex RNA profiling (MERFISH) can be used to measure the degree of associations among transcripts. Numerous RNA species have been identified, counted, and localized in single cells using MERFISH, a single-molecule imaging approach that uses combinatorial labeling and sequential imaging with an encoding scheme capable of detection and/or correction of errors. This multiplexed measurement of individual RNAs can be used to measure the gene expression profile and noise, along with covariation in expression among different genes, and spatial distribution of RNAs within single cells.

3.1.1. Localization of small RNAs

For miRNAs, ISH is exceptionally challenging because of miRNA features such as small size, sequence similarity among various miRNA family members, and low tissue-specific or development-specific expression levels. Standard ISH protocols can be modified to improve miRNA detection [45]. Locked nucleic acid (LNA/DNA) probes have great utility in miRNA detection because of short hybridization time, high efficiency, discriminatory power, and high melting temperature of the miRNA/probe complex [46]. Minimal length of LNA/DNA probes was found to be 12 nt with probes usually containing 30% LNA nucleotides [46]. A mixture of 2′-OMe RNA and LNA modifications in a 2:1 ratio resulted in improved specificity and stability of the probe/RNA duplex in comparison to LNA/DNA probes [47]. Experiment specificity was found to be further improved by lengthening the probe length to 19 nt [48].

3.1.2. Localization by MERFISH

Chen et al. [33] used array-synthesized oligopools as templates to make encoding probes in the MERFISH protocol. An oligopaint approach developed by Beliveau et al. [49] can generate a large number of oligonucleotide probes to label chromosome DNA. Inspired by this approach, Chen et al. [33] designed a two-step labeling scheme to encode and read out cellular RNAs. They labeled a target set of cellular RNAs with a set of encoding probes, each probe comprising a RNA targeting sequence and two flanking readout sequences. Four readout sequences were assigned to each target RNA species based on error-correction optimized code words.

http://dx.doi.org/10.5772/intechopen.69452

They identified these readout sequences with complementary FISH probes via rounds of hybridization and imaging; each round using a different readout probe. To increase the signal-to-background ratio, each cellular RNA is labeled with ∼192 encoding probes.

3.2. RNA diffusion

Brownian effects are ubiquitous in numerous examples of soft condensed matter physics [20] in which the system can be modeled as a set of interacting degrees of freedom in contact with a heat reservoir. Brownian motion plays an important role when one infers macroscopic behaviors from mesoscopic levels of description, frequently a desire in the study of complex systems. Dynamics at the mesoscopic level is governed by a set of Langevin processes or equivalently by the corresponding N-particle Fokker–Planck equation. This scheme applies nonequilibrium thermodynamics to derive the kinetic equations describing the evolution of an N-particle probability distribution function [20]. One then considers a system of N Brownian particles diluted in a solvent, which acts as a thermal reservoir. Particle velocities are then modeled as internal thermodynamic variables and permit an analysis in the phase space of the Brownian particles. A local equilibrium hypothesis constrains the phase space level and from it one derives the thermodynamic entropy balance equation. Entropy production accounts for irreversible processes taking place in the phase space, then quantifying fluxes and forces can be done in a similar manner as in the thermodynamics of irreversible processes [20]. A general thermodynamic treatment of systems of N interacting Brownian motion particles as described by Fokker-Planck equations is detailed by Savel'ev et al. [16].

4. Resilience as a systems biology measure from transcriptome model

Development of a resilience measure from transcriptome RNAs could improve basic knowledge of the transcriptome and responses to stress. Transcriptome size and overall variation have been documented across cell cycle stages, tissue types, developmental stages, diurnal cycles, sexes, and environment [50]. Despite the ubiquity of transcriptome size variation, its potential to introduce systematic bias into expression profiling has been largely overlooked and this study uncovers responses of the transcriptome to stress.

4.1. Formalization of metric for resilience in biological systems using STIC metrics

Insight into structural determinants of robustness and resilience can guide the understanding of systems that go through transitions. Systems engineering research has developed methodologies to measure the functionality and complexity of engineered systems for designing and assessing system resilience. While system functions, resilience, functionality, and complexity are widely used concepts in systems engineering, there is significant diversity in definitions and no unified approach to measurement in the systems biology area [51]. One method for measuring impacts on functionality in dynamic engineered systems is based on changes in kinetic energy [52]. This metric can be applied at particular levels of abstraction and system scales, consistent with the established multiscale nature of biological systems.

4.2. Measuring complexity

A difficulty in complexity theory is the lack of a clear definition for complexity, particularly one that is measurable [53]. Underlying cause for this lack of a unified complexity definition is that there are numerous conceptual types of complexity. The first formal treatment of complexity focused on algorithmic complexity, which reflects the computation requirements for a mathematical process [54]. Senge [55] and Sterman [56] expand the scope of definition to include dynamic complexity, which is primarily characterized by difficult-to-discern and hard-to-measure cause-effect relations. A recent workable definition is that of thermodynamic depth, which essentially asserts that complexity is a "measure of how hard it is to put something together" [57]. Several variations on this approach share the commonality that complexity should disappear for both ordered and purely stochastic systems [58]. Additionally, Bar-Yam [59] defined complexity as the length of the shortest string that can represent the properties of a physical system. This string could be the result of measurements and observations over time.

An energy-based metric was proposed by Chaisson [60] measuring the energy rate density, where Φm is energy rate density, E is energy flow through a system, τ is the time frame, and m is system mass. Chaisson obtains results that correlate well with other notions of complexity, and below we add our proposed relation from this transcriptome model framework

$$\Phi m = E/\tau m \text{ or which we propose is} : \alpha(\Sigma^S\text{NAM} + \Sigma^S\text{RCM})/N \quad (5)$$

A practical difficulty in using the Φm metric is determining the appropriate mass and energy. In measuring the Φm of a transcriptome, we can use the mass of RNA production and the total energy processed by the system. Energy in this framework could be the total sum of all possible RNA-RNA interactions, which is just the count of all NAM and RCM in W as a sum of overall transcript sequences S. However, the total energy of a transcriptome does not flow just through its cell, but also exported to the extracellular space and captured from that external source of transcripts, the mass of which is difficult to measure.

While higher functionality can be associated with increased resiliency and robustness, the concepts are not synonymous. As defined by the INCOSE Resilient Systems Working Group, "Resilience is the capability of a system with specific characteristics before, during, and after a disruption to absorb the disruption, recover to an acceptable level of performance, and sustain that level for an acceptable period of time" [61]. Robustness is the ability of a system to reject disturbances without altering its state. A system is robust when it can continue functioning in the presence of internal and external challenges without fundamental changes to the original system. In relation to previous section on energy availability, robustness is the ability for a system to retain reachable states in the event of falling available energy.

4.3. Framework for measuring resilience

Instead, complexity in the presented framework can be derived from properties of W or T as in **Figure 3**. Consider a transcriptome from a cell type alpha to be represented as T_α, such that it is the sum of all RNAs, including mRNA, miRNA, lncRNA, and rRNA within the cell (**Table 1**). This set is the result of transcripts produced from the cellular DNA, $T_\alpha{}^0$, transcripts captured

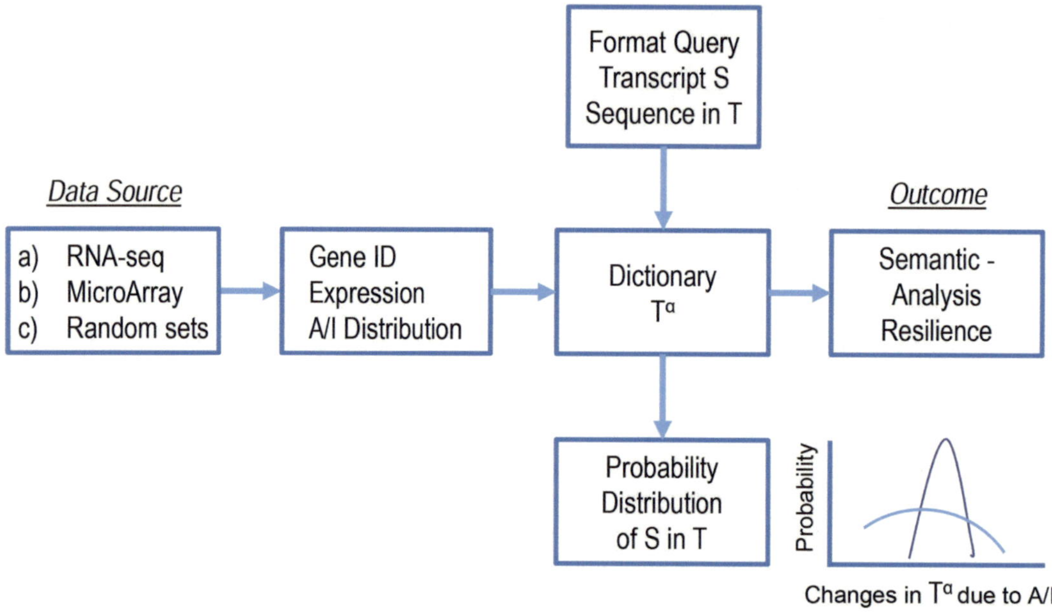

Figure 3. Framework for deriving transcriptome interactions and resilience. Data source is from RNA expression experiments using RNA-seq or microarray values, or randomized sets for controls. From input sets, the aligned gene ID and frequency of the extracted words are populated into a dictionary. Gene ID is used to calculate solvent-accessible (A) and inaccessible (I) word probabilities from full length transcripts *in silico*. The dictionary can be queried for any sequence S to find probability distribution of S in the dictionary. Changes in the transcriptome will change the distribution due to changes in A/I for affected words. Overall metrics of the dictionary measure resilience using Eq. (8) in the text.

from the extracellular space (EC) in the form of microparticles and exosomes $T_{EC}{}^{IN}$, and depletion as microparticle or exosome export to the extracellular space with $T_\alpha{}^{OUT}$. Or,

$$T_\alpha = T_\alpha^0 + T_{EC}^{IN} - T_\alpha^{OUT} \tag{6}$$

with

$$T_\alpha{}^{OUT} = T_\alpha * \mathfrak{F}[S,\ RC, n] \approx T_\alpha *\ [a * f_S(S)/(f_{RC}(S, RC)\ * n)] \tag{7}$$

where $\mathfrak{F}$ is a filter function with parameters S (transcript sequence), RC (reverse complement of transcript sequence), n sequence length of S, and "a" is a fitting parameter with suitable dimensions, derived from: $\mathfrak{F}\ \alpha$ NAM/(RCM * n) proportionality. Thus the extracellular pool is composed of transcripts with greater similarity S, and less reverse complementarity RC to the transcriptome of origin and also have smaller size n. The filter functions $f_S(S)$ and $f_{RC}(S,RC)$ operate on sequences S and RC, and essentially is a semantic selection filter on transcripts by affecting diffusion. We propose that resilience of the cell is proportional to size of the transcriptome filter $\mathfrak{F}$, then resilience $\alpha\ |\mathfrak{F}|$, where $|\mathfrak{F}| = |f_S| + |f_{RC}|$, or normalized for transcriptome size,

$$\text{Resilience} = (|f_S| + |f_{RC}|)/N \tag{8}$$

such that $|f_S|$ is sum of all similarity matches, $|f_{RC}|$ is sum of all reverse complement interactions, and N is the total nucleotide size of the transcriptome.

5. Discussion

The concept of resilience is receiving increasing attention in chronic stress-related diseases. Resilience has been shown in clinical studies to play a protective role in patients with chronic conditions including osteoarthritis, breast and ovarian cancer, diabetes, and cardiovascular disease related to psychosocial dimensional levels. The purpose of this study is to explore the relationships between RNA-RNA interactions and to devise a measure of resilience at the cellular level.

5.1. Prospects, challenges, and limitations for resilience measure by variance in RNA-seq

Although research on empirical indicators of robustness and resilience is rudimentary, there is already a fast-growing body of engineering modeling as well as empirical work in ecology. Nonetheless, major challenges remain in developing robust procedures for assessment of the transcriptome. A goal of systems biology is to analyze large-scale multidomain networks to reveal relationships between network structures and their biological function. While generally, it is not feasible to visualize and understand whole networks, a common analysis is to partition the network into subnetworks responsible for specific biological functions. Since biological functions can be carried out by particular groups of molecules, dividing networks into naturally grouped clusters can help investigate the relationships between function and topology of system networks or reveal hidden knowledge behind them. The expression in Eq. (8) for resilience is a measure of the size of network interactions possible within a transcriptome.

5.2. Notion of the transcriptome as an information system

The body of this work considers the transcriptome as an information system modeling a dynamic system. A dynamic system is characterized by two concerns: the static structure and dynamic behavior. The structural elements of dynamic systems are those elements which may be identified from static snapshots of the problem space; while dynamic aspects involve those semantic elements of the system that exist over the time domain. While modeling the static aspects of an information system like RNA expression data, an understanding of the dynamic nature of information systems in the cell is low. Behavioral issues of large information systems are usually complex, consisting of many interactive sessions with the outside environment, tasks like coordination and collaboration among different entities. Dynamic systems can exhibit emergent properties that result from the dynamics, and which cannot be attributed to static structural factors. However, given any real world information system consisting of many multistream interactive processes, emergent properties are usually complex, without a common characteristic structure. Such emergent properties are beginning to be addressed with the transcriptome.

6. Conclusion

We show that the transcriptome can be modeled as an information system with emergent dynamic properties. The term *nebula* regulation is introduced to consider the regulatory effects

of the whole transcriptome acting locally through RNA-RNA interactions and shifts between accessible and inaccessible stretches of RNA sequence. Described as a network of interactions from semantic analysis of similarity and reverse complementarity, together with the size of a transcript, affect the diffusion of transcripts in a cell, and hence the distribution of RNAs. A measure to represent resilience is proposed as the sum of the component elements (similarity, reverse complementarity, and normalized by total nucleotides) of this transcriptome filter.

Acknowledgements

This work is supported in part by 8U54MD007588, G12MD007602, P50 HL117929, and P30 HL107238 grants from NIH/National Institute on Minority Health and Health Disparities. The content is solely the responsibility of the author and does not necessarily represent official views of the respective institutions.

Author details

William Seffens

Address all correspondence to: wseffens@msm.edu

Department of Physiology, Morehouse School of Medicine, Atlanta, GA, USA; Seftec, Inc., Atlanta, GA USA

References

[1] Tian B, Manley JL. Alternative polyadenylation of mRNA precursors. Nature Reviews Molecular Cell Biology. 2017;**18**(1):18–30

[2] Misteli T. Physiological importance of RNA and protein mobility in the cell nucleus. Histochemistry and Cell Biology. 2008;**129**(1):5–11. [Epub 2007 Nov 10]

[3] Trovato F, Tozzini V. Diffusion within the cytoplasm: A mesoscale model of interacting macromolecules. Biophysical Journal. 2014;**107**(11):2579–2591

[4] Ben-Ari Y, Brody Y, Kinor N, Mor A, Tsukamoto T, Spector D, Singer R, Shav-Tal Y. The life of an mRNA in space and time. Journal of Cell Science. 2010;**123**:1761–1774

[5] Hopper AK. Cellular dynamics of small RNAs. Critical Reviews in Biochemistry and Molecular Biology. 2006;**41**(1):3–19

[6] Jalali S, Bhartiya D, Lawani M, Sivasubbu S, Scaria V. Systematic transcriptome wide analysis of lncRNA-miRNA interactions. PLoS One. 2013;**8**:e53823

[7] Collins LJ. The RNA infrastructure: An introduction to ncRNA networks. Advances in Experimental Medicine and Biology. 2011;**722**:1–19. DOI: 10.1007/978-1-4614-0332-6_1

[8] Jeggari A, Marks DS, Larsson E. miRcode: A map of putative microRNA target sites in the long non-coding transcriptome. Bioinformatics. 2012;**28**:2062–2063. DOI: 10.1093/bioinformatics/bts344

[9] Salmena L, Poliseno L, Tay Y, Kats L, Pandolfi P. A ceRNA hypothesis: The rosetta stone of a hidden RNA language? Cell. 2011;**146**:353–358

[10] Crooke ST, Wang S, Vickers TA, Shen W, Liang XH. Cellular uptake and trafficking of antisense oligonucleotides. Nature Biotechnology. 2017;**35**(3):230–237

[11] Bonnici V, Manca V. Informational laws of genome structures. Scientific Reports. 2016;**6**:28840. DOI: 10.1038/srep28840

[12] Shannon CE. A mathematical theory of communication. The Bell System Technical Journal. 1948;**27**:623–656

[13] Shannon CE. An algebra for theoretical genetics [PhD thesis]. Massachusetts Institute of Technology, 1940. MIT-THESES//1940–3 Online text at MIT. Contains a biography on pp. 64–65

[14] Lockhart E, Lucas M, Yoo J, Seffens W. Codon usage pattern detection in human, mouse, zebrafish and chicken genes using artificial neural networks. In: IEEE Symposium on Computational Intelligence in Bioinformatics and Computational Biology (CIBCB); 2009; TN

[15] Wang X-Q, Abebe F, Seffens W. Dynamic system modeling the whole transcriptome in a eukaryotic cell. In: Proceedings of Dynamic Systems and Applications; 2015; Atlanta, GA. Dynamic Publishers, Inc.

[16] Savel'ev S, Marchesoni F, Taloni A, Nori F. Diffusion of interacting Brownian particles: Jamming and anomalous diffusion. Physical Review. 2006;**74**:021119

[17] Seffens W, Abebe F, Evans C, Wang X-Q. Spatial Partitioning of miRNAs is related to sequence similarity in overall transcriptome. International Journal of Molecular Sciences. 2016;**17**:830. DOI: 10.3390/ijms17060830

[18] Wang X. Composition of seed sequence is a major determinant of microRNA targeting patterns. Bioinformatics. 2014;**30**(10):1377–1383

[19] Regner B, Vucinic D, Domnisoru C, Bartol T, Hetzer M, Tartakovsky D, Sejnowski T. Anomalous diffusion of single particles in cytoplasm. Biophysical Journal. 2013;**104**: 1652–1660

[20] Mayorga M, Romero-Salazar L, Rubi J. Stochastic model for the dynamics of interacting Brownian particles. Physica. 2002;**307**:297–314

[21] Yeh I-C, Hummer G. Diffusion and electrophoretic mobility of single-stranded RNA from molecular dynamics simulations. Biophysical Journal. 2004;**86**(2):681–689

[22] Singh YH, Andrabi M, Kahali B, Ghosh C, Mizuguchi K, Kochetov A, Ahmad S. On nucleotide solvent accessibility in RNA structure. Gene. 2010;**463**:41–48

[23] Seffens W, Digby D. mRNAs have greater calculated folding free energies than shuffled or codon choice randomized sequences. Nucleic Acids Research. 1999;**27**:1578–1584

[24] Yoo J-K, Digby D, Davis A, and Seffens W. Whole transcriptome mRNA secondary structure analysis using distributed computation. In: Zhang Y-Q, Lin T, editors. Proceedings of International IEEE-Granular Computing. Atlanta, GA: Georgia State University; 2006. pp. 647–650

[25] Bernhart SH, Hofacker IL, Stadler PF. Local base pairing probabilities in large sequences. Bioinformatics. 2006;**22:**614–615

[26] Lange S, Maticzka D, Mohl M, Gagnon J, Brown C, Backofen R. Global or local? Predicting secondary structure and accessibility in mRNAs. Nucleic Acids Research. 2012;**40**(12):5215–5226

[27] Walia R, Caragea C, Lewis B, Towfic F, Terriblini M, El-Manzalawy Y, Dobbs D, Honavar V. Protein-RNA interface residue prediction using machine learning: an assessment of the state of the art. BMC Bioinformatics. 2012;**13**:89

[28] Hubbard S, Thornton JM. NACCESS. Department of Biochemistry and Molecular Biology, University College London; 1993

[29] Tang Y, Bouvier E, Kwok CK, Ding Y, Nekrutenko A, Bevilacqua PC, Assmann SM. Structure fold: Genome-wide RNA secondary structure mapping and reconstruction in vivo. Bioinformatics. 2015;**31**(16):2668–2675. DOI: 10.1093/bioinformatics/btv213

[30] Ding Y, Kwok CK, Tang Y, Bevilacqua PC, Assmann SM. Genome-wide profiling of in vivo RNA structure at single-nucleotide resolution using structure-seq. Nature Protocols. 2015;**10**(7):1050–1066. DOI: 10.1038/nprot.2015.064

[31] Ding Y, Tang Y, Kwok CK, Zhang Y, Bevilacqua PC, Assmann SM. In vivo genome-wide profiling of RNA secondary structure reveals novel regulatory features. Nature. 2014;**505** (7485):696–700. DOI: 10.1038/nature12756

[32] Kwok CK, Tang Y, Assmann SM, Bevilacqua PC. The RNA structurome: Transcriptome-wide structure probing with next-generation sequencing. Trends in Biochemical Sciences. 2015;**40**(4):221–232. DOI: 10.1016/j.tibs.2015.02.005

[33] Chen KH, Boettiger AN, Moffitt JR, Wang S, Zhuang X. Spatially resolved, highly multiplexed RNA profiling in single cells. Science. 2015;**348**:aaa6090

[34] Friedel CC, Dolken L, Ruzsics Z, Koszinowski UH, Zimmer R. Conserved principles of mammalian transcriptional regulation revealed by RNA half-life. Nucleic Acids Research. 2009;**37**(17):e115

[35] Villarroya-Beltri C, Gutiérrez-Vázquez C, Sánchez-Cabo F, Pérez-Hernández D, Vázquez J, Martin-Cofreces N, Martinez-Herrera DJ, Pascual-Montano A, Mittelbrunn M, Sánchez-

Madrid F. Sumoylated hnRNPA2B1 controls the sorting of miRNAs into exosomes through binding to specific motifs. Nature Communications. 2013;**4**:2980. DOI: 10.1038/ncomms3980 l

[36] Park CW, Zeng Y, Zhang X, Subramanian S, Steer C. Mature microRNAs identified in highly purified nuclei from HCT116 colon cancer cells. RNA Biology. 2010;7(5):606–614

[37] Huang X, Yuan T, Tschannen M, Sun Z, Jacob H, Du M, Liang M, Dittmar RL, Liu Y, Liang M, Kohli M, Thibodeau SN, Boardman L, Wang L. Characterization of human plasma-derived exosomal RNAs by deep sequencing. BMC Genomics. 2013;**14**:319

[38] Cheng L, Sharples RA, Scicluna BJ, Hill AF. Exosomes provide a protective and enriched source of miRNA for biomarker profiling compared to intracellular and cell-free blood. Journal of Extracellular Vesicles. 2014;**3**:23743

[39] Guduric-Fuchs J, O'Connor A, Camp B, O'Neill CL, Medina RJ, Simpson DA. Selective extracellular vesicle-mediated export of an overlapping set of microRNAs from multiple cell types. BMC Genomics. 2012;**13**:357

[40] Bullard J, Purdom E, Hansen K, Dudoit, S. Evaluation of statistical methods for normalization and differential expression in mRNA-Seq experiments. BMC Bioinformatics. 2010;**11**:94

[41] Anders S, Huber W. Differential expression analysis for sequence count data. Genome Biology. 2010;**11**:R106

[42] Dillies M-A, Rau A, Aubert J, Hennequet-Antier C, Jeanmougin M, Servant N, Keime C, Marot G, Castel D, Estelle J, Guernec G, Jagla B, Jouneau L, Laloe D, Gall CL, Schaeffer B, Crom SL, Guedj M, Jaffrezic F. A comprehensive evaluation of normalization methods for Illumina high-throughput RNA sequencing data analysis. Briefings in Bioinformatics. 2013;**14**, 671–683

[43] Risso D, Ngai J, Speed TP, Dudoit S. Normalization of RNA-seq data using factor analysis of control genes or samples. Nature Biotechnology. 2014;**32**:896–902

[44] Wu D, Hu Y, Tong S, Gantier M. The use of miRNA microarrays for the analysis of cancer samples with global miRNA decrease. RNA. 2013;**19**:876–888

[45] Urbanek M, Nawrocka A, Krzyzosiak W. Small RNA detection by in situ hybridization methods. International Journal of Molecular Sciences. 2015;**16**:13259–13286

[46] Kloosterman WP, Wienholds E, de Bruijn E, Kauppinen S, Plasterk RH. In situ detection of miRNAs in animal embryos using LNA-modified oligonucleotide probes. Nature Methods. 2006;**3**:27–29

[47] Soe MJ, Moller T, Dufva M, Holmstrom K. A sensitive alternative for microRNA in situ hybridizations using probes of 2′-O-methyl RNA + LNA. Journal of Histochemistry and Cytochemistry. 2011;**59**:661–672

[48] Majlessi M, Nelson NC, Becker MM. Advantages of 2′-O-methyl oligoribonucleotide probes for detecting RNA targets. Nucleic Acids Research. 1998;**26**:2224–2229

[49] Beliveau BJ, Joyce EF, Apostolopoulos N, Yilmaz F, Fonseka CY, McCole RB, Chang Y, Li JB, Senaratne TN, Williams BR, Rouillard J-M, Wu C-t. Versatile design and synthesis platform for visualizing genomes with Oligopaint FISH probes. Proceedings of the National Academy of Sciences of the United States of America. 2012;**109**:21301–21306

[50] Coate J, Doyle J. Chromosome size: Are we getting the message?. Chromosoma. 2015;**124**: 27–43

[51] Scheffer M, Carpenter SR, Lenton TM, Bascompte J, Brock W, Dakos V, van de Koppel J, van de Leeput IA, Levin SA, van Nes EH, Pascual M, Vandermeer J. Anticipating critical transitions. Science. 2012;**338**(6105):344–348

[52] Clark J. Functionality, Complexity, and Approaches to Assessment of Resilience Under Constrained Energy and Information. Ohio: Air Force Institute of Technology, Wright-Patterson AFB; 2015. AFIT-ENV-DS-15-M-159. Accession number ADA619053

[53] Lloyd S, Pagels H. Complexity as thermodynamic depth. Annals of Physics. 1988;**188**: 186–213

[54] Corning PA. Complexity is just a word!. Technological Forecasting and Social Change. 1998;**58**:1–4

[55] Senge P. The Fifth Discipline: The Art and Practice of the Learning Organization. New York: Doubleday; 1990

[56] Sterman J. Business Dynamics: Systems Thinking and Modeling for a Complex World. Boston: McGraw-Hill, Irwin; 2000

[57] Crutchfield JP, Shalizi CR. Thermodynamic depth of causal states: When paddling around in Occam's pool shallowness is a virtue. Physical Review E. 1999;**59**(1):275–283

[58] Li W. On the relationship between complexity and entropy for Markov chains and regular languages. Complexity. 1991;**5**:381–399

[59] Bar-Yam Y. Multiscale complexity/entropy. Advances in Complex Systems. 2004;**7**:47–63

[60] Chaisson EJ. Energy rate density as a complexity metric and evolutionary driver. Complexity. 2011;**16**:27–40

[61] INCOSE. INCOSE Resilient Systems Working Group (RSWG) Charter [Internet]. 2011. Available from: URL http://www.incose.org/about/organization/pdf/RSWG_Charter.pdf

Chapter 5

Transcriptome Analysis of Non-Coding RNAs in Livestock Species: Elucidating the Ambiguity

Duy N. Do, Pier-Luc Dudemaine,
Bridget Fomenky and Eveline M. Ibeagha-Awemu

Additional information is available at the end of the chapter

http://dx.doi.org/10.5772/intechopen.69872

Abstract

The recent remarkable development of transcriptomics technologies, especially next generation sequencing technologies, allows deeper exploration of the hidden landscapes of complex traits and creates great opportunities to improve livestock productivity and welfare. Non-coding RNAs (ncRNAs), RNA molecules that are not translated into proteins, are key transcriptional regulators of health and production traits, thus, transcriptomics analyses of ncRNAs are important for a better understanding of the regulatory architecture of livestock phenotypes. In this chapter, we present an overview of common frameworks for generating and processing RNA sequence data to obtain ncRNA transcripts. Then, we review common approaches for analyzing ncRNA transcriptome data and present current state of the art methods for identification of ncRNAs and functional inference of identified ncRNAs, with emphasis on tools for livestock species. We also discuss future challenges and perspectives for ncRNA transcriptome data analysis in livestock species.

Keywords: bioinformatics, genome editing, livestock species, long non-coding RNA, non-coding RNA, microRNA, transcriptome

1. Introduction

A vast portion of the mammalian transcriptome is composed of non-protein coding transcripts or non-coding RNA (ncRNA). Some ncRNAs are processed into functionally important transcripts such as microRNA (miRNA), transfer RNA (tRNA), ribosomal RNA (rRNA), small nucleolar RNA (snoRNA), small nuclear RNA (snRNA), small interfering RNA (siRNA), PIWI-interacting RNA (piRNA), circular RNA (circRNA), long non-coding RNA (lncRNA)

and several classes with limited information about their functions. In addition to the well described ncRNA classes, clusters of ncRNA (22–200 nucleotides (nt)) were detected at the 5, and 3′end of human and mouse genes, and named promoter-associated short RNAs (PASRs) and termini-associated short RNAs (TASRs) [1]. Mercer et al. [2] described a class of ncRNA, about 50–200 nt, that are processed from the 3′UTRs of protein-coding genes (uaRNAs). The uaRNAs are in sense direction to the protein-coding gene and show stage, sex and sub-cellular specific expression. A class of ncRNA derived from tRNA precursors and named tRNA-derived RNA fragments (tRF) or tRNA-derived small RNAs (tsRNAs) appear to be processed by Dicer while others are Dicer independently processed [3, 4]. Small nucleolar RNAs (snoRNA) can also be processed into small miRNA-like molecules called sno-derived RNAs or sdRNAs [5, 6] which play roles in guiding enzymes to target RNAs for modification [7]. In this chapter, only the main classes of functional ncRNAs (miRNA, snoRNA, siRNA, piRNA and lncRNA), not considering the translation related ncRNAs (rRNA and tRNA), will be further discussed. NcRNAs have been implicated in many biological processes including transcriptional inference, translational modifications, mRNA cleavage, epigenetic modifications, regulation of structural organization, and modulation of alternative splicing, small RNA precursor, and endo or secondary siRNA generation [7–10].

2. Transcriptome analysis of non-coding RNA

2.1. Platforms for transcriptome analysis of non-coding RNA

Transcriptome analysis reached a turning point in its history with the arrival of high throughput next-generation sequencing technologies like RNA-Sequencing (RNA-Seq) [11, 12]. Before this time, microarray was the gold standard for transcript profiling or simultaneous measurement of the expression level of thousands of genes in a given sample [13, 14]. Microarray technology however has major drawbacks like non-specific probe hybridization signals and errors in background level measurements [15], as well as limited gene diversity since probes are designed to represent only a set of preselected genes. Unique hybridization properties of each probe may affect their dynamic range and thus create bias in data processing algorithms [16]. The flexibility offered by RNA-Seq technology enables detection of unknown splice junctions [17], novel transcripts [18], new single nucleotide polymorphisms (SNPs) [19] and many other features all in the same assay. RNA-Seq technology has taken the possibility of fine tuning our knowledge of the transcriptome to a much higher level. In recent years, RNA-Seq has proved its worth as a technology that will replace microarray in whole-genome transcript profiling [20–22]. Correlation of RNA-Seq to RNA-Seq differential gene expression data resulted in good overlap than RNA-Seq to microarray data [23, 24], thus confirming that RNA-Seq is the preferred method to analyze the transcriptome. Moreover, correlation of transcriptome quantification by the two methods versus transcript level measured by shotgun mass spectroscopy showed better estimation with RNA-Seq analysis [25]. Through the evolution process of RNA-Seq technology, other new aspects have been included such as allele specific transcriptome analysis. Moreover, since the RNA-Seq procedure does not rely

on known genome annotation, but rather on all the information available in a given sample, there is clear opportunity to make discoveries at a rate never expected before.

A diversity of platforms offer a wide range of RNA-sequencing possibilities[12]. For example, Illumina HiSeq and MiSeq technologies offer short sequence reads (36–300 base pairs (bp)) while Oxford Nanopore can reach sequence lengths of greater than 150 kilo base pairs (kb) [26]. The sequencing techniques could be DNA-polymerase dependent (i.e. sequencing-by-synthesis (e.g. Illumina MiSeq/HiSeq)) while others like PacBio and Oxford Nanopore are single-molecule sequencers. The sequencing error rate ranges from 0.1% (Illumina MiSeq/HiSeq) to about 1.3% (PacBio RSII single pass). An overview of sequencing platforms and their characteristics is shown in **Table 1**. The error rate between platforms varies [27], so it is important to consider this especially when the goal is to sequence short read transcripts like miRNA.

The challenges of managing RNA-Seq data are considerable in terms of data storage and analysis as well as algorithm development. Since the technology is not yet fully matured, shortcomings exist at every step of sequence analysis. Various tools are available for alignment of reads, transcript construction, quantification, differential gene expression, pathways and correlation analyses [28] (**Tables 2** and **3**). Nonetheless, the use and specificity of the softwares differ highly from one type of analysis to another and the hardest part is making sure that the right tool is chosen at every step. A review of best practices for RNA-Seq data analysis was published recently [29]. The gap between the rapid evolution of RNA-Seq technology and the development of data analysis tools is hindering wide application in livestock species. Most data analysis tools are developed for use with genomes of human and common model organisms (mouse, rat) and require tweaking before use with livestock genomes. For example, when performing target prediction analysis for newly discovered transcripts, it is the practise to use human/mouse databases as it brings a lot of power to the analysis. However, there is great bias coming from the assumption that livestock biological systems are identical to human or mouse.

2.2. Generation of ncRNA sequence data and pre-mapping quality control

2.2.1. Generation of ncRNA sequence data

The choice of the sequencing platform is critical to attain the goals of a study. Numerous protocols and commercial kits to generate cDNA libraries from RNA samples are available and they are mostly based on the same principles (e.g. fragmentation, reverse-transcription, adapter ligation and amplification). The steps in library preparation for lncRNA are the same as for mRNA since they share similar biogenesis pathways. The starting material for lncRNA library preparation is total RNA. Majority of lncRNA transcripts have poly-A tails while a small proportion do not. Library preparation methods based on poly-A tail selection are cheaper but less robust since non-poly-A tail transcripts are lost. An ideal but more expensive method involves depletion of rRNA (constitutes ~90% of total RNA). Library preparation with rRNA depleted total RNA is robust as it allows quantification of all other RNA transcripts including lowly expressed transcripts. Thus, the first step in lncRNA library preparation is to consider whether to perform poly-A tail selection or to deplete rRNA (**Figure 1**). The next dilemma is deciding whether or not

Platform	Read length[1] (base pair)	Throughput[2]	Number of reads[3]	Error profile
Illumina MiniSeq (high output)	75 (SE)	1.6–1.8 Gb	22–25 M	<1%, substitution
	75 (PE)	3.3–7.5 Gb	44–50 M	<1%, substitution
	150 (PE)	6.6–7.5 Gb	44–50 M	
Illumina MiniSeq (mid output)	75 (SE)	2.1–2.4 Gb	14–16 M	<1%, substitution
Illumina MiSeq v2	36 (SE)	540–610 Mb	12–15 M	<0.1%, substitution
	25 (PE)	750–850 Mb	24–30 M	<0.1%, substitution
	150 (PE)	4.5–5.1 Gb	24–30 M	<0.1%, substitution
	250 (PE)	7.5–8.5 Gb	24–30 M	<0.1%, substitution
Illumina MiSeq v3	75 (PE)	3–4 Gb	44–50 M	<0.1%, substitution
	300 (PE)	13–15 Gb	44–50 M	<0.1%, substitution
Illumina NextSeq 500/550 (high output)	75 (SE)	25–30 Gb	400 M	<1%, substitution
	75 (PE)	50–60 Gb	800 M	<1%, substitution
	150 (PE)	100–120 Gb	800 M	<1%, substitution
Illumina NextSeq 500/550 (mid output)	75 (PE)	16–20 Gb	~260 M	<1%, substitution
	150 (PE)	32–40 Gb	~260 M	<1%, substitution
Illumina HiSeq250v2 Rapid run	36 (SE)	9–11 Gb	300 M	0.1%, substitution
	50 (PE)	25–30 Gb	600 M	0.1%, substitution
	100 (PE)	50–60 Gb		0.1%, substitution
	150 (PE)	75–90 Gb		0.1%, substitution
	250 (PE)	125–150 Gb		0.1%, substitution
Illumina HiSeq250v3	36 (SE)	47–52 Gb	1.5 B	0.1%, substitution
	50 (PE)	135–150 Gb	3 B	0.1%, substitution
	100 (PE)	270–300 Gb		0.1%, substitution
Illumina HiSeq250v4	36 (SE)	64–72 Gb	2 B	0.1%, substitution
	50 (PE)	180–200 Gb	4 B	0.1%, substitution
	100 (PE)	360–400 Gb		0.1%, substitution
	125 (PE)	450–500 Gb		0.1%, substitution
Illumina HiSeq3000/4000	50 (SE)	105–125 Gb	2.5 B	0.1%, substitution
	75 (PE)	325–375 Gb		0.1%, substitution
	150 (PE)	650–750 Gb		0.1%, substitution
Illumina HiSeqX	150 (PE)	800–900 Gb	2.6–3 B	0.1%, substitution
	150 (PE)	1.6–20 B	167 Gb–6 Tb	

http://dx.doi.org/10.5772/intechopen.69872

Platform	Read length[1] (base pair)	Throughput[2]	Number of reads[3]	Error profile
Ion Proton	200 (SE)	Up to 10 Gb	60 M	1% indel
Ion PGM 318	200 or 400 (SE)	0.6–2 Gb	4–5.5 M	1% indel
Ion PGM 316	200 or 400 (SE)	0.3–1 Gb	2–3 M	1% indel
Ion PGM 314	200 or 400 (SE)	30–100 Mb	0.4–0.5 M	1% indel
PacBio Sequel	8–12 kb (SE)	3.5–7 Gb	>100,000	N/A
PacBio RS II	~20 kb	0.5–1Gb	~55,000	~13%, indel
454 GS Junior	~400 (SE, PE)	35 Mb	~0.1 M	1%, indel
454 GS Junior+	~700 (SE, PE)	70 Mb	~0.1 M	1%, indel
454 GS FLX Titanium XLR70	Up to 600; 450 mode (SE, PE)	450 Mb	~1 M	1%, indel
454 GS FLX Titanium XL+	Up to 1000; 700 mode (SE, PE)	700 Mb	~1 M	1%, indel
SOLiD 5500 xl	50 or 75 (SE)	160–320 Gb	~1.4 B	≤0.1%, AT bias
SOLiD 5500 Wildfire	50 or 75 (SE)	80–160 Gb	700 M	≤0.1%, AT bias
Oxford Nanopore MK1 MinION	Up to 200 Kb	~1.5 Gb		~12%, indel
Oxford Nanopore GridION X5	~Hundreds of Kb	100 Gb		
Oxford Nanopore PromethION		~4 Tb		

[1]SE: single end, PE: paired end, Kb, Kilo base pair.
[2]Mb: Megabyte, Gb: Gigabyte, TB: Terabyte.
[3]M: Million, B: Billion.

Table 1. Overview of some sequencing platforms for transcriptome analysis and their characteristics.

to preserve strand information during library preparation. As lncRNA annotation is still in the initial phase, it is crucial to preserve strand information to enable correct genome localization of novel transcripts. Paired-end sequencing is to be considered over single end sequencing for lncRNA characterization to facilitate construction of transcripts with clear-cut exon boundaries. Paired-end sequencing also allows accurate detection of splicing position. Sequencing long fragments (>100 bp) is also desired to get adequate coverage of the genome and consequently, better transcript construction. The number of multiplexed samples on each sequencing lane affects lncRNA sequence depth. Reducing cost by multiplexing more samples than necessary reduces quality of results obtained. It has been demonstrated that the depth of sequencing is relative to the nature of the expected results [30, 31]. To accomplish lncRNA discovery with confidence, a minimum of 100 million reads per sample is suggested to enable *de novo* transcript assembly.

The procedure for the generation of miRNA sequence data differs slightly from the procedure for lncRNA analysis. First of all, miRNAs are small (18–24 bp) in size and do not require RNA

Step	Tools	Application/Web link	References
Trimming*	Trimmomatic	Illumina single end and paired end quality and adapter trimming. http://www.usadellab.org/cms/?page=trimmomatic	[39]
	PEAT	Specific for paired end sequencing quality and adapter trimming. https://github.com/jhhung/PEAT	[50]
	Trim Galore	Quality and adapter trimming with some extra functionality for Bisulfite-Seq. https://www.bioinformatics.babraham.ac.uk/projects/trim_galore	[51]
	Skewer	Adapter trimming, can take into account indels. https://github.com/relipmoc/skewer	[52]
	AlienTrimmer	Detect and remove alien k-mers in both ends of sequence reads. ftp://ftp.pasteur.fr/pub/gensoft/projects/AlienTrimmer/.	[53]
	Cutadapt	Finds and remove adapter, primers, poly-A and other types of unwanted sequences. https://github.com/marcelm/cutadapt	
	NxTrim	Discard as little sequence as possible from Illumina Nextera Mate Pair reads, single end and paired end reads. https://github.com/sequencing/NxTrim	[54]
	SeqPurge	Can detect very short adapter sequences. https://github.com/imgag/ngs-bits/blob/master/doc/tools/SeqPurge.md	[55]
Alignment**	STAR	Align RNA-Seq reads to a reference genome, detect splice junctions. https://github.com/alexdobin/STAR	[45]
	Bowtie / Bowtie2	Align short DNA sequences to genomes with Burrows-Wheeler index. bowtie-bio.sourceforge.net/bowtie2	[56, 57]
	BWA	Mapping low-divergent sequences against large reference genome. bio-bwa.sourceforge.net	[58]
	TopHat2	Use Bowtie for alignment. TopHat analyzes results to identify splice junctions. https://ccb.jhu.edu/software/tophat	[59]
	Rockhopper	Specific for bacterial RNA-Seq data. It supports de novo and reference based transcript assembly. cs.wellesley.edu/~btjaden/Rockhopper	[60]
	SpliceMap	De novo splice junction discovery and alignment tool. https://web.stanford.edu/group/wonglab/SpliceMap	[61]
	StringTie	De novo transcript assembly. Quantitation of full-length transcripts representing multiple splice variants for each gene locus. https://ccb.jhu.edu/software/stringtie	[47]
	Trinity	De novo reconstruction of transcriptomes from RNA-seq data. https://github.com/trinityrnaseq/trinityrnaseq/wiki	[62]

*Further trimming tools are available at: https://omictools.com/adapter-trimming-category/

**Further alignment tools are available at: https://omictools.com/read-alignment-category/

Table 2. Frequently used tools for trimming and alignment.

Names	Major purpose[1]	Known miRNA annotation[2]	Novel miRNA discovery	DE analyses	Target prediction	Pathway enrichment	Livestock Species	References
miRDeep	miRNA identification	+	+	–	–	–	+	[74]
mirTools	miRNA identification	+	+	+	+	–	+	[71]
UEA sRNA Workbench	miRNA identification	+	+	+	+	–	+	[76]
sRNAtoolbox	miRNA identification	+	+	+	+	–	+	[77]
MIReNA	miRNA identification	+	–	–	–	–	+	[81]
miRExpress	miRNA identification	–	+	–	–	–	+	[93]
DARIO	miRNA identification	+	+	–	+	–	–	[94]
Target scan	Target prediction	–	–	–	+	–	+	[95]
DIANA-microT-CDS	Target prediction	–	–	–	+	+	–	[96]
miRanda	Target prediction	–	–	–	+	–	+	[97]
miRDB	Target prediction	–	–	–	+	–	+	[98]
miRTar	Target prediction	–	–	–	+	–	–	[99]
mirWIP	Target prediction	–	–	–	+	–	–	[100]
MMIA	Target prediction	–	–	–	+	+	–	[101]
PITA	Target prediction	–	–	–	+	–	+	[102]
psRNATarget	Target prediction	–	–	–	+	–	–	[103]
RNA22	Target prediction	–	–	–	+	–	+	[104]
RNAhybrid	Target prediction	–	–	–	+	–	+	[105]

Names	Major purpose[1]	Known miRNA annotation[2]	Novel miRNA discovery	DE analyses	Target prediction	Pathway enrichment	Livestock Species	References
TargetRank	Target prediction	–	–	–	+	–	–	[106]
DIANA-mirPath v3	Down-stream miRNA analyses	–	–	–	+	+	+	[107]
miRGator	Integrated tools	–	–	+	+	+	–	[108]
MAGIA	Down-stream miRNA analyses	–	–	–	–	+	–	[109]
miRNet	Down-stream miRNA analyses	–	–	–	–	+	+	[110]
miRSystem	Down-stream miRNA analyses	–	–	–	–	+	+	[111]
miRNAMap	Integrated tools	+	+	–	+	+	+	[112]
miRTarBase	Integrated tools	+	+	+	+	+	+	[113]
TransmiR	Down-stream miRNA analyses	–	–	–	–	+	+	[114]
PicTar	Target prediction	–	–	–	+	–	+	[115]
miRWalk	Integrated tools	+	+	+	–	–	+	[116]
MiRecords	Integrated tools	+	+	+	–	–	+	[117]
multiMiR	Integrated tools	+	+	+	–	–	+	[118]
miRconnX	Integrated tools	+	+	+	+	+	–	[119]
DIANA-mirExTra	Down-stream miRNA analyses	–	–	–	–	+	–	[120]
TarBase	Database	+	+	+	–	+	+	[121]

[1]Further tools for miRNA annotation are available at: https://tools4mirs.org/software/known_mirna_identification/; Further tools for novel miRNA discovery and miRNA precursor prediction are available at: https://tools4mirs.org/software/precursor_prediction/; Further tools for miRNA target prediction are available at: https://tools4mirs.org/software/target_prediction; https://omictools.com/mirna-target-prediction-category

[2]"+" Function is included, "–" Function is not included.

Table 3. Overview of tools used for the analysis of miRNA sequence data.

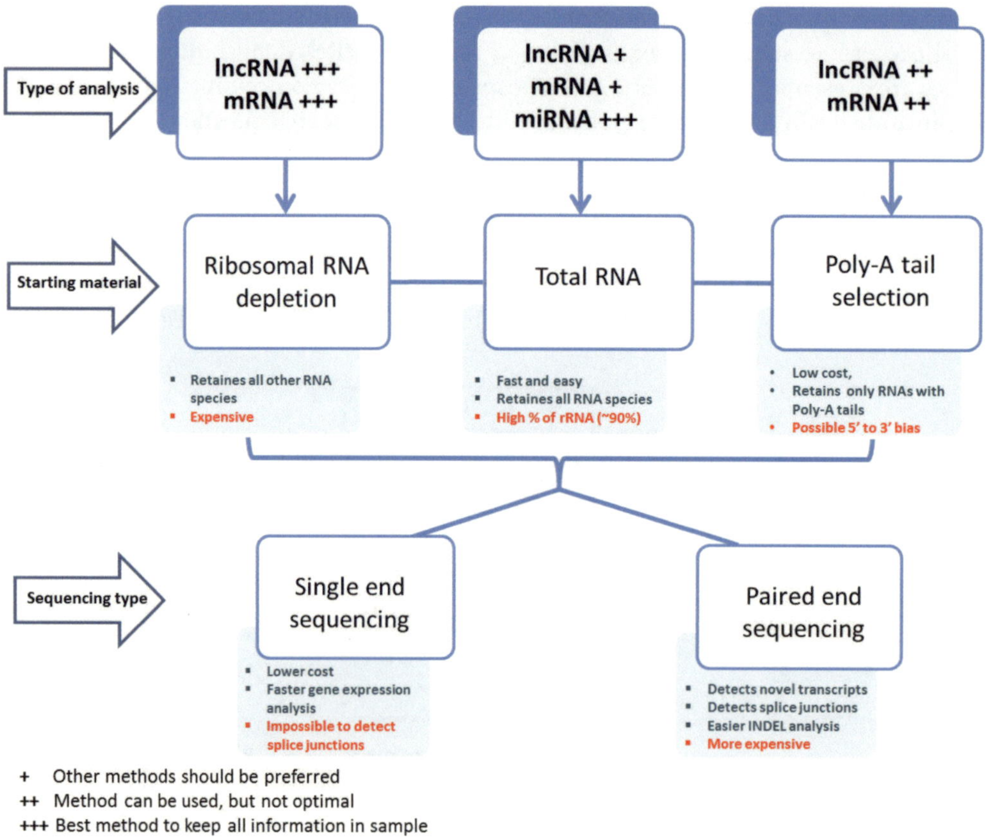

Figure 1. Starting material and sequencing method considerations according to RNA species to be analyzed.

fragmentation prior to library construction. Total RNA is the recommended starting material for miRNA library preparation (**Figure 1**). Although some commercial kits provide the option to enrich the miRNA fraction prior to library preparation, there is evidence that some small RNA species are lost during enrichment [32]. The protocols for miRNA library preparation are generally similar to lncRNA and include adapter ligation step, reverse transcription and amplification followed by size selection and purification of the cDNA. Fifty bp single end sequencing is sufficient for miRNA libraries since miRNAs are generally small. Thus, Illumina platforms are well suited for sequencing miRNA libraries. Studies showed that approximately 2 million reads are sufficient for differential expression analysis while 8 million reads are sufficient for discovery analysis [33, 34]. Considering that over 150 million reads are available per lane on HiSeq machines, sample multiplexing can be as high as 18 to 20 libraries per lane.

2.2.2. Common data processing steps

Upon availability of sequence data, many bioinformatics tools are used in the analytical procedures. Some processing steps are optional but strongly recommended; while others are required before the next step can be performed. Many pipelines have been developed to

answer specific questions, but the softwares used can be very different. A global view of the general processing steps and frequently used tools for lncRNA and miRNA sequence data analyses are presented in **Figures 2** and **3**, respectively. These processing steps can be modified to include desired or specific tools depending on the research question.

2.2.3. Raw data quality control

Sequence data generated by Illumina platforms and most platforms is in FASTQ format. The FASTQ format is a text file consisting of the nucleic acid sequence (read) and base calling accuracy score (Phred score) attributed to each base pair of the sequence. FastQC [35], Picard

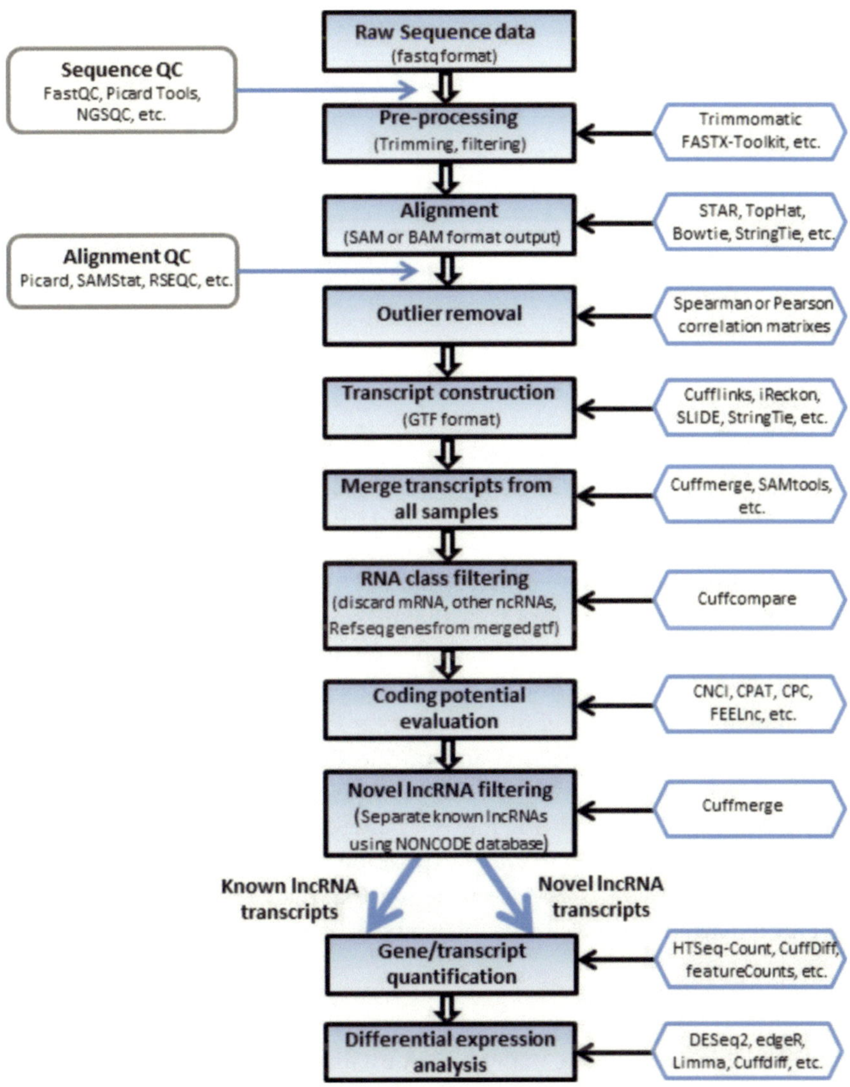

Figure 2. General processing steps and tools used in lncRNA sequence analysis.

http://dx.doi.org/10.5772/intechopen.69872

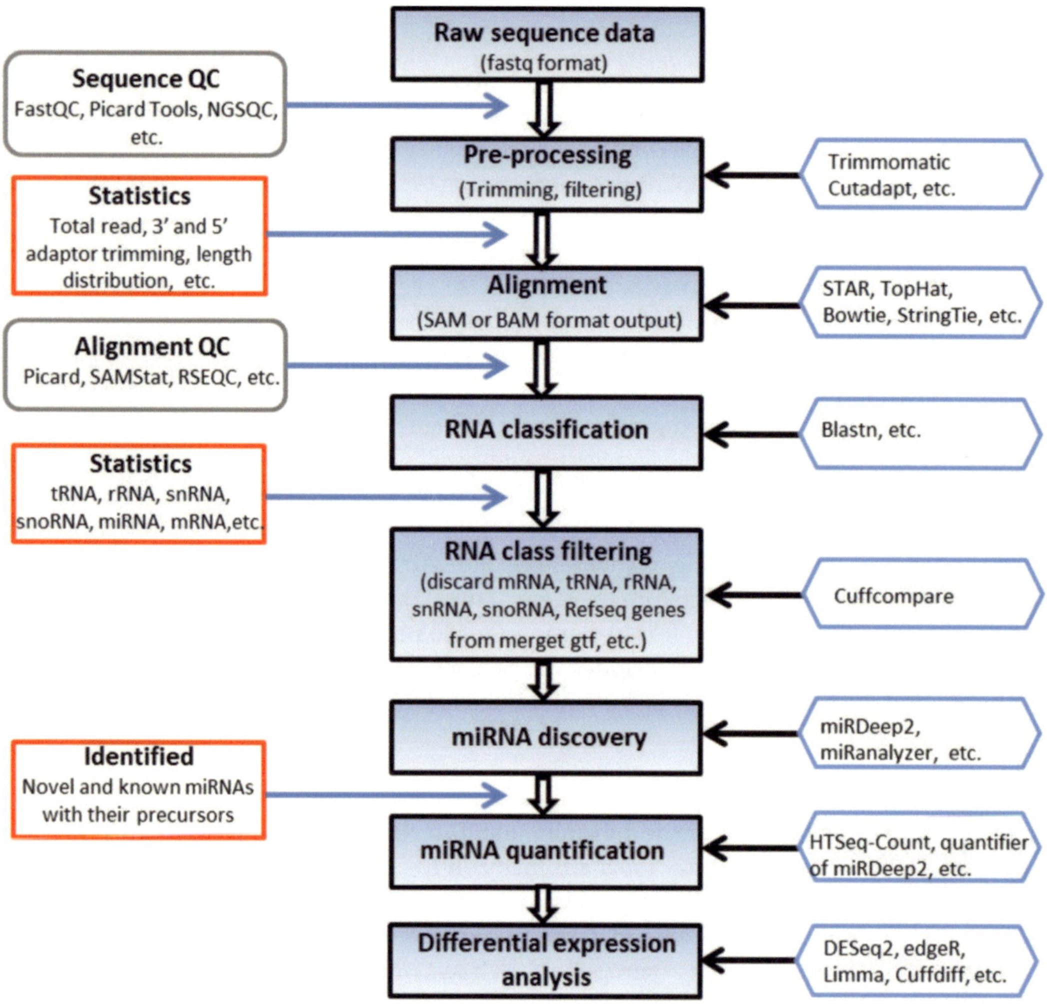

Figure 3. General processing steps and tools used in miRNA sequence analysis.

tools (https://broadinstitute.github.io/picard/) and NGS QC tool kit [36] are often used to assess the quality of raw sequence reads. This step is necessary to determine if the sequencing outcome is as expected. These tools inform on the total number of reads, the overall quality of base call according to the position, GC percentage and other features. Care should be taken when interpreting the results because GC content is species specific and some softwares evaluate GC content according to the human genome. In order to avoid bias in the mapping step, a quality trimming is necessary to get rid of low quality base pairs and remaining adapter sequences. A recent study showed that incorrect trimming can lead to generation of short reads impairing the capacity to correctly predict differences in expression changes [37]. Several trimming tools are available [38] (https://omictools.com/adapter-trimming-category) including Trimmomatic [39], FASTX-Toolkit [40], CutAdapt [41], etc.(**Table 2**). Following trimming, filtering of reads is necessary to get rid of very short and overall low quality reads to keep bias level as low as possible.

2.2.4. *Alignment*

After trimming and filtering, reads are ready for alignment or *de novo* construction. Alignment consists of mapping reads to a reference genome. Various alignment tools have been developed [42, 43] (https://omictools.com/read-alignment-category) including frequently used tools like TopHat [44], STAR [45], Bowtie [46], StringTie [47], etc. (**Table 2**). These softwares have their own specifications highlighting the importance of understanding the utility of each tool and the options they offer. The alignment tool used can have great impact on the end results. It has been observed that the choice of aligner and specific options can affect results of differential gene expression analysis [48]. Aligners can be grouped in two types, gapped (also known as split, e.g. STAR, BWA, etc.) and ungapped (e.g. Bowtie, etc.). Bowtie (ungapped group) can easily map reads to a genome, but is less effective at finding spliced junctions. Aligners in the gapped group are able to align reads and detect spliced variants. In the absence of a reference genome, *de novo* assembly aligners (e.g. Trinity [49]) can be used. In the context of lncRNA read alignment, gapped softwares are preferred since the transcripts are not all annotated and portions of the reads of the same transcript may align to one position of the genome and the remaining to another position. Alignment is one of the longest steps in RNA-Seq sequence analysis therefore selection of the right tool might have significant impact on the outcome of the analysis. It is also important to perform mapping quality control following alignment. Quality check includes the percentages of mapped and unmapped reads, the location of the reads (intronic and exonic) and the 5′–3′ coverage.

2.2.5. *Transcript construction and quantification*

RNA-Seq transcript construction and the alignment steps can demand considerable computing time. Transcript construction tools are many (https://omictools.com/transcript-quantification-category) including commonly used tools like Cufflinks [63], iReckon [64], StringTie [47], etc. This step requires paired-end data and high sequence coverage to reconstruct lowly expressed transcripts. With the assumption that transcripts are species specific, raw data or alignment files from all samples from the same population can be merged to increase coverage [65]. This modification will help clarify transcript boundaries in case of *de novo* transcript assembly. Particular considerations for lncRNA transcript construction include sample pooling according to species and tissue type. LncRNA expression is known to demonstrate tissue specificity [66–68].

2.2.6. *miRNA processing steps*

Overall, the procedures for miRNA identification and discovery are less time consuming and do not include as many steps as for mRNA and lncRNA identification. The global process includes quality and adaptors trimming with quality checkpoints before and after each step. A size selection to keep sequences between 17 and 30 nt (sometimes up to 35 nt) is often performed right after the quality and adaptors trimming step. This is followed by read mapping and filtering of other RNA sequences (rRNA, tRNA, snRNA, mRNA, lncRNA, etc.). The reads thought to represent miRNA are analyzed with miRNA prediction tools like miRDeep2 [69],

miRanalyzer [70], mirTools 2.0 [71], etc. (**Table 3**). Subsequent interrogation of miRBase database enables classification of retained miRNAs as known or novel miRNAs. A tool like miRDeep2 has a quantifier module that generates a read count table for each miRNA using precursor and mature sequence files as input. An overview of tools for miRNA identification are presented in **Table 3** and further discussed in the next section.

3. Tools for ncRNA identification

3.1. Tools for miRNA identification

The identification of miRNAs can be either annotation of known miRNAs or discovery of novel miRNAs. A variety of algorithms and bioinformatics tools are applied to annotate known miRNAs as well as to discover new miRNAs from sequence data. These tools can use several features such as sequence conservation among species, structural features like hairpin and minimal folding free energy [72]. Many tools are available for miRNA annotation (https://tools4mirs.org/software/known_mirna_identification/) [73] including frequently used tools like miRdeep [74], miRanalyzer [75], mirTools 2.0[71], UEA sRNA Workbench [76], sRNAtoolbox [77], and SeqBuster [78] (**Table 3**). Many more tools have been developed for novel miRNA discovery and miRNA precursor prediction (https://tools4mirs.org/software/precursor_prediction/)[73] including frequently used tools like MiPred [79], miRanalyzer [75], miR-Abela [80], MiReNA [81], UEA sRNA Workbench [76] and mirDeep [74] (**Table 3**). Major features of miRNA discovery tools have been reviewed [82–84]. Regarding livestock species, the choice of methods for miRNA discovery and novel miRNA annotation vary among studies and species. For example, De Vliegher et al. [85] used miRbase [86] and UNAFold [87] for miRNA annotation and discovery in bovine mammary gland tissues while Peng et al [88] used miRbase [86] and RNAfold [89] for these purposes in porcine mammary glands. In our own studies, miRbase [86] and mirDeep2 [74] were used to identify miRNAs in various tissues including bovine mammary gland tissues [90], milk fat [90–92], milk whey and cells [90].

3.2. Tools for lncRNA identification

To date, a large number of lncRNA genes have been identified in the genomes of human (141,353), cow (23,896) and chicken (13,085) (http://www.bioinfo.org/noncode/analysis.php, accessed on 24-03-2017). Several methodologies have been described to identify/distinguish lncRNAs from mRNAs and successfully applied to livestock species such as coding potential calculator (CPC) [122], PhyLoCSF [123], coding-non-coding index (CNCI) [124], coding potential assessment tool (CPAT) [125], Predictor of Long non-coding RNAs and mRNAs based on an improved k-mer scheme (PLEK) [126] and Flexible Extraction of LncRNAs (FEELnc) [127], etc. The FEELnc program developed by the functional annotation of animal genome project consortium (FAANG) [128] is recommended as a standardized protocol for lncRNA analyses in animal species. In order to distinguish lncRNAs from mRNAs, FEELnc program uses a machine-learning method for estimation of a protein-coding score according to the

RNA size, open reading frame coverage and multi k-mer usage [127]. The FEELnc program can derive an automatically computed cut-off so it maximizes the lncRNA prediction sensitivity and specificity. An overview of tools for lncRNA identification/characterization is listed in **Table 4**.

Tools	Type	Major Function/web link	References
ChIPBase	Database	Identifies binding motif matrices and their binding sites. Predicts transcriptional regulatory relationships between transcription factors and genes. http://rna.sysu.edu.cn/chipbase/.	[129]
LNCipedia	Database	Provides basic transcript information and structure, human lncRNA transcripts and genes. http://www.lncipedia.org/.	[130]
lncRNAdb	Database	Provides comprehensive annotation of eukaryotic lncRNAs. Offers an improved user interface enabling greater accessibility to sequence information, expression data and the literature. http://www.lncrnadb.org/.	[131]
LNCat	Database	Stores the information of 24 lncRNA annotation resources. Allows achieving refined annotation of lncRNAs within the interested region. http://biocc.hrbmu.edu.cn/LNCat/	[132]
LncRNASNP	Database	Provide comprehensive resources of single nucleotide polymorphisms (SNPs) in human/mouse lncRNAs. bioinfo.life.hust.edu.cn/lncRNASNP/	[133]
lncRNAWiki	Database	Provide open-content and publicly editable curation and collection of information on human lncRNAs. http://lncrna.big.ac.cn/index.php/Main_Page	[134]
NONCODE	Database	Presents the most complete collection and annotation of non-coding RNAs (excluding tRNAs and rRNAs) for 18 species including human, mouse, cow, rat, chicken, pig, fruitfly, zebrafish, *Caenorhabditis elegans* and yeast. www.noncode.org/	[135]
ALDB	Database	Enables the exploration and comparative analysis of lncRNAs in domestic animals. Offers information on genome-wide expression profiles and animal quantitative trait loci (QTLs) of domestic animals. http://res.xaut.edu.cn/aldb/index.jsp	[136]
GENCODE	Database	Presents all gene features in the human genome. Contains annotation of lncRNA loci publicly available with the predominant transcript form consisting of two exons. https://www.gencodegenes.org	[137]

http://dx.doi.org/10.5772/intechopen.69872

Tools	Type	Major Function/web link	References
ncRDeathDB	Database	Present a comprehensive bioinformatics resource to ncRNA-associated cell death interactions. www.rna-society.org/ncrdeathdb	[138]
LncVar	Database	Presents genetic variation associated with long noncoding genes. bioinfo.ibp.ac.cn/LncVar	[139]
IRNdb	Database	Combines microRNA, PIWI-interacting RNA, and lncRNA information with immunologically relevant target genes. http://irndb.org	[140]
AnnoLnc	Annotation	Presents online portal for systematically annotating newly identified human lncRNAs.	[141]
LongTarget	Target prediction	Present a computational method and program to predict lncRNA DNA-binding motifs and binding sites. lncrna.smu.edu.cn	[142]
LncRNA2Function	Functional inferences	Facilitates search for the functions of a specific lncRNA or the lncRNAs associated with a given functional term, or annotate functionally a set of human lncRNAs of interest. http://mlg.hit.edu.cn/lncrna2function	[143]
Co-LncRNA	Function inference	Presents a web-based computational tool that allows users to identify GO annotations and KEGG pathways that may be affected by co-expressed protein-coding genes of single or multiple lncRNAs. www.bio-bigdata.com/Co-LncRNA/	[144]
LncReg	Function inference	Provides regulatory information about lncRNAs, such as targets, regulatory mechanisms, and experimental evidence for regulation and key molecules participating in regulation. bioinformatics.ustc.edu.cn/lncreg/	[145]
Linc2GO	Function inference	Provides comprehensive functional annotations for human lincRNA. http://www.bioinfo.tsinghua.edu.cn/~liuke/Linc2GO	[146]
FARNA	Function annotation	Integrates ncRNA information related to expression, pathways and diseases in a large number of human tissues and primary cells. www.cbrc.kaust.edu.sa/farna/	[147]
ViRBase	Database	Provides the scientific community with a resource for efficient browsing and visualization of virus-host ncRNA-associated interactions and interaction networks in viral infection. http://www.rna-society.org/virbase	[148]

Tools	Type	Major Function/web link	References
LncRNA2Target	Database	Stores lncRNA-to-target genes. Provides a web interface for searching targets of a particular lncRNA or for the lncRNAs that target a particular gene. https://www.lncrna2target.org/	[149]
Lncin	Function annotation	Identifies lncRNAs-associated modules from protein interaction networks and predicts the function of lncRNAs based on the protein functions in the modules. lncin.ym.edu.tw	[150]
NPInter	Function annotation	Integrates experimentally verified functional interactions between noncoding RNAs (excluding tRNAs and rRNAs) and other biomolecules (proteins, RNA and genomic DNA). www.bioinfo.org.cn/NPInter	[151]
CPC	Coding potential assessment	Distinguishes between coding and noncoding RNA. Uses a Support Vector Machine-based classifier to assess the protein-coding potential of a transcript. cpc.cbi.pku.edu.cn/	[122]
CNCI	Coding potential assessment	Distinguishes between protein-coding and non-coding sequences independent of known annotations. Applies to a variety of species without whole-genome sequence or with poorly annotated information. https://github.com/www-bioinfo-org/CNCI	[124]
CPAT	Coding potential assessment	Distinguishes between coding and noncoding RNA. Uses a logistic regression model to assess the protein coding potential. rna-cpat.sourceforge.net/	[125]
FEELnc	LncRNA prediction	Derives an automatically computed cut-off so it maximizes the lncRNA prediction sensitivity and specificity. https://github.com/tderrien/FEELnc	[127]
PLEK	lncRNA prediction	Uses k-mer scheme and a support vector machine (SVM) algorithm to distinguish lncRNAs from mRNAs. http://www.ibiomedical.net/plek/	[126]

Table 4. Overview of tools for the analysis of lncRNA sequence data.

3.3. Tools for identification of other non-coding RNA

Currently, few tools have been developed for the identification of groups of ncRNAs other than miRNAs and lncRNAs. The popular tools for piRNA identification include ProTRAC [152], piClust [153], piRNAQuest [154], etc. (**Table 5**). proTRAC detects piRNA clusters based on a probabilistic analysis with assumption of a uniform distribution while piClust uses a density based clustering approach for the detection of piRNAs. piRNAQuest allows a search of the piRNome for silencers [154]. Another notable framework is SeqCluster [155], a python pipeline for the annotation and classification of non-miRNA small ncRNAs. The pipeline permits a

highly versatile and user-friendly interaction with data in order to easily classify small RNA sequences with putative functional importance [155]. For other small RNAs, ncPRO-seq [156] allows the discovery of unknown ncRNA or siRNA-coding regions from small RNA sequence data. DARIO [94] is a web-tool that allows annotation and detection of ncRNAs from various species but not livestock species. CoRAL [157] is a machine learning method that classifies ncRNAs by relying on biologically interpretable features. Several tools also have been developed for predicting circRNAs such as PredicircRNATool [158] and PredcircRNA [159] which apply a machine learning approach to distinguish circRNAs from other ncRNAs (**Table 5**).

Tools	Types	Main Features/web link	References
ProTRAC	piRNA prediction	Detects and analyses piRNA clusters based on quantifiable deviations from a hypothetical uniform distribution regarding the decisive piRNA cluster characteristics. https://sourceforge.net/projects/protrac/	[152]
piClust	piRNA prediction	Finds piRNA clusters and transcripts from small RNA-seq data using a density based clustering approach. http://epigenomics.snu.ac.kr/piclustweb	[153]
piRNAQuest	piRNA database	Provides annotation of piRNAs based on their genomic location in gene, intron, intergenic, CDS, UTR, repeat elements, pseudogenes and syntenic regions. bicresources.jcbose.ac.in/zhumur/pirnaquest	[154]
SeqCluster	ncRNA classification	A framework python for the annotation and classification of the non-miRNA small RNA transcriptome. http://seqcluster.readthedocs.io/#	[155]
ncPRO-seq	ncRNA discovery	Allows the discovery of unknown ncRNA- or siRNA-coding regions from sRNA sequence data. http://ncpro.curie.fr/.	[156]
DARIO	ncRNA discovery	Allows annotation and detection of ncRNAs from various species but not livestock species. http://dario.bioinf.uni-leipzig.de/index.py	[94]
CoRAL	ncRNA classification	A machine learning method that classifies ncRNA by relying on biologically interpretable features. http://wanglab.pcbi.upenn.edu/coral	[157]
DASHR	Database	Stores human small ncRNAs: miRNAs, piRNAs, snRNAs, snoRNAs, scRNAs (small cytoplasmic RNAs), tRNAs, and rRNAs information. lisanwanglab.org/DASHR	[160]
Sno/scaRNAbase	Database	A curated database for small nucleolar RNAs (snoRNAs) and small cajal body-specific RNAs (scaRNAs). gene.fudan.edu.cn/snoRNAbase.nsf	[161]

Tools	Types	Main Features/web link	References
snoRNA	Database	Contains over 1000 snoRNA sequences from Bacteria, Archaea, and Eukaryotes. http://evolveathome.com/snoRNA/snoRNA.php	[162]
CircNet		Provides the following resources: (i) novel circRNAs, (ii) integrated miRNA-target networks, (iii) expression profiles of circRNA isoforms, (iv) genomic annotations of circRNA isoforms, and (v) sequences of circRNA isoforms. circnet.mbc.nctu.edu.tw	[163]
PredicircRNATool	circRNA prediction	Uses a machine learning method for predicting circRNAs from those of non-circularized, expressed exons based on conformational and thermodynamic properties in the flanking introns. https://sourceforge.net/projects/predicircrnatool	[158]
circRNADb	circRNA database	Contains 32,914 human circular RNAs. http://reprod.njmu.edu.cn/circrnadb	[164]
PredcircRNA	cirRNA prediction	Applies a machine learning approach to predict circRNA. https://github.com/xypan1232/PredcircRNA	[159]
CirsBase	Database	Provides scripts to identify known and novel circRNAs in sequence data. circbase.org	[165]
Circ2Traits	Database	Contains a database of potential association of circular RNAs with diseases in human. http://gyanxet-beta.com/circdb	[166]
CircInteractome	Database	Provides a web tool for mapping (RNA Binding Proteins (RBP)- and miRNA-binding sites on human circRNAs. Allows to (i) identify potential circRNAs which can act as RBP sponges, (ii) design junction-spanning primers for specific detection of circRNAs of interest, (iii) design siRNAs for circRNA silencing, and (iv) identify potential internal ribosomal entry sites. https://circinteractome.nia.nih.gov	[167]
tRNAdb	Database	Contains 12,000 tRNA genes from 577 species and 623 tRNA sequences from 104 species, provides various services such as graphical representations of tRNA secondary structures. trnadb.bioinf.uni-leipzig.de	[168]

Table 5. Overview of tools and databases for sequence analysis of other small ncRNAs.

http://dx.doi.org/10.5772/intechopen.69872

4. Tools for differential expression analysis of non-coding RNA

Various tools allow for the detection of genes (mRNA or ncRNA) differentially expressed (DE) between two or more conditions or states from sequence data. The major differences among tools are their implemented statistical methods, input and output file formats as well as filtering steps for DE analyses. Many tools such as DESeq [169], edgeR [170], NBPSeq [171], TSPM [172], baySeq [173], EBSeq [174], NOISeq [175], SAMseq [176] and ShrinkSeq [177] use count data as input file, while others like limma [178] and Cufflinks use transformed data or BAM files (the binary version of sequence alignment data) as input, respectively. Tools that use count data can be divided in to two groups; parametric (DESeq [169], edgeR [170], NBPSeq [171], TSPM [172], baySeq [173], EBSeq [174]) and non-parametric methods (NOISeq [175], SAMseq [176]). For parametric methods, most softwares (baySeq [173], DESeq [169], NBPSeq [171], edgeR [170], EBSeq [174] and NBPSeq) use a negative binomial model to account for over dispersion except ShrinkSeq which has two options for distribution, either negative binomial or a zero-inflated negative binomial distribution. These methods also implement different statistical test approaches; DESeq, edgeR and NBPSeq perform a classical hypothesis testing approach while baySeq, EBSeq and ShrinkSeq apply Bayesian methods. The comparison of methods and performances have been done and reviewed by many authors [29, 179–183]. In general, no single method performs well for all datasets. In a survey of performance of DE analyses methods, Conesa et al. [29] observed that limma package [178] performed well under many conditions. Many studies observed similar performances by DESeq and edgeR in ranking genes [29, 179–183]. However, DESeq is more conservative while edgeR is more liberal in controlling false discovery rate (FDR) [29]. Other tools such as SAMseq is better in controlling FDR while NOISeq is efficient in avoiding false positives [29].

5. Bioinformatics tools for target prediction and functional inference of non-coding RNA

Following discovery and detection of important ncRNAs from RNA sequence data, the important next steps are to understand their regulatory roles. Since ncRNAs commonly act by interacting with target genes (mostly inhibit expression), various tools have been developed to predict their target genes and to infer their functions (**Tables 3** and **4**). A simple work flow for inferring the functions of miRNAs is shown in **Figure 4**.

5.1. Functional inference of miRNAs

5.1.1. Bioinformatics tools for target prediction and functional inference of miRNAs

Inferring individual targets for a given miRNA can be done either by computational or experimental methods. Computational target prediction is coordinated in a sequence-specific manner and the target genes are normally predicted based on information derived from the

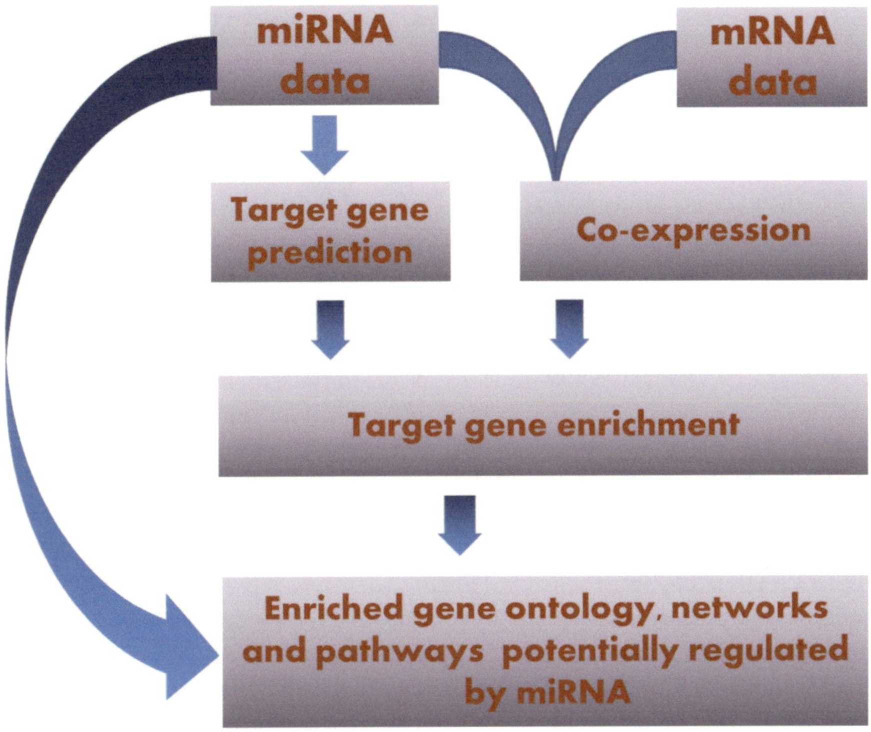

Figure 4. A simple work flow for inference of miRNA function.

potency of binding between miRNA and putative targets. Generally, the methods for computational prediction of miRNA targets can be grouped in single platforms such as TargetScan [95], PicTar [115], RNAhybrid [105] or multiple platforms such as miRwalk [116], TarBases [121], miRecords [117] as well as integrative platforms which include downstream analyses of putative target genes such as DIANA-microT-CDS [96], miRPathDB [184], etc. A collection of tools for miRNA target prediction are available at https://omictools.com/mirna-target-prediction-category and https://tools4mirs.org/software/target_prediction/ [185] (**Table 3**). Among the prediction tools, the major differences in principles are in the algorithm applied and in filtering steps considering the secondary structure of the target mRNA (reviewed in [83, 115, 186]). Consequently, the specificity, sensitivity and accuracy of prediction are different among tools. Additionally, the performances of tools also differ based on the skills of the user (such as formatting of input and output, programming skills, web interface and so on). Taken together, all these factors affect popularity of tools [72, 187]. A word cloud plot of the popularity of tools based on their citation per year is shown in **Figure 5**.

5.1.2. Popular single platforms for miRNA target prediction

TargetScan can be accessed via the web interface or by running a perl script (local run) [95]. The software detects targets in the 3'UTR of protein-coding transcripts by base-pairing rules (seed complementarity) and predicts miRNAs for miRNA families instead of individual

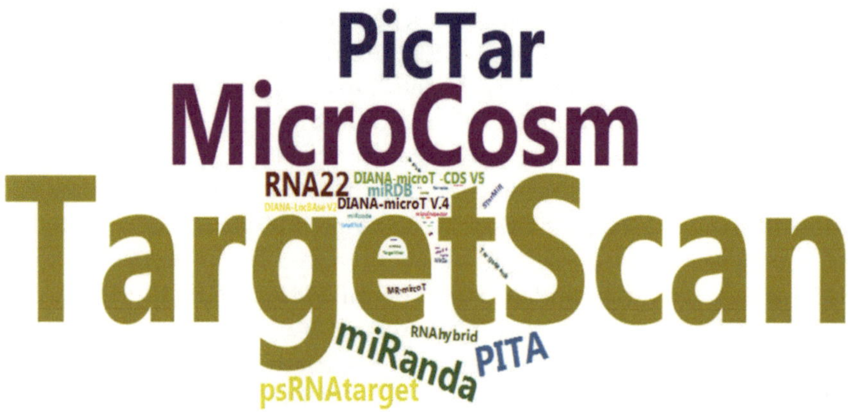

Figure 5. Word cloud for relative use of miRNA target prediction tools (based on number of citations per year).

miRNAs. To assess important miRNA-target interaction, TargetScan outputs two matrices: probability of conserved targeting (Pct) and total contextual score (TCS). Pct corresponds to a Bayesian estimate of the probability that a miRNA site on the 3′ UTR of a mRNA is conserved due to miRNA targeting while TCS represents the strength of the sequential features (site-type, 3′ pairing contribution, local AU contribution, position contribution, target site abundance and seed-pairing stability) that facilitate miRNA-target hybridization/cleavage. PicTar also searches for identical seed sequences to predict miRNA-mRNA interaction [115]. PicTar derives an overall score to assess the strength of the miRNA-target interaction. PicTar computes a score based on the maximum likelihood that a given 3′ UTR sequence is targeted by a fixed set of miRNAs. The PicTar algorithm scores any 3′ UTR that has at least one aligned conserved predicted binding site for a miRNA, and then incorporates all possible binding sites into the score. RNAhybrid computes target genes based on the free energy of hybridization of a long and a short RNA [105]. Hybridization is performed in a kind of domain mode; for example the short sequence is hybridized to the best fitting part of the long one. Rna22 [104] is a pattern-based approach to find miRNA binding sites and corresponding miRNA:mRNA complexes without a cross-species sequence conservation filter. Rna22 is resilient to noise and does not rely upon cross-species conservation. Unlike previous methods, Rna22 starts by finding putative miRNA binding sites in the sequence of interest followed by identification of the targeting miRNA. It can identify putative miRNA binding sites even though the targeting miRNA is unknown. miRanda was the first bioinformatics tool to predict the target genes of miRNAs. The miRanda algorithm is based on a comparison of miRNAs complementarity to 3′UTR of genes [97]. miRanda calculates the binding energy of the duplex structure, evolutionary conservation of the whole target site and its position within the 3′UTR and accounts for a weighted sum of match and mismatch scores for base pairs and gap penalties.

5.1.3. Portals for miRNA target prediction

miRWalk, a comprehensive database developed by Dweep et al [116] documents miRNA binding sites within the complete sequence of a gene and combines this information with predicted

binding sites data resulting from 12 target prediction programs (DIANA-microTv4.0, DIANA-microT-CDS, miRanda-rel2010, mirBridge, miRDB4.0, miRmap, miRNAMap, doRiNA, PicTar2, PITA, RNA22v2, RNAhybrid2.1 and Targetscan6.2) to build platforms of binding sites for the promoter, coding (5 prediction datasets), 5′ and 3′UTR regions. It also contains experimentally verified miRNA-target interaction information collected via text-mining search and data from existing resources (miRTarBase, PhenomiR, miR2Disease and HMDD). MirRecords is a resource for animal miRNA-target interactions developed at the University of Minnesota [117]. MiRecords integrates predicted miRNA targets produced by 10 miRNA target prediction programs (DIANA-microTv4.0, miRanda-rel2010, miRDB4.0, PicTar2, PITA, RNAhybrid2.1, Targetscan6.2, miRTarget2, microinspector, NBmiRTar). It also contains information on experimentally validated miRNA targets obtained from the literature. mirDIP integrates 12 miRNA prediction datasets from miRNA prediction databases (DIANA-microTv4.0, miRanda-rel2010, miRDB4.0, PicTar2, PITA, RNAhybrid2.1, Targetscan6.2 and microCosm) allowing to customize miRNA target searches. multiMiR contains a collection of nearly 50 million records from 14 different databases [118]. It allows user-defined cut-offs for predicted binding strength to provide the most confident selection.

5.1.4. *Integrated tools for miRNA analysis*

Various integrated tools as well as work flow for miRNA analysis have been developed to perform downstream analyses of putative target genes (e.g. gene ontology, pathways enrichments of target genes, etc.) such as MMIA [101], MAGIA [109] and miRconnX [119], to link miRNA to transcription factors or to analyze the effect of several miRNAs such as DIANA-mirExTra v2.0 [120] and TransMIR [114]. Typically, predicted target genes are used as input for functional enrichment to infer the potential functions of miRNAs. Furthermore, several tools are also used to correlate the expression levels of miRNAs with mRNA in a particular experiment to infer miRNA function such as miRnet [110], miRSystem [111] and DIANA-miRPath v3.0 [107]. Several tools have also been developed to directly link miRNAs to biological processes such as DMirNet [188], miRnet [110] and DIANA-miRPath v3.0 [107]. Many tools and resources have also been developed to link miRNAs to specific phenotypes/environments including diseases such as miRNAs in obsessive-compulsive disorder [189], autophagy in gerontology [190], epilepsy [191] and cancer [192]. Among the most popular integrated tools, DIANA-tools (www.microrna.gr) covers a wide scope and research scenarios integrating several tools such as DIANA-microT-CDS, DIANA-TarBase v7.0, DIANA-miRGen v3.0, DIANA-miRPath v3.0, and DIANA-mirExTra v2.0. DIANA-microT-CDS uses different thresholds and meta-analysis followed by pathway enrichment to perform miRNA target prediction [96]. DIANA-TarBase is a manually curated target database with more than half a million miRNA-target interactions curated from published experiments performed with 356 different cell types from 24 species. DIANA-miRPath is an online software suite dedicated to the assessment of miRNA regulatory roles and the identification of controlled pathways [107]. DIANA-mirExTra performs combined differential expression analysis of mRNAs and miRNAs to uncover miRNAs and transcription factors that play important regulatory roles between two investigated state [193]. miRNet is an easy-to-use web-based tool for statistical analysis and functional interpretation of various datasets generated in miRNAs studies in

various species. Moreover, it also allows users to explore the results of miRNA-target interaction [110]. MMIA is a web tool for integration of miRNA and mRNA expression data with predicted miRNA target information for analyzing miRNA-associated phenotypes and biological functions by gene set enrichment analyses [101].

5.2. Functional inference of lncRNA

Compared to miRNAs, fewer bioinformatics tools have been developed for functional inference of lncRNAs. Several databases have been developed to curate computationally predicted and experimentally verified lncRNAs, such as LncRNAdb [194], GENCODE [137], lncRNAtor [7], lncRNome [195], NONCODE [135], lncRNAWiki [134], LncRNA2Function [143] and starBase v2.0 [196]. LncRNAdb was the first lncRNA database [194] and its updated version (LncRNAdb v2.0) integrates lncRNAs reported in livestock species (cattle, sheep, pig, horse and chicken) [131]. DeepBase database is an online platform for annotation and discovery of lncRNAs from RNA-seq data and it contains a large number of transcript entries for bovine (43,156) and chicken (47,004) lncRNAs. Other databases for livestock species are RNAcentral [197] which currently houses information from 23 ncRNA databases (http://rnacentral.org/, access March, 2017) but only contains a small number of lncRNAs from livestock species (cattle, pig, horse and chicken). NONCODE [135] contains lncRNAs for 16 species including cattle and chicken in the latest version. The first lncRNA database with a particular focus on domesticated animals was ALDB [136]. ALDB contains 12,103 pig lincRNAs (long intergenic non-coding RNA), 8923 chicken lincRNAs, and 8250 cow lincRNAs (http://www.ibiomedical.net/aldb/, access March, 2017). However, no comprehensive database currently covers available information on lncRNAs from livestock species, therefore the availability of a comprehensive tool will be valuable and helpful for subsequent genomic and functional annotation of lncRNAs and comparative interspecies analyses [198]. Inference of lncRNAs functions can also be done by connecting their expression patterns with specific cell types or biological processes to draw possible conclusions on their potential roles. LncRNAs can act in cis and/or trans manner to influence or interact with nearby or distant genes, respectively [2, 199]. For cis-regulation, the genomic location can be used as a guide for guilt-by-association analysis which allows global understanding of lncRNAs and protein coding genes that are tightly co-expressed and thus presumably co-regulated. Cis-relationships can foreseeably arise through complementary sequence motifs, tethering, blocking, and product-independent transcription [2]. For example, the human HOTTIP lncRNA is a cis-acting lncRNA expressed in the HOXA cluster that activates transcription of flanking genes [200]. The bioinformatics tools for cis-regulation prediction include ncFANs (http://www.ebiomed.org/ncFANs) [201] which uses a coding-non-coding gene co-expression network to infer lncRNA function.

6. Emerging platforms and technologies for understanding and using ncRNAs

Efficient and reliable techniques for accurate detection of genome information are important for productivity and health of livestock species [202]. The introduction of next generation

sequencing technologies has increased throughput studies of ncRNAs considerably. Consequently, studies on ncRNAs have contributed toward better understanding of disease resistance, productivity, breeding and meat quality in livestock species [203]. Although the numbers of detected ncRNA transcripts are increasing continuously, the ncRNAs identified and annotated in livestock species are still very scanty, compared with human data. Therefore, there is need to continue to explore the ncRNA transcriptome of livestock species [204]. The ability to explore and modify the genomes of livestock species could be beneficial in improving disease resistance, productivity, breeding capability as well as generation of new biomedical models [205].

Genome editing tools have emerged that allow efficient and precise genome manipulation of many organisms including livestock. The genome editing technique is built on engineered, programmable and highly specific nucleases that induce site-specific changes in the genomes of cellular organisms [206]. Subsequent cellular DNA repair processes generates desired insertions, deletions or substitutions at the loci of interest establishing linkages between genetic variations and biological phenotypes [207]. Presently, four artificially engineered nuclease systems have been developed for genome editing: meganucleases derived from microbial mobile elements, zinc finger nucleases (ZFNs) based on eukaryotic transcription factor DNA binding motif, transcription activator-like effector-based nucleases (TALEN) derived from a plan-invasive bacterial protein, and clustered regularly interspaced short palindromic repeats (CRISPR)-CRISPR associated protein 9 (Cas9) system [208]. Centromere and Promoter Factor 1 (Cpf1) is used as an alternative to Cas9 nuclease which requires only a single CRISPR RNA (crRNA) for targeting [209]. CRISPR/Cas9 is easily applicable and has developed really fast over the past years since only programmable RNA is required to generate sequence specificity [210].

CRISPR–Cas9 system is based on a bacterial CRISPR-Cas9 nuclease from *Streptococcus pyogenes* enabling inexpensive and high-throughput interrogation of gene function [211]. CRISPR-based screening can be used to study non-coding sequences, characterize enhancer elements and regulatory sequences crucial to elucidate the roles of ncRNA [212]. With the CRISPR–Cas9 system, the genome can be sliced at specific sites [213]. Genome editing techniques have been modified and used to alter the genomes of many organisms, thus offering opportunities for generation of genetically modified farm animals [214]. CRISPR offers the ability to target and study particular DNA sequences in the vast expanse of a genome [215]. There are two chief ingredients in the CRISPR–Cas9 system: a Cas9 enzyme that snips through DNA like a pair of molecular scissors, and a small RNA molecule that directs the scissors to a specific sequence of DNA to make the cut. The genome can be edited as desired at nearly any site if a template is provided [216].

In order to adapt this far-reaching application of gene-editing technology to agricultural improvement, various approaches have been applied to a number of livestock species. In pigs, direct cytoplasmic injection of Cas9 mRNA and single-guide RNA into zygotes generated biallelic knockout piglets [217]. The CRISPR-Cas9 system was used to generate gene-edited pigs protected from porcine reproductive and respiratory syndrome virus [218] and to genetically modify single blastocyst inducing indel mutations in a given gene locus[219]. Both Talen and ZNF have been injected directly into pig zygotes to produce live genome edited pigs [220]. Similarly, the porcine myostatin (MSTN) gene, which functions as a negative regulator of muscle growth, was

disrupted using CRISPR/Cas9 system to efficiently generate biologically safe genetically modified pigs [221]. Similarly, zygote injection of TALEN mRNA targeting MSTN gene led to production of gene-edited cattle and sheep [205]

In cattle, the CRISPR/Cas9 system was successfully used to clone embryos that could be used to develop livestock transgenes for agricultural science [222]. Hornlessness was introduced into dairy cattle by genome editing and reproductive cloning providing the potential to improve the welfare of millions of cattle [223]. In the cattle industry, gene-edited calves have been produced with specified genetics by ovum pickup, *in vitro* fertilization and zygote microinjection (OPU-IVF-ZM). The CRISPR/Cas9 system has also been used efficiently to generate gene knock out sheep [224].

In livestock, CRISPR-Cas9 has been greatly enhanced by single-guide RNA generating site-specific DNA breaks through homology-directed repair and used for diverse applications, from disease modelling of individual loci to parallelized loss-of-function screens of thousands of regulatory elements [225]. Equally, bioinformatics designs for CRISPR deletions are now possible with a tool known as CRISPETa developed with efficient CRISPR deletion of an enhancer and exonic fragment of MALAT1, a lncRNA. CRISPETa can be used for single target regions or thousands of targets and has high-coverage library designs for entire classes of non-coding elements which can be adopted for use in livestock species [226]. CRISPR-Cas9 may be used with a gene drive incorporated with genome edit to investigate the control of any biological process and can be used to accelerate livestock breeding [225]. Gene drives can be constructed with the use of CRISPR-Cas9 tool that can favour the inheritance of edited alleles possible to modify a whole population [227]. In the DNA, a double strand break can be initiated by a gene drive during the copying process. Using the sequence of the chromosome containing the gene drive elements as a repair template, the DNA break could be repaired by cellular pathways such as homology-directed repair [228]. Editing the genomic DNA elements targeting non-coding regions is vital since silencing of ncRNA genes using RNA interference tools still presents major challenges. An improved vector system adapted to delete non-protein-coding regulatory elements; double excision CRISPR Knockout (DECKO) using two-step cloning to produce vectors (lentivirus) with two guide RNAs concurrently [229], has been used effectively to silenced five ncRNAs (miRNAs-miR21, miR29a and lncRNAs-UCA1 and MALAT1) [230]. The use of genome editing technologies will create novel viewpoints for enquiry to advance our knowledge on biological function of ncRNAs in livestock species and facilitate creating animals with precise alterations.

7. Conclusion and remarks

With the application of next generation sequencing technologies, the number of ncRNAs reported in livestock species has increased dramatically in the last 5 years. Various tools and pipelines have been introduced to make sense out of ncRNA sequence data. This chapter has provided a comprehensive overview of the current and emerging tools and methods for generating and analyzing ncRNA (miRNA, lncRNA as well as other small ncRNAs) sequence

data (transcriptome) with special emphases on the tools that can be applied to livestock species. While bioinformatics tools for miRNA analyses are quite mature, there is a general lack of comprehensive bioinformatics tools for lncRNA and other small ncRNAs. It is our belief that comprehensive "omics" databases that integrate existing and future ncRNA transcriptome databases in the framework of livestock species will contribute towards elucidation of the ambiguity surrounding RNA sequence data. Moreover, given the fact that several emerging platforms (such as genome editing tools) for understanding ncRNAs have been introduced recently, these tools certainly bring great opportunities for broader and also deeper exploration of ncRNA functions. In addition, meticulous *in silico* prediction and careful interpretation of results are critical when handling ncRNA sequence data. Finally, wet-lab validation of the results of transcriptome data will be vital to confirm the functions of ncRNAs in livestock species.

Acknowledgements

We acknowledge financial support from Agriculture and Agri-Food Canada.

Author details

Duy N. Do[1,2], Pier-Luc Dudemaine[1], Bridget Fomenky[1,3] and Eveline M. Ibeagha-Awemu[1]*

*Address all correspondence to: eveline.ibeagha-awemu@agr.gc.ca

1 Agriculture and Agri-Food Canada, Sherbrooke Research and Development Centre, Sherbrooke, Quebec, Canada

2 Department of Animal Science, McGill University, Ste-Anne-de Bellevue, Quebec, Canada

3 Département des Sciences Animales, Université Laval, Québec, QC, Canada

References

[1] Mercer TR, Wilhelm D, Dinger ME, Solda G, Korbie DJ, Glazov EA, Truong V, Schwenke M, Simons C, Matthaei KI. Expression of distinct RNAs from 3′ untranslated regions. Nucleic Acids Research. 2011;**39**(6):2393-2403

[2] Mercer TR, Dinger ME, Mattick JS. Long non-coding RNAs: Insights into functions. Nature Reviews Genetics. 2009;**10**(3):155-159

[3] Haussecker D, Huang Y, Lau A, Parameswaran P, Fire AZ, Kay MA. Human tRNA-derived small RNAs in the global regulation of RNA silencing. RNA. 2010;**16**(4):673-695

[4] Lee YS, Shibata Y, Malhotra A, Dutta A. A novel class of small RNAs: tRNA-derived RNA fragments (tRFs). Genes & Development. 2009;**23**(22):2639-2649

[5] Ender C, Krek A, Friedländer MR, Beitzinger M, Weinmann L, Chen W, Pfeffer S, Rajewsky N, Meister G. A human snoRNA with microRNA-like functions. Molecular Cell. 2008;**32**(4): 519-528

[6] Taft RJ, Glazov EA, Lassmann T, Hayashizaki Y, Carninci P, Mattick JS. Small RNAs derived from snoRNAs. RNA. 2009;**15**(7):1233-1240

[7] Matera AG, Terns RM, Terns MP. Non-coding RNAs: Lessons from the small nuclear and small nucleolar RNAs. Nature Reviews Molecular Cell Biology. 2007;**8**(3):209-220

[8] Fatica A, Bozzoni I. Long non-coding RNAs: new players in cell differentiation and development. Nature Reviews Genetics. 2014;**15**(1):7-21

[9] Stefani G, Slack FJ. Small non-coding RNAs in animal development. Nature Reviews Molecular Cell Biology. 2008;**9**(3):219-230

[10] Taft RJ, Pang KC, Mercer TR, Dinger M, Mattick JS. Non-coding RNAs: Regulators of disease. The Journal of Pathology. 2010;**220**(2):126-139

[11] Wang Z, Gerstein M, Snyder M. RNA-Seq: A revolutionary tool for transcriptomics. Nature Reviews Genetics. 2009;**10**(1):57-63

[12] Goodwin S, McPherson JD, McCombie WR. Coming of age: Ten years of next-generation sequencing technologies. Nature reviews Genetics. 2016;**17**(6):333-351

[13] Schena M, Shalon D, Davis RW, Brown PO. Quantitative monitoring of gene expression patterns with a complementary DNA microarray. Science. 1995;**270**(5235):467-470

[14] Tarca AL, Romero R, Draghici S. Analysis of microarray experiments of gene expression profiling. American Journal of Obstetrics and Gynecology. 2006;**195**(2):373-388

[15] Kroll KM, Barkema GT, Carlon E. Modeling background intensity in DNA microarrays. Physical Review. E, Statistical, Nonlinear, and Soft Matter Physics. 2008;**77**(6 Pt 1):061915

[16] Wu Z, Irizarry RA, Gentleman R, Martinez-Murillo F, Spencer F. A model-based background adjustment for oligonucleotide expression arrays. Journal of the American Statistical Association. 2004;**99**(468):909-917

[17] Schreiber K, Csaba G, Haslbeck M, Zimmer R. Alternative splicing in next generation sequencing data of *Saccharomyces cerevisiae*. PLoS One. 2015;**10**(10):e0140487

[18] Roberts A, Pimentel H, Trapnell C, Pachter L. Identification of novel transcripts in annotated genomes using RNA-Seq. Bioinformatics. 2011;**27**(17):2325-2329

[19] Piskol R, Ramaswami G, Li JB. Reliable identification of genomic variants from RNA-seq data. American Journal of Human Genetics. 2013;**93**(4):641-651

[20] Cloonan N, Forrest AR, Kolle G, Gardiner BB, Faulkner GJ, Brown MK, Taylor DF, Steptoe AL, Wani S, Bethel G et al. Stem cell transcriptome profiling via massive-scale mRNA sequencing. Nature Methods. 2008;**5**(7):613-619

[21] Morin R, Bainbridge M, Fejes A, Hirst M, Krzywinski M, Pugh T, McDonald H, Varhol R, Jones S, Marra M. Profiling the HeLa S3 transcriptome using randomly primed cDNA and massively parallel short-read sequencing. Biotechniques. 2008;**45**(1):81-94

[22] Wang Y, Xue S, Liu X, Liu H, Hu T, Qiu X, Zhang J, Lei M. Analyses of Long Non-Coding RNA and mRNA profiling using RNA sequencing during the pre-implantation phases in pig endometrium. Scientific Report. 2016;**6**:20238

[23] Bottomly D, Walter NA, Hunter JE, Darakjian P, Kawane S, Buck KJ, Searles RP, Mooney M, McWeeney SK, Hitzemann R. Evaluating gene expression in C57BL/6J and DBA/2J mouse striatum using RNA-Seq and microarrays. PLoS One. 2011;**6**(3):e17820

[24] Sirbu A, Kerr G, Crane M, Ruskin HJ. RNA-Seq vs dual- and single-channel microarray data: Sensitivity analysis for differential expression and clustering. PLoS One. 2012;**7**(12):e50986

[25] Fu X, Fu N, Guo S, Yan Z, Xu Y, Hu H, Menzel C, Chen W, Li Y, Zeng R et al. Estimating accuracy of RNA-Seq and microarrays with proteomics. BMC Genomics. 2009;**10**:161

[26] Jain M, Olsen HE, Paten B, Akeson M. The Oxford Nanopore MinION: Delivery of nanopore sequencing to the genomics community. Genome Biology. 2016;**17**(1):239

[27] Chu Y, Corey DR. RNA sequencing: Platform selection, experimental design, and data interpretation. Nucleic Acid Therapeutics. 2012;**22**(4):271-274

[28] Garber M, Grabherr MG, Guttman M, Trapnell C. Computational methods for transcriptome annotation and quantification using RNA-seq. Nature Methods. 2011;**8**(6):469-477

[29] Conesa A, Madrigal P, Tarazona S, Gomez-Cabrero D, Cervera A, McPherson A, Szcześniak MW, Gaffney DJ, Elo LL, Zhang X. A survey of best practices for RNA-seq data analysis. Genome Biology. 2016;**17**(1):13

[30] Liu Y, Ferguson JF, Xue C, Silverman IM, Gregory B, Reilly MP, Li M. Evaluating the impact of sequencing depth on transcriptome profiling in human adipose. PLoS One. 2013;**8**(6):e66883

[31] Liu Y, Zhou J, White KP. RNA-seq differential expression studies: More sequence or more replication? Bioinformatics. 2014;**30**(3):301-304

[32] Podolska A, Kaczkowski B, Litman T, Fredholm M, Cirera S. How the RNA isolation method can affect microRNA microarray results. Acta Biochimica Polonica. 2011;**58**(4):535-540

[33] Campbell JD, Liu G, Luo L, Xiao J, Gerrein J, Juan-Guardela B, Tedrow J, Alekseyev YO, Yang IV, Correll M et al. Assessment of microRNA differential expression and detection in multiplexed small RNA sequencing data. RNA. 2015;**21**(2):164-171

[34] Metpally RP, Nasser S, Malenica I, Courtright A, Carlson E, Ghaffari L, Villa S, Tembe W, Van Keuren-Jensen K. Comparison of analysis tools for miRNA high throughput sequencing using nerve crush as a model. Frontiers in Genetics. 2013;**4**:20

[35] Andrews S. FastQC: A quality control tool for high throughput sequence data. 2010. Available online at: http://www.bioinformatics.babraham.ac.uk/projects/fastqc

[36] Patel RK, Jain M. NGS QC Toolkit: A toolkit for quality control of next generation sequencing data. PloS One. 2012;**7**(2):e30619

[37] Williams CR, Baccarella A, Parrish JZ, Kim CC. Trimming of sequence reads alters RNA-Seq gene expression estimates. BMC Bioinformatics. 2016;**17**:103

[38] Chen C, Khaleel SS, Huang H, Wu CH. Software for pre-processing Illumina next-generation sequencing short read sequences. Source Code for Biology and Medicine. 2014;**9**:8-8

[39] Bolger AM, Lohse M, Usadel B. Trimmomatic: A flexible trimmer for Illumina sequence data. Bioinformatics. 2014;**30**(15):2114-2120

[40] Gordon A, Hannon G. Fastx-toolkit. FASTQ/A short-reads preprocessing tools (unpublished). http://hannonlab *cshl edu/fastx_toolkit*; 2010

[41] Martin M. Cutadapt removes adapter sequences from high-throughput sequencing reads. EMBnetjournal. 2011;**17**(1): Next Generation Sequencing Data Analysis

[42] Mielczarek M, Szyda J. Review of alignment and SNP calling algorithms for next-generation sequencing data. Journal of Applied Genetics. 2016;**57**(1):71-79

[43] Shang J, Zhu F, Vongsangnak W, Tang Y, Zhang W, Shen B. Evaluation and comparison of multiple aligners for next-generation sequencing data analysis. BioMed Research International. 2014;**2014**:309650

[44] Trapnell C, Pachter L, Salzberg SL. TopHat: Discovering splice junctions with RNA-Seq. Bioinformatics. 2009;**25**(9):1105-1111

[45] Dobin A, Davis CA, Schlesinger F, Drenkow J, Zaleski C, Jha S, Batut P, Chaisson M, Gingeras TR. STAR: Ultrafast universal RNA-seq aligner. Bioinformatics. 2013;**29**(1):15-21

[46] Langmead B. Aligning short sequencing reads with Bowtie. Current Protocols in Bioinformatics. 2010, Chapter 11:Unit 11 17

[47] Pertea M, Pertea GM, Antonescu CM, Chang TC, Mendell JT, Salzberg SL. StringTie enables improved reconstruction of a transcriptome from RNA-seq reads. Nature Biotechnology. 2015;**33**(3):290-295

[48] Yang C, Wu PY, Tong L, Phan JH, Wang MD. The impact of RNA-seq aligners on gene expression estimation. ACM BCB. 2015;**2015**:462-471

[49] Haas BJ, Papanicolaou A, Yassour M, Grabherr M, Blood PD, Bowden J, Couger MB, Eccles D, Li B, Lieber M, et al. De novo transcript sequence reconstruction from RNA-seq using the Trinity platform for reference generation and analysis. Nature Protocols. 2013;**8**(8):1494-1512

[50] Li YL, Weng JC, Hsiao CC, Chou MT, Tseng CW, Hung JH. PEAT: An intelligent and efficient paired-end sequencing adapter trimming algorithm. BMC Bioinformatics. 2015;**16(**Suppl 1):S2

[51] Wu Z, Wang X, Zhang X. Using non-uniform read distribution models to improve isoform expression inference in RNA-Seq. Bioinformatics. 2011;**27**(4):502-508

[52] Jiang H, Lei R, Ding SW, Zhu S. Skewer: A fast and accurate adapter trimmer for next-generation sequencing paired-end reads. BMC Bioinformatics. 2014;**15**:182

[53] Criscuolo A, Brisse S. AlienTrimmer: A tool to quickly and accurately trim off multiple short contaminant sequences from high-throughput sequencing reads. Genomics. 2013;**102**(5-6):500-506

[54] O'Connell J, Schulz-Trieglaff O, Carlson E, Hims MM, Gormley NA, Cox AJ. NxTrim: Optimized trimming of Illumina mate pair reads. Bioinformatics. 2015;**31**(12):2035-2037

[55] Sturm M, Schroeder C, Bauer P. SeqPurge: Highly-sensitive adapter trimming for paired-end NGS data. BMC Bioinformatics. 2016;**17**:208

[56] Langmead B, Salzberg SL. Fast gapped-read alignment with Bowtie 2. Nature Methods. 2012;**9**(4):357-359

[57] Langmead B, Trapnell C, Pop M, Salzberg SL. Ultrafast and memory-efficient alignment of short DNA sequences to the human genome. Genome Biology. 2009;**10**(3):R25

[58] Li H, Durbin R. Fast and accurate long-read alignment with Burrows-Wheeler transform. Bioinformatics. 2010;**26**(5):589-595

[59] Kim D, Pertea G, Trapnell C, Pimentel H, Kelley R, Salzberg SL. TopHat2: Accurate alignment of transcriptomes in the presence of insertions, deletions and gene fusions. Genome Biology. 2013;**14**(4):R36

[60] McClure R, Balasubramanian D, Sun Y, Bobrovskyy M, Sumby P, Genco CA, Vanderpool CK, Tjaden B. Computational analysis of bacterial RNA-Seq data. Nucleic Acids Research. 2013;**41**(14):e140

[61] Au KF, Jiang H, Lin L, Xing Y, Wong WH. Detection of splice junctions from paired-end RNA-seq data by SpliceMap. Nucleic Acids Research. 2010;**38**(14):4570-4578

[62] Haas BJ, Papanicolaou A, Yassour M, Grabherr M, Blood PD, Bowden J, Couger MB, Eccles D, Li B, Lieber M et al. De novo transcript sequence reconstruction from RNA-Seq: Reference generation and analysis with Trinity. Nature Protocols. 2013;**8**(8):1494-1512. DOI: 10.1038/nprot.2013.1084

[63] Trapnell C, Williams BA, Pertea G, Mortazavi A, Kwan G, van Baren MJ, Salzberg SL, Wold BJ, Pachter L. Transcript assembly and quantification by RNA-Seq reveals unannotated transcripts and isoform switching during cell differentiation. Nature Biotechnology. 2010;**28**(5):511-515

[64] Mezlini AM, Smith EJ, Fiume M, Buske O, Savich GL, Shah S, Aparicio S, Chiang DY, Goldenberg A, Brudno M. iReckon: Simultaneous isoform discovery and abundance estimation from RNA-seq data. Genome Research. 2013;**23**(3):519-529

[65] Liu NY, Xu W, Papanicolaou A, Dong SL, Anderson A. Identification and characterization of three chemosensory receptor families in the cotton bollworm *Helicoverpa armigera*. BMC Genomics. 2014;**15**:597

[66] Tsoi LC, Iyer MK, Stuart PE, Swindell WR, Gudjonsson JE, Tejasvi T, Sarkar MK, Li B, Ding J, Voorhees JJ et al. Analysis of long non-coding RNAs highlights tissue-specific expression patterns and epigenetic profiles in normal and psoriatic skin. Genome Biology. 2015;**16**:24

[67] Amin V, Harris RA, Onuchic V, Jackson AR, Charnecki T, Paithankar S, Lakshmi Subramanian S, Riehle K, Coarfa C, Milosavljevic A. Epigenomic footprints across 111 reference epigenomes reveal tissue-specific epigenetic regulation of lincRNAs. Nature Communications. 2015;**6**:6370

[68] Koufariotis LT, Chen Y-PP, Chamberlain A, Vander Jagt C, Hayes BJ. A catalogue of novel bovine long noncoding RNA across 18 tissues. PLoS One. 2015;**10**(10):e0141225

[69] Friedlander MR, Mackowiak SD, Li N, Chen W, Rajewsky N. miRDeep2 accurately identifies known and hundreds of novel microRNA genes in seven animal clades. Nucleic Acids Research. 2012;**40**(1):37-52

[70] Hackenberg M, Rodriguez-Ezpeleta N, Aransay AM. miRanalyzer: An update on the detection and analysis of microRNAs in high-throughput sequencing experiments. Nucleic Acids Research. 2011;**39**(Web Server issue):W132-W138

[71] Wu J, Liu Q, Wang X, Zheng J, Wang T, You M, Sheng Sun Z, Shi Q. mirTools 2.0 for non-coding RNA discovery, profiling, and functional annotation based on high-throughput sequencing. RNA Biology. 2013;**10**(7):1087-1092

[72] Akhtar MM, Micolucci L, Islam MS, Olivieri F, Procopio AD: Bioinformatic tools for microRNA dissection. Nucleic Acids Research. 2016;**44**(1):24-44

[73] Shukla V, Varghese VK, Kabekkodu SP, Mallya S, Satyamoorthy K. A compilation of Web-based research tools for miRNA analysis. Briefings in Functional Genomics. 2017. https://doi.org/10.1093/bfgp/elw042

[74] Friedländer MR, Mackowiak SD, Li N, Chen W, Rajewsky N. miRDeep2 accurately identifies known and hundreds of novel microRNA genes in seven animal clades. Nucleic Acids Research. 2012;**40**(1):37-52

[75] Hackenberg M, Sturm M, Langenberger D, Falcon-Perez JM, Aransay AM. miRanalyzer: A microRNA detection and analysis tool for next-generation sequencing experiments. Nucleic Acids Research. 2009;**37**(suppl 2):W68-W76

[76] Stocks MB, Moxon S, Mapleson D, Woolfenden HC, Mohorianu I, Folkes L, Schwach F, Dalmay T, Moulton V. The UEA sRNA workbench: A suite of tools for analysing and visualizing next generation sequencing microRNA and small RNA datasets. Bioinformatics. 2012;**28**(15):2059-2061

[77] Rueda A, Barturen G, Lebrón R, Gómez-Martín C, Alganza Á, Oliver JL, Hackenberg M. sRNAtoolbox: An integrated collection of small RNA research tools. Nucleic Acids Research. 2015;**43**(W1):W467-W473

[78] Pantano L, Estivill X, Martí E. SeqBuster, a bioinformatic tool for the processing and analysis of small RNAs datasets, reveals ubiquitous miRNA modifications in human embryonic cells. Nucleic Acids Research. 2010;**38**(5):e34-e34

[79] Jiang P, Wu H, Wang W, Ma W, Sun X, Lu Z. MiPred: Classification of real and pseudo microRNA precursors using random forest prediction model with combined features. Nucleic Acids Research. 2007;**35**(Suppl 2):W339-W344

[80] Sewer A, Paul N, Landgraf P, Aravin A, Pfeffer S, Brownstein MJ, Tuschl T, van Nimwegen E, Zavolan M. Identification of clustered microRNAs using an ab initio prediction method. BMC Bioinformatics. 2005;**6**(1):267

[81] Mathelier A, Carbone A. MIReNA: Finding microRNAs with high accuracy and no learning at genome scale and from deep sequencing data. Bioinformatics. 2010;**26**(18):2226-2234

[82] Gomes CPC, Cho J-H, Hood L, Franco OL, Pereira RW, Wang K. A review of computational tools in microRNA discovery. Frontiers in Genetics. 2013;**4**:81

[83] Peterson SM, Thompson JA, Ufkin ML, Sathyanarayana P, Liaw L, Congdon CB. Common features of microRNA target prediction tools. Frontiers in Genetics. 2014;**5**:23

[84] Chiang HR, Schoenfeld LW, Ruby JG, Auyeung VC, Spies N, Baek D, Johnston WK, Russ C, Luo S, Babiarz JE. Mammalian microRNAs: Experimental evaluation of novel and previously annotated genes. Genes & Development. 2010;**24**(10):992-1009

[85] Li Z, Liu H, Jin X, Lo L, Liu J. Expression profiles of microRNAs from lactating and non-lactating bovine mammary glands and identification of miRNA related to lactation. BMC Genomics. 2012;**13**(1):731

[86] Kozomara A, Griffiths-Jones S. miRBase: Annotating high confidence microRNAs using deep sequencing data. Nucleic Acids Research. 2014;**42**(D1):D68-D73

[87] Markham NR, Zuker M. UNAFold: Software for nucleic acid folding and hybridization. Bioinformatics: Structure, Function and Applications. 2008:3-31

[88] Peng J, Zhao J-S, Shen Y-F, Mao H-G, Xu N-Y. MicroRNA expression profiling of lactating mammary gland in divergent phenotype swine breeds. International Journal of Molecular Sciences. 2015;**16**(1):1448-1465

[89] Gruber AR, Lorenz R, Bernhart SH, Neuböck R, Hofacker IL. The vienna RNA websuite. Nucleic Acids Research. 2008;**36**(suppl 2):W70-W74

[90] Li R, Dudemaine P-L, Zhao X, Lei C, Ibeagha-Awemu EM. Comparative analysis of the miRNome of bovine milk fat, whey and cells. PloS One. 2016;**11**(4):e0154129

[91] Schroeder DI, Jayashankar K, Douglas KC, Thirkill TL, York D, Dickinson PJ, Williams LE, Samollow PB, Ross PJ, Bannasch DL. Early developmental and evolutionary origins of gene body DNA methylation patterns in mammalian placentas. PLoS Genetics. 2015;**11**:e1005442

[92] Do DN, Li R, Dudemaine P-L, Ibeagha-Awemu EM. MicroRNA roles in signalling during lactation: An insight from differential expression, time course and pathway analyses of deep sequence data. Scientific Reports. 2017;**7**:44605

[93] Wang W-C, Lin F-M, Chang W-C, Lin K-Y, Huang H-D, Lin N-S. miRExpress: Analyzing high-throughput sequencing data for profiling microRNA expression. BMC Bioinformatics. 2009;**10**(1):328

[94] Fasold M, Langenberger D, Binder H, Stadler PF, Hoffmann S. DARIO: A ncRNA detection and analysis tool for next-generation sequencing experiments. Nucleic Acids Research. 2011;**39**(Web Server issue):W112-W117: gkr357

[95] Lewis BP, Shih I-h, Jones-Rhoades MW, Bartel DP, Burge CB. Prediction of mammalian microRNA targets. Cell. 2003;**115**(7):787-798

[96] Paraskevopoulou MD, Georgakilas G, Kostoulas N, Vlachos IS, Vergoulis T, Reczko M, Filippidis C, Dalamagas T, Hatzigeorgiou AG. DIANA-microT web server v5. 0: Service integration into miRNA functional analysis workflows. Nucleic Acids Research. 2013;**41**(W1):W169-W173

[97] Enright AJ, John B, Gaul U, Tuschl T, Sander C, Marks DS. MicroRNA targets in Drosophila. Genome Biology. 2003;**5**(1):R1

[98] Wong N, Wang X. miRDB: An online resource for microRNA target prediction and functional annotations. Nucleic Acids Research. 2014;**43**(D1):D146-D152. gku1104

[99] Hsu JBK, Chiu CM, Hsu SD, Huang WY, Chien CH, Lee TY, Huang HD. miRTar: An integrated system for identifying miRNA-target interactions in human. BMC Bioinformatics. 2011;**12**(1):300

[100] Hammell M, Long D, Zhang L, Lee A, Carmack CS, Han M, Ding Y, Ambros V. mirWIP: microRNA target prediction based on microRNA-containing ribonucleoprotein–enriched transcripts. Nature Methods. 2008;**5**(9):813-819

[101] Nam S, Li M, Choi K, Balch C, Kim S, Nephew KP. MicroRNA and mRNA integrated analysis (MMIA): A web tool for examining biological functions of microRNA expression. Nucleic Acids Research. 2009;**37**(suppl 2):W356-W362

[102] Kertesz M, Iovino N, Unnerstall U, Gaul U, Segal E. The role of site accessibility in microRNA target recognition. Nature Genetics. 2007;**39**(10):1278-1284

[103] Dai X, Zhao PX. psRNATarget: A plant small RNA target analysis server. Nucleic Acids Research. 2011;**39**(suppl 2):W155-W159

[104] Miranda KC, Huynh T, Tay Y, Ang Y-S, Tam W-L, Thomson AM, Lim B, Rigoutsos I. A pattern-based method for the identification of MicroRNA binding sites and their corresponding heteroduplexes. Cell. 2006;**126**(6):1203-1217

[105] Krüger J, Rehmsmeier M. RNAhybrid: microRNA target prediction easy, fast and flexible. Nucleic Acids Research. 2006;**34**(Suppl 2):W451-W454

[106] Nielsen CB, Shomron N, Sandberg R, Hornstein E, Kitzman J, Burge CB. Determinants of targeting by endogenous and exogenous microRNAs and siRNAs. RNA. 2007;**13**(11): 1894-1910

[107] Vlachos IS, Zagganas K, Paraskevopoulou MD, Georgakilas G, Karagkouni D, Vergoulis T, Dalamagas T, Hatzigeorgiou AG. DIANA-miRPath v3.0: Deciphering microRNA function with experimental support. Nucleic Acids Research. 2015;**43**(W1):W460-W466

[108] Nam S, Kim B, Shin S, Lee S. miRGator: An integrated system for functional annotation of microRNAs. Nucleic Acids Research. 2008;**36**(suppl 1):D159-D164

[109] Sales G, Coppe A, Bisognin A, Biasiolo M, Bortoluzzi S, Romualdi C. MAGIA, a web-based tool for miRNA and genes integrated analysis. Nucleic Acids Research. 2010;**38**(Web Server issue):W352-W359. gkq423

[110] Fan Y, Siklenka K, Arora SK, Ribeiro P, Kimmins S, Xia J. miRNet-dissecting miRNA-target interactions and functional associations through network-based visual analysis. Nucleic Acids Research. 2016;**44**(W1):W135-W141

[111] Lu TP, Lee CY, Tsai MH, Chiu YC, Hsiao CK, Lai LC, Chuang EY. miRSystem: An integrated system for characterizing enriched functions and pathways of microRNA targets. PloS One. 2012;**7**(8):e42390

[112] Hsu SD, Chu CH, Tsou AP, Chen SJ, Chen HC, Hsu PWC, Wong YH, Chen YH, Chen GH, Huang HD. miRNAMap 2.0: Genomic maps of microRNAs in metazoan genomes. Nucleic Acids Research. 2008;**36**(Suppl 1):D165-D169

[113] Hsu SD, Lin FM, Wu WY, Liang C, Huang WC, Chan WL, Tsai WT, Chen GZ, Lee CJ, Chiu CM. miRTarBase: A database curates experimentally validated microRNA–target interactions. Nucleic Acids Research. 2010;**39**(Database issue):D163-D169. gkq1107

[114] Wang J, Lu M, Qiu C, Cui Q. TransmiR: A transcription factor–microRNA regulation database. Nucleic Acids Research. 2010;**38**(suppl 1):D119-D122

[115] Krek A, Grün D, Poy MN, Wolf R, Rosenberg L, Epstein EJ, MacMenamin P, Da Piedade I, Gunsalus KC, Stoffel M. Combinatorial microRNA target predictions. Nature Genetics. 2005;**37**(5):495-500

[116] Dweep H, Sticht C, Pandey P, Gretz N. miRWalk–database: Prediction of possible miRNA binding sites by "walking" the genes of three genomes. Journal of Biomedical Informatics. 2011;**44**(5):839-847

[117] Xiao F, Zuo Z, Cai G, Kang S, Gao X, Li T. miRecords: An integrated resource for microRNA–target interactions. Nucleic Acids Research. 2009;**37**(suppl 1):D105-D110

[118] Ru Y, Kechris KJ, Tabakoff B, Hoffman P, Radcliffe RA, Bowler R, Mahaffey S, Rossi S, Calin GA, Bemis L. The multiMiR R package and database: Integration of microRNA–target interactions along with their disease and drug associations. Nucleic Acids Research. 2014;**42**(17):e133-e133

[119] Huang GT, Athanassiou C, Benos PV. mirConnX: Condition-specific mRNA-microRNA network integrator. Nucleic Acids Research. 2011;**39**(suppl 2):W416-W423

[120] Vlachos IS, Vergoulis T, Paraskevopoulou MD, Lykokanellos F, Georgakilas G, Georgiou P, Chatzopoulos S, Karagkouni D, Christodoulou F, Dalamagas T. DIANA-mirExTra v2. 0: Uncovering microRNAs and transcription factors with crucial roles in NGS expression data. Nucleic Acids Research. 2016;**44**(Web Server issue):W128-W134. gkw455

[121] Vergoulis T, Vlachos IS, Alexiou P, Georgakilas G, Maragkakis M, Reczko M, Gerangelos S, Koziris N, Dalamagas T, Hatzigeorgiou AG. TarBase 6.0: Capturing the exponential growth of miRNA targets with experimental support. Nucleic Acids Research. 2012;**40**(D1):D222-D229

[122] Kong L, Zhang Y, Ye Z-Q, Liu X-Q, Zhao S-Q, Wei L, Gao G. CPC: Assess the protein-coding potential of transcripts using sequence features and support vector machine. Nucleic Acids Research. 2007;**35**(suppl 2):W345-W349

[123] Lin MF, Jungreis I, Kellis M. PhyloCSF: A comparative genomics method to distinguish protein coding and non-coding regions. Bioinformatics. 2011;**27**(13):i275-i282

[124] Sun L, Luo H, Bu D, Zhao G, Yu K, Zhang C, Liu Y, Chen R, Zhao Y. Utilizing sequence intrinsic composition to classify protein-coding and long non-coding transcripts. Nucleic Acids Research. 2013;**41**(17):e166-e166

[125] Wang L, Park HJ, Dasari S, Wang S, Kocher J-P, Li W. CPAT: Coding-Potential Assessment Tool using an alignment-free logistic regression model. Nucleic Acids Research. 2013;**41**(6):e74-e74

[126] Li A, Zhang J, Zhou Z. PLEK: A tool for predicting long non-coding RNAs and messenger RNAs based on an improved k-mer scheme. BMC Bioinformatics. 2014;**15**(1):311

[127] Wucher V, Legeai F, Hedan B, Rizk G, Lagoutte L, Leeb T, Jagannathan V, Cadieu E, David A, Lohi H. FEELnc: A tool for long non-coding RNA annotation and its application to the dog transcriptome. Nucleic Acids Research. 2017;**45**(8):e57. gkw1306

[128] Andersson L, Archibald AL, Bottema CD, Brauning R, Burgess SC, Burt DW, Casas E, Cheng HH, Clarke L, Couldrey C et al. Coordinated international action to accelerate genome-to-phenome with FAANG, the Functional Annotation of Animal Genomes project. Genome Biology. 2015;**16**(1):57

[129] Yang J-H, Li J-H, Jiang S, Zhou H, Qu L-H. ChIPBase: A database for decoding the transcriptional regulation of long non-coding RNA and microRNA genes from ChIP-Seq data. Nucleic Acids Research. 2013;**41**(D1):D177-D187

[130] Volders PJ, Helsens K, Wang X, Menten B, Martens L, Gevaert K, Vandesompele J, Mestdagh P. LNCipedia: A database for annotated human lncRNA transcript sequences and structures. Nucleic Acids Research. 2013;**41**(D1):D246-D251

[131] Quek XC, Thomson DW, Maag JL, Bartonicek N, Signal B, Clark MB, Gloss BS, Dinger ME. lncRNAdb v2. 0: Expanding the reference database for functional long noncoding RNAs. Nucleic Acids Research. 2014;**43**(Database issue):D168-D173. gku988

[132] Xu J, Bai J, Zhang X, Lv Y, Gong Y, Liu L, Zhao H, Yu F, Ping Y, Zhang G. A comprehensive overview of lncRNA annotation resources. Briefings in bioinformatics. 2016;**18**(2):236-249. bbw015

[133] Gong J, Liu W, Zhang J, Miao X, Guo A-Y. lncRNASNP: A database of SNPs in lncRNAs and their potential functions in human and mouse. Nucleic Acids Research. 2015;**43**(D1):D181-D186

[134] Ma L, Li A, Zou D, Xu X, Xia L, Yu J, Bajic VB, Zhang Z. LncRNAWiki: Harnessing community knowledge in collaborative curation of human long non-coding RNAs. Nucleic Acids Research. 2014;**43**(Database issue):D187-D192. gku1167

[135] Xie C, Yuan J, Li H, Li M, Zhao G, Bu D, Zhu W, Wu W, Chen R, Zhao Y. NONCODEv4: Exploring the world of long non-coding RNA genes. Nucleic Acids Research. 2014;**42**(D1):D98-D103

[136] Cao J, Wei C, Liu D, Wang H, Wu M, Xie Z, Capellini TD, Zhang L, Zhao F, Li L. DNA methylation Landscape of body size variation in sheep. Scientific Reports. 2015;**5**

[137] Derrien T, Johnson R, Bussotti G, Tanzer A, Djebali S, Tilgner H, Guernec G, Martin D, Merkel A, Knowles DG. The GENCODE v7 catalog of human long noncoding RNAs: Analysis of their gene structure, evolution, and expression. Genome Research. 2012;**22**(9):1775-1789

[138] Wu D, Huang Y, Kang J, Li K, Bi X, Zhang T, Jin N, Hu Y, Tan P, Zhang L. ncRDeathDB: A comprehensive bioinformatics resource for deciphering network organization of the ncRNA-mediated cell death system. Autophagy. 2015;**11**(10):1917-1926

[139] Chen X, Hao Y, Cui Y, Fan Z, He S, Luo J, Chen R. LncVar: A database of genetic variation associated with long non-coding genes. Bioinformatics. 2017;**33**(1):112-118

[140] Denisenko E, Ho D, Tamgue O, Ozturk M, Suzuki H, Brombacher F, Guler R, Schmeier S. IRNdb: The database of immunologically relevant non-coding RNAs. Database. 2016;**2016**. baw138

[141] Hou M, Tang X, Tian F, Shi F, Liu F, Gao G. AnnoLnc: A web server for systematically annotating novel human lncRNAs. BMC Genomics. 2016;**17**(1):931

[142] He S, Zhang H, Liu H, Zhu H. LongTarget: A tool to predict lncRNA DNA-binding motifs and binding sites via Hoogsteen base-pairing analysis. Bioinformatics. 2015;**31**(2):178-186

[143] Jiang Q, Ma R, Wang J, Wu X, Jin S, Peng J, Tan R, Zhang T, Li Y, Wang Y. LncRNA2Function: A comprehensive resource for functional investigation of human lncRNAs based on RNA-seq data. BMC Genomics. 2015;**16**(3):S2

[144] Zhao Z, Bai J, Wu A, Wang Y, Zhang J, Wang Z, Li Y, Xu J, Li X. Co-LncRNA: Investigating the lncRNA combinatorial effects in GO annotations and KEGG pathways based on human RNA-Seq data. Database. 2015;**2015**. bav082

[145] Zhou Z, Shen Y, Khan MR, Li A. LncReg: A reference resource for lncRNA-associated regulatory networks. Database. 2015;**2015**. bav083

[146] Liu K, Yan Z, Li Y, Sun Z. Linc2GO: A human LincRNA function annotation resource based on ceRNA hypothesis. Bioinformatics. 2013;**29**(17):2221-2222

[147] Alam T, Uludag M, Essack M, Salhi A, Ashoor H, Hanks JB, Kapfer C, Mineta K, Gojobori T, Bajic VB. FARNA: Knowledgebase of inferred functions of non-coding RNA transcripts. Nucleic Acids Research. 2016;**45**(5):2838-2848. gkw973

[148] Li Y, Wang C, Miao Z, Bi X, Wu D, Jin N, Wang L, Wu H, Qian K, Li C. ViRBase: A resource for virus–host ncRNA-associated interactions. Nucleic Acids Research. 2014;**43**(Database issue):D578-D582. gku903

[149] Jiang Q, Wang J, Wu X, Ma R, Zhang T, Jin S, Han Z, Tan R, Peng J, Liu G. LncRNA2Target: A database for differentially expressed genes after lncRNA knockdown or overexpression. Nucleic Acids Research. 2015;**43**(D1):D193-D196

[150] Wu CH, Hsu CL, Lu PC, Lin WC, Juan HF, Huang HC. Identification of lncRNA functions in lung cancer based on associated protein-protein interaction modules. Scientific Reports. 2016;**6**:35959

[151] Wu T, Wang J, Liu C, Zhang Y, Shi B, Zhu X, Zhang Z, Skogerbø G, Chen L, Lu H. NPInter: The noncoding RNAs and protein related biomacromolecules interaction database. Nucleic Acids Research. 2006;**34**(suppl 1):D150-D152

[152] Rosenkranz D, Zischler H. proTRAC-a software for probabilistic piRNA cluster detection, visualization and analysis. BMC Bioinformatics. 2012;**13**(1):5

[153] Jung I, Park JC, Kim S. piClust: A density based piRNA clustering algorithm. Computational Biology and Chemistry. 2014;**50**:60-67

[154] Sarkar A, Maji RK, Saha S, Ghosh Z. piRNAQuest: Searching the piRNAome for silencers. BMC Genomics. 2014;**15**(1):555

[155] Pantano L, Estivill X, Martí E. A non-biased framework for the annotation and classification of the non-miRNA small RNA transcriptome. Bioinformatics. 2011;**27**(22):3202-3203

[156] Chen C-J, Servant N, Toedling J, Sarazin A, Marchais A, Duvernois-Berthet E, Cognat V, Colot V, Voinnet O, Heard E et al. ncPRO-seq: A tool for annotation and profiling of ncRNAs in sRNA-seq data. Bioinformatics. 2012;**28**(23):3147-3149

[157] Leung YY, Ryvkin P, Ungar LH, Gregory BD, Wang L-S. CoRAL: Predicting non-coding RNAs from small RNA-sequencing data. Nucleic Acids Research. 2013;**41**(14):e137. gkt426

[158] Liu Z, Han J, Lv H, Liu J, Liu R. Computational identification of circular RNAs based on conformational and thermodynamic properties in the flanking introns. Computational Biology and Chemistry. 2016;**61**:221-225

[159] Pan X, Xiong K. PredcircRNA: Computational classification of circular RNA from other long non-coding RNA using hybrid features. Molecular Biosystems. 2015;**11**(8):2219-2226

[160] Leung YY, Kuksa PP, Amlie-Wolf A, Valladares O, Ungar LH, Kannan S, Gregory BD, Wang LS. DASHR: Database of small human noncoding RNAs. Nucleic Acids Research. 2015;**44**(D1):D216-D222. gkv1188

[161] Xie J, Zhang M, Zhou T, Hua X, Tang L, Wu W. Sno/scaRNAbase: A curated database for small nucleolar RNAs and cajal body-specific RNAs. Nucleic Acids Research. 2007;**35**(suppl 1):D183-D187

[162] Ellis JC, Brown DD, Brown JW. The small nucleolar ribonucleoprotein (snoRNP) database. RNA. 2010;**16**(4):664-666

[163] Liu Y-C, Li J-R, Sun C-H, Andrews E, Chao R-F, Lin F-M, Weng S-L, Hsu S-D, Huang C-C, Cheng C. CircNet: A database of circular RNAs derived from transcriptome sequencing data. Nucleic Acids Research. 2015;**44**(D1):D209-D215. gkv940

[164] Chen X, Han P, Zhou T, Guo X, Song X, Li Y. circRNADb: A comprehensive database for human circular RNAs with protein-coding annotations. Scientific Reports. 2016;**6**:34985

[165] Glazar P, Papavasileiou P, Rajewsky N. circBase: A database for circular RNAs. RNA. 2014;**20**(11):1666-1670

[166] Ghosal S, Das S, Sen R, Basak P, Chakrabarti J. Circ2Traits: A comprehensive database for circular RNA potentially associated with disease and traits. Frontiers in Genetics. 2013;**4**:283

[167] Dudekula DB, Panda AC, Grammatikakis I, De S, Abdelmohsen K, Gorospe M. CircInteractome: A web tool for exploring circular RNAs and their interacting proteins and microRNAs. RNA Biology. 2016;**13**(1):34-42

[168] Juhling F, Morl M, Hartmann RK, Sprinzl M, Stadler PF, Putz J. tRNAdb 2009: Compilation of tRNA sequences and tRNA genes. Nucleic Acids Research. 2009;**37** (Database issue):D159-D162

[169] Anders S, Huber W. Differential expression analysis for sequence count data. Genome Biology. 2010;**11**

[170] Robinson MD, McCarthy DJ, Smyth GK. EdgeR: A bioconductor package for differential expression analysis of digital gene expression data. Bioinformatics. 2010;**26**(1):139-40

[171] Di Y, Schafer DW, Cumbie JS, Chang JH. The NBP negative binomial model for assessing differential gene expression from RNA-seq. Statistical Applications in Genetics and Molecular Biology. 2011;**10**(1): 1-28

[172] Auer PL, Doerge RW. A two-stage Poisson model for testing RNA-seq data. Statistical Applications in Genetics and Molecular Biology. 2011;**10**(1):1-26

[173] Hardcastle TJ, Kelly KA. baySeq: Empirical Bayesian methods for identifying differential expression in sequence count data. BMC Bioinforma. 2010;**11**:442

[174] Leng, Ning, John A. Dawson, James A. Thomson, Victor Ruotti, Anna I. Rissman, Bart MG Smits, Jill D. Haag, Michael N. Gould, Ron M. Stewart, and Christina Kendziorski. EBSeq: an empirical Bayes hierarchical model for inference in RNA-seq experiments. Bioinformatics.2013;**29**(8):1035-1043

[175] Tarazona S, García-Alcalde F, Dopazo J, Ferrer A, Conesa A. Differential expression in RNA-seq: A matter of depth. Genome Research. 2011;**21**(12):2213-2223

[176] Li J, Tibshirani R. Finding consistent patterns: A nonparametric approach for identifying differential expression in RNA-seq data. Statistical Methods in Medical Research. 2013;**22**(5):519-536

[177] Van de Wiel MA, Leday GGR, Pardo L, Rue H, Van der Vaart AW, Van Wieringen WN. Bayesian analysis of RNA sequencing data by estimating multiple shrinkage priors. Biostatistics. 2012;**14**(1):113-128

[178] Ritchie ME, Phipson B, Wu D, Hu Y, Law CW, Shi W, Smyth GK. limma powers differential expression analyses for RNA-sequencing and microarray studies. Nucleic Acids Research. 2015;**43**(7):e47. gkv007

[179] Soneson C, Delorenzi M. A comparison of methods for differential expression analysis of RNA-seq data. BMC Bioinformatics. 2013;**14**(1):91

[180] Seyednasrollah F, Laiho A, Elo LL. Comparison of software packages for detecting differential expression in RNA-seq studies. Briefings in Bioinformatics. 2015;**16**(1):59-70

[181] Zhang ZH, Jhaveri DJ, Marshall VM, Bauer DC, Edson J, Narayanan RK, Robinson GJ, Lundberg AE, Bartlett PF, Wray NR. A comparative study of techniques for differential expression analysis on RNA-Seq data. PloS One. 2014;**9**(8):e103207

[182] Robles JA, Qureshi SE, Stephen SJ, Wilson SR, Burden CJ, Taylor JM. Efficient experimental design and analysis strategies for the detection of differential expression using RNA-Sequencing. BMC Genomics. 2012;**13**(1):484

[183] Rapaport F, Khanin R, Liang Y, Pirun M, Krek A, Zumbo P, Mason CE, Socci ND, Betel D. Comprehensive evaluation of differential gene expression analysis methods for RNA-seq data. Genome Biology. 2013;**14**(9):3158

[184] Backes C, Kehl T, Stöckel D, Fehlmann T, Schneider L, Meese E, Lenhof H-P, Keller A. miRPathDB: A new dictionary on microRNAs and target pathways. Nucleic Acids Research. 2017;**45**(D1):D90-D96

[185] Lukasik A, Wójcikowski M, Zielenkiewicz P. Tools4miRs–one place to gather all the tools for miRNA analysis. Bioinformatics. 2016;**32**(17):2722-2724

[186] Rajewsky N. microRNA target predictions in animals. Nature Genetics. 2006; **38**:S8-S13

[187] Moore AC, Winkjer JS, Tseng TT. Bioinformatics resources for microRNA discovery. Biomarker Insights. 2015;**10**(Suppl 4):53

[188] Lee M, Lee H. DMirNet: Inferring direct microRNA-mRNA association networks. BMC Systems Biology. 2016;**10**(5):51

[189] Privitera AP, Distefano R, Wefer HA, Ferro A, Pulvirenti A, Giugno R. OCDB: A database collecting genes, miRNAs and drugs for obsessive-compulsive disorder. Database: The Journal of Biological Databases and Curation. 2015;**2015**. bav069

[190] Zhang L, Xie T, Tian M, Li J, Song S, Ouyang L, Liu B, Cai H. GAMDB: A web resource to connect microRNAs with autophagy in gerontology. Cell Proliferation. 2016;**49**(2):246-251

[191] Mooney C, Becker BA, Raoof R, Henshall DC. EpimiRBase: A comprehensive database of microRNA-epilepsy associations. Bioinformatics. 2016;**32**(9):1436-1438

[192] Dong L, Luo M, Wang F, Zhang J, Li T, Yu J. TUMIR: An experimentally supported database of microRNA deregulation in various cancers. Journal of Clinical Bioinformatics. 2013;**3**(1):7

[193] Iftikhar H, Schultzhaus JN, Bennett CJ, Carney GE. The in vivo genetic toolkit for studying expression and functions of *Drosophila melanogaster* microRNAs. RNA Biology. 2016 (just-accepted):00-00

[194] Amaral PP, Clark MB, Gascoigne DK, Dinger ME, Mattick JS. lncRNAdb: A reference database for long noncoding RNAs. Nucleic Acids Research. 2011;**39**(Suppl 1):D146-D151

[195] Bhartiya D, Pal K, Ghosh S, Kapoor S, Jalali S, Panwar B, Jain S, Sati S, Sengupta S, Sachidanandan C et al. lncRNome: A comprehensive knowledgebase of human long noncoding RNAs. Database. 2013;bat034

[196] Li J-H, Liu S, Zhou H, Qu L-H, Yang J-H. starBase v2.0: Decoding miRNA-ceRNA, miRNA-ncRNA and protein–RNA interaction networks from large-scale CLIP-Seq data. Nucleic Acids Research. 2014;**42**(D1):D92-D97

[197] Consortium TR. RNAcentral: A comprehensive database of non-coding RNA sequences. Nucleic Acids Research. 2017;**45**(D1):D128-D134

[198] Weikard R, Demasius W, Kuehn C. Mining long noncoding RNA in livestock. Animal Genetics. 2016

[199] Wang KC, Chang HY. Molecular mechanisms of long noncoding RNAs. Molecular Cell. 2011;**43**(6):904-914

[200] Quagliata L, Matter MS, Piscuoglio S, Arabi L, Ruiz C, Procino A, Kovac M, Moretti F, Makowska Z, Boldanova T. Long noncoding RNA HOTTIP/HOXA13 expression is associated with disease progression and predicts outcome in hepatocellular carcinoma patients. Hepatology. 2014;**59**(3):911-923

[201] Liao Q, Xiao H, Bu D, Xie C, Miao R, Luo H, Zhao G, Yu K, Zhao H, Skogerbø G et al. ncFANs: A web server for functional annotation of long non-coding RNAs. Nucleic Acids Research. 2011;**39**(Suppl 2):W118-W124

[202] Laible G, Wei J, Wagner S. Improving livestock for agriculture - technological progress from random transgenesis to precision genome editing heralds a new era. Biotechnology Journal. 2015;**10**(1):109-120

[203] Anamika K, Verma S, Jere A, Desai A. Transcriptomic Profiling Using Next Generation Sequencing—Advances, Advantages, and Challenges. In: Kulski JK, editor. Next Generation Sequencing - Advances, Applications and Challenges. 2016. Rijeka: InTech. Ch. 04

[204] Veneziano D, Nigita G, Ferro A. Computational approaches for the analysis of ncRNA through deep sequencing techniques. Frontiers in Bioengineering and Biotechnology. 2015;**3**:77

[205] Proudfoot C, Carlson DF, Huddart R, Long CR, Pryor JH, King TJ, Lillico SG, Mileham AJ, McLaren DG, Whitelaw CB et al. Genome edited sheep and cattle. Transgenic Research. 2015;**24**(1):147-153

[206] Zhang F, Wen Y, Guo X. CRISPR/Cas9 for genome editing: Progress, implications and challenges. Human Molecular Genetics. 2014;**23**(R1):R40-R46

[207] Yu L, Batara J, Lu B. Application of Genome Editing Technology to MicroRNA Research in Mammalians. In: Modern Tools for Genetic Engineering, Michael Kormann (Ed.), InTech, Ch. 7, DOI: 10.5772/64330

[208] Cox DBT, Platt RJ, Zhang F. Therapeutic genome editing: Prospects and challenges. Nature Medicine. 2015;**21**(2):121-131

[209] Kevan MA Gartland MD, Tommaso B, Mariapia VM and Jill SG. Advances in biotechnology: Genomics and genome editing. The EuroBiotech Journal. 2017;**1**(1):3-10

[210] Shen S, Loh TJ, Shen H, Zheng X, Shen H. CRISPR as a strong gene editing tool. BMB Reports. 2017;**50**(1):20-24

[211] Hsu PD, Lander ES, Zhang F. Development and applications of CRISPR-Cas9 for genome engineering. Cell. 2014;**157**(6):1262-1278

[212] Zhuo C, Hou W, Hu L, Lin C, Chen C, Lin X. Genomic editing of non-coding RNA genes with CRISPR/Cas9 ushers in a potential novel approach to study and treat schizophrenia. Frontiers in Molecular Neuroscience. 2017;**10**:28

[213] West J, Gill WW. Genome Editing in Large Animals. Journal of Equine Veterinary Science. 2016;**41**:1-6

[214] Petersen B, Niemann H. Molecular scissors and their application in genetically modified farm animals. Transgenic Research. 2015;**24**(3):381-396

[215] Tan WS, Carlson DF, Walton MW, Fahrenkrug SC, Hackett PB. Precision editing of large animal genomes. Advances in Genetics. 2012;**80**:37-97

[216] Zhang JH, Adikaram P, Pandey M, Genis A, Simonds WF. Optimization of genome editing through CRISPR-Cas9 engineering. Bioengineered. 2016;**7**(3):166-174

[217] Wang X, Zhou J, Cao C, Huang J, Hai T, Wang Y, Zheng Q, Zhang H, Qin G, Miao X et al. Efficient CRISPR/Cas9-mediated biallelic gene disruption and site-specific knockin after rapid selection of highly active sgRNAs in pigs. Scientific Reports. 2015;**5**:13348

[218] Whitworth KM, Rowland RRR, Ewen CL, Trible BR, Kerrigan MA, Cino-Ozuna AG, Samuel MS, Lightner JE, McLaren DG, Mileham AJ et al. Gene-edited pigs are protected from porcine reproductive and respiratory syndrome virus. Nature Biotechnology. 2016;**34**(1):20-22

[219] Butler JR, Ladowski JM, Martens GR, Tector M, Tector AJ. Recent advances in genome editing and creation of genetically modified pigs. International Journal of Surgery (London, England). 2015;**23**(Pt B):217-222

[220] Lillico SG, Proudfoot C, Carlson DF, Stverakova D, Neil C, Blain C. Live pigs produced from genome edited zygotes. Scientific Report. 2013;**3**:2847

[221] Wang K, Ouyang H, Xie Z, Yao C, Guo N, Li M, Jiao H, Pang D. Efficient generation of myostatin mutations in pigs using the CRISPR/Cas9 system. Scientific Report. 2015;**5**:16623

[222] Choi W, Yum S, Lee S, Lee W, Lee J, Kim S, Koo O, Lee B, Jang G. Disruption of exogenous eGFP gene using RNA guided endonuclease in bovine transgenic somatic cells. Zygote (Cambridge, England). 2015;**23**(6):916-923

[223] Carlson DF, Lancto CA, Zang B, Kim E-S, Walton M, Oldeschulte D, Seabury C, Sonstegard TS, Fahrenkrug SC. Production of hornless dairy cattle from genome-edited cell lines. Nature Biotechnology. 2016;**34**(5):479-481

[224] Crispo M, Mulet AP, Tesson L, Barrera N, Cuadro F, dos Santos-Neto PC, Nguyen TH, Creneguy A, Brusselle L, Anegon I et al. Efficient Generation of Myostatin Knock-Out Sheep Using CRISPR/Cas9 Technology and Microinjection into Zygotes. PLoS One. 2015;**10**(8):e0136690

[225] Barrangou R, Doudna JA. Applications of CRISPR technologies in research and beyond. Nature Biotechnology. 2016;**34**(9):933-941

[226] Pulido-Quetglas C, Aparicio-Prat E, Arnan C, Polidori T, Hermoso T, Palumbo E, Ponomarenko J, Guigo R, Johnson R. Scalable design of paired CRISPR guide RNAs for genomic deletion. PLOS Computational Biology. 2017;**13**(3):e1005341

[227] Wu B, Luo L, Gao XJ. Cas9-triggered chain ablation of cas9 as a gene drive brake. Nature Biotechnology. 2016;**34**(2):137-138

[228] Gonen S, Jenko J, Gorjanc G, Mileham AJ, Whitelaw CBA, Hickey JM. Potential of gene drives with genome editing to increase genetic gain in livestock breeding programs. Genetics Selection Evolution. 2017;**49**(1):3

[229] Aparicio-Prat E, Arnan C, Sala I, Bosch N, Guigó R, Johnson R. DECKO: Single-oligo, dual-CRISPR deletion of genomic elements including long non-coding RNAs. BMC Genomics. 2015;**16**(1):846

[230] Hilton IB, D'Ippolito AM, Vockley CM, Thakore PI, Crawford GE, Reddy TE, Gersbach CA. Epigenome editing by a CRISPR-Cas9-based acetyltransferase activates genes from promoters and enhancers. Nature Biotechnology. 2015;**33**(5):510-517

Chapter 6

Transcriptome Sequencing for Precise and Accurate Measurement of Transcripts and Accessibility of TCGA for Cancer Datasets and Analysis

Bijesh George, Vivekanand Ashokachandran, Aswathy Mary Paul and Reshmi Girijadevi

Additional information is available at the end of the chapter

http://dx.doi.org/10.5772/intechopen.70026

Abstract

Next-generation sequencing (NGS) technologies are now well established and have become a routine analysis tool for its depth, coverage, and cost. RNA sequencing (RNA-Seq) has readily replaced the conventional array-based approaches and has become method of choice for qualitative and quantitative analysis of transcriptome, quantification of alternative spliced isoforms, identification of sequence variants, novel transcripts, and gene fusions, among many others. The current chapter discusses the multi-step transcriptome data analysis processes in detail, in the context of re-sequencing (where a reference genome is available). We have discussed the processes including quality control, read alignment, quantification of gene from read level, visualization of data at different levels, and the identification of differentially expressed genes and alternatively spliced transcripts. Considering the data that are freely available to the public, we also discuss The Cancer Genome Atlas (TCGA), as a resource of RNA-Seq data on cancer for selection and analysis in specific contexts of experimentation. This chapter provides insights into the applicability, data availability, tools, and statistics for a beginner to get familiar with RNA-Seq data analysis and TCGA.

Keywords: RNA-Seq, transcriptome data analysis, NGS data analysis, TCGA

1. Introduction

Genetic and epigenetic features encompassed in the genome are the basic determinants of fate and functions of cells. At the human interface, qualitative and/or quantitative differences in transcripts are the first level readout of these features in any specific context of their identification

[1]. These contexts may refer to a diseased state or the influence of stimulation such as intrinsic ligands or response to immunogens. With the total transcripts often referred to as transcriptome, the stage-specific or cell type-specific transcriptome of cells are valuable to evaluate the genetic and epigenetic features characteristic to them. From high- to low-input RNA, the RNA sequencing methods have considerably improved to appreciate the inter- and intra-level population heterogeneity of cells. Not restricted to messenger RNA (mRNA), these technologies are also being increasingly exploited to analyze other transcription-based products such as microRNAs and lncRNAs, reaching out to the identification of over 10–30 pg of a human cell or tissue [2]. RNA or transcripts are of two categories, protein coding mRNAs which synthesize protein and non-coding RNAs involved in regulating gene expression and in cell structure maintenance. mRNA makes up only 6% of the total RNA content of a cell or tissue; a number of methods and kits are available for RNA extraction from the cell [2, 3].

The human genome has more than 99.5% sequence identity to each other at the genomic level when analyzed in toto. However, they are also paradoxically personalized and are amenable to somatic variations. Hence, the cells could also be heterogeneous at genome level within an individual, and the genomic sequence variations are necessary to be accounted whenever they are analyzed at the transcriptome level. Toward this, the sequence obtained by RNA sequencing also reflects their coding sequence in the genome, kept aside, the RNA editing. Further, there are a plethora of other sequence determinants that could also be analyzed by sequence-based identification of transcripts. These determinants include the isoforms, gene fusions and identification of transcripts from putative pseudogenes. Unarguably, human cancer cells or tissues of diverse origins and stages in different populations are the most explored differential genome and transcriptome to date accounting the amount of data derived by RNA sequencing [4]. The Cancer Genome Atlas (TCGA) is probably the most extensive resource of providing access to cancer data especially from next-generation sequencing (NGS) platform. TCGA provides a number of options to perform analysis on cancer-related experimental data and stands as a major data repository for cancer data.

2. Transcriptomics

2.1. Gene expression

Gene expression at transcript level is a temporal dynamics event that involves turn "on" or "off" mechanism constituted by the coordinated action of epigenetic factors and transcriptional regulators. Since gene products are part of metabolic pathways in the organism, the inefficiency of protein synthesis control mechanism can lead to an abnormal behavior of metabolic pathways and then lead to diseases [5]. Determining or quantifying the amount of transcripts in a biological condition provides a clear picture about the involvement of that gene in a particular condition. It is necessary to use the quantitative methods to understand normal cell development, disease mechanisms and to determine when, where, and how much a gene is showing divergence with different biological condition [1]. Identification of key genetic factors/marker/a set of genes responsible for a certain biological process can make a sizable change to existing treatment mechanism approach [6].

2.2. Applicability of transcriptome data

Functions of each gene are not completely defined, information about the involvement of genes in functional pathways is identified and available from biological databases which provide clues on how each gene behaves in different metabolic pathways. Estimating the genes expressed in a particular biological condition allows comparing with the existing annotations. Only a small percentage of the genome is expressed in each cell, and a portion of the RNA synthesized in the cell is specific for that cell type [4], identifying the genes which are differentially expressed in similar tissue, but different context has therapeutic significance. Moreover, transcriptome sequencing allows identifying transcript level variations such as cassette exon, mutually exclusive exons, intron retentions, indels, alternative splice junctions, alternative promoters (**Figure 1**), and isoform-specific expression profiles [7].

2.3. Requirements

The number of biological/technical replicates, adequate sequencing depth, and essentially, the sequencing qualities are the major factors that should be accounted in a sequencing-based

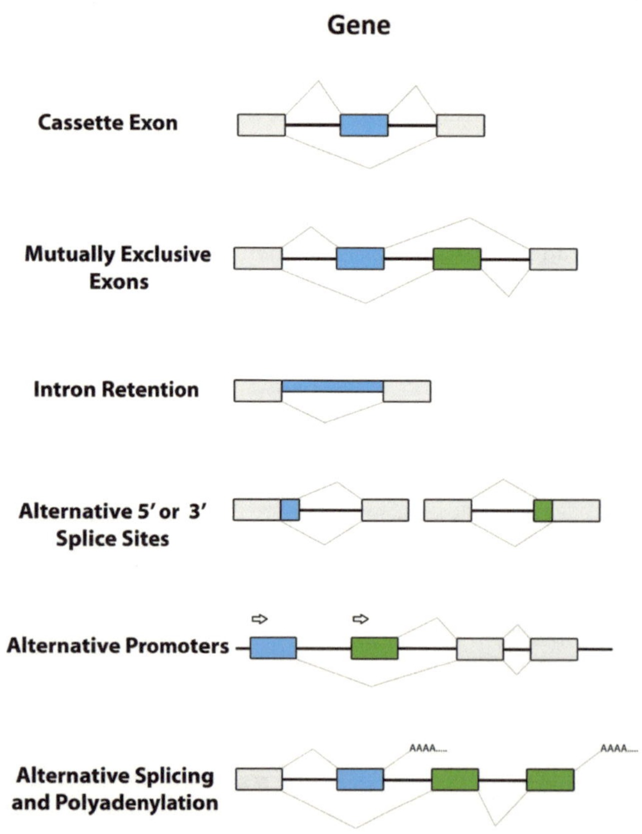

Figure 1. Alternative splicing. Here exons are boxes and lines are introns. Promoters represented by arrows and polyadenylation sites with AAA.

study. The parameters such as the availability of reference genome for the organism from which the sample is analyzed, information about the sequencer quality encoding, and whether multiplexing has been performed are also critical for the analysis. One should have a clear understanding of the biological sample, experimental conditions, and the biological questions that are in pursuit before starting a bioinformatics analysis of any transcriptome data [9].

Computational specifications have to be taken care to perform a genome assembly in a reasonable time without interruption. At least 8 core processor with 16 GB of RAM and enough fast storage system is required to perform a genome alignment within a reasonable time [7]. Genome assembly or alignment is the most computational resource consuming process, and the further downstream analysis such as variant calling or differential expression analysis can be performed using a desktop with an appreciable configuration.

Computational biologists prefer to use UNIX-based systems/servers for NextGen sequence analysis as large data can be handled more comfortably through command line by UNIX than a Windows OS [10].

2.4. Software requirements

A number of established and easily accessible one-shop sequence analysis tools [7, 11] are available online. However, it is important that one should understand the different steps involved in the analysis pipeline that are rather similar across them. There are various pieces of software in the pipeline, and each of them produces a number of output files. These include the main output file that can be used for further analysis and other supporting information such as the statistics of mapping, indicating the fraction of input data that had been successfully utilized by the algorithm (always get a higher fraction for good quality experiment) [7]. One should be aware of the files generated during each of the analysis steps that is fed into the next algorithm in the pipeline.

2.5. Precautions

A number of algorithms have been developed in recent years, and most of them are available as open-source algorithms. It is important to understand that the transcriptome analysis can be completed using open-source software and tools. Before starting the bioinformatics analysis on transcriptome data, one should decide the algorithms that can be used (**Figure 2**) including its release/version information in each successive step in the pipeline. Following the review articles that compare multiple algorithms and the research publications that have used specific algorithms, appropriate algorithms can be selected in each step [12]. Now, the next step is to select the annotation files to be used for the analysis.

Even though the information is same, data representation varies between annotation files from different biological data resources. An example given below represents human chromosome 22 from various biological data resources. Hence, one should confirm the annotation files such as genome file (.fasta) and gene transfer format (.gtf) files are compactible to each other.

Resource	Representation
NCBI reference genome GRCh38.p7	>gi|568801992|ref|NT_167212.2| chromosome 22 genomic scaffold, GRCh38.p7 primary assembly HSCHR22_CTG1_1
UCSC latest version GRCh38/hg38	>chr22
Ensembl	>22

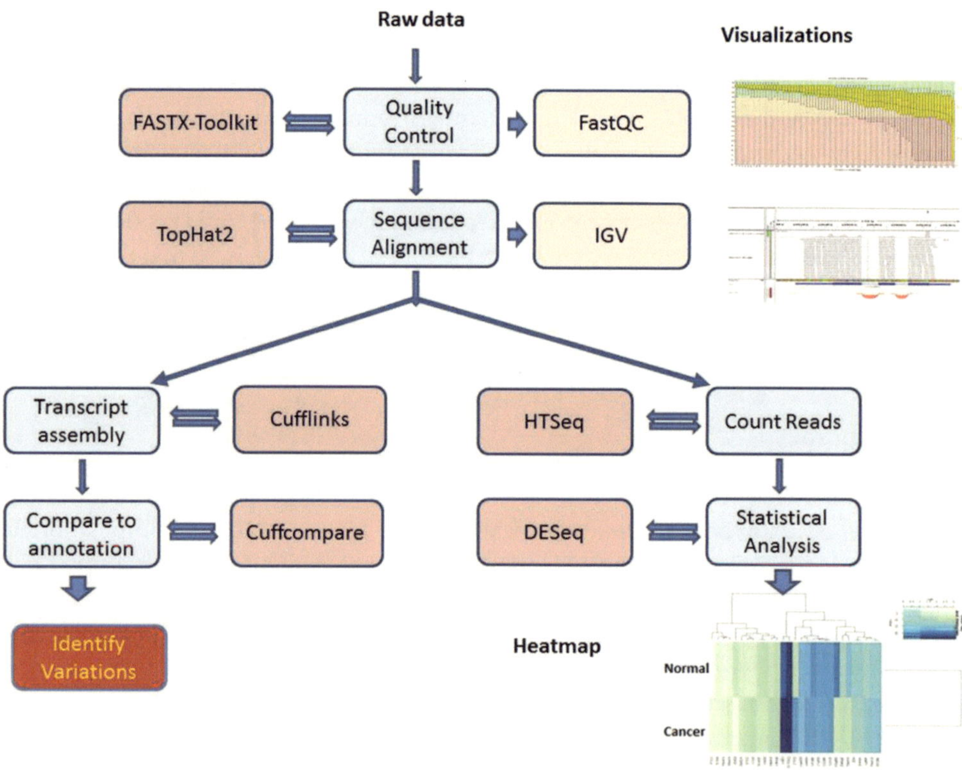

Figure 2. Transcriptomics workflow.

2.6. File formats

In each step of the analysis pipeline, multiple file formats are generated or used. It is necessary to know the information contained in each type of files. Here, we discuss file types classified into three categories. The first category is the raw files that contain the information adopted from the sequencer to represent the raw sequences with a quality score for each base-pair identification [13]. The file formats can be .sff, .csfasta + .qual, .fastq, etc. The most common file format is the .fastq extension. Second file category is the alignment files that represent the information on how each read or the fragment had been aligned to the reference genome [14], these files can be in .sam, .bam, and .bed formats. The third category is the annotated data files that represent data readily available from standard biological databases such as reference

genome sequences (in .fasta format) and the annotated gene information (.gtf, .gff formats). Apart from all the standard file formats listed above, there are algorithm specific files which contain additional information about the specific run of the each algorithm in the pipeline.

3. Transcriptome data analysis

The high-throughput methods previously described (RNA-Seq) are done by direct sequencing of complementary DNA (cDNA) and as a result gives insights into the gene expression profiling [12, 15–17], quantification of alternative splicing [8, 9, 18, 19], variant calling [20–23], novel transcripts [14, 24, 25], and several others. These quantitative measurements are done by the final data produced by each sequencing platforms. However, the process of sequencing involves different steps (reverse transcription, amplification, fragmentation, purification, adaptor ligation, and sequencing that the chance of error in any step is highly likely and could result in faulty outputs. It makes the data in the worst case not suitable for further analysis, so that the experiment may have to be repeated. Nonetheless, these errors can be monitored and necessary actions can be undertaken to rectify the errors prior to analysis. Such preliminary steps are often referred to as quality control analysis of sequencing data.

3.1. Quality control

This section of the chapter will discuss various reasons and statistical assessment of errors such as sequence read quality, read duplication, GC bias, nucleotide composition bias, adapter contamination, flow cell contamination, enrichment, and false positive errors [26, 27], and how those can be tackled using available tools. The data used for the analysis in this chapter are mainly in the ".fastq" format, the most common format output of runs on many platforms. However, there are many quality control analysis tools available that either come aligned with the machine itself or as standalone software (commercial and open source). The quality control analysis can be done using many software tools, and one of the popular open-source software is FastQC [28].

Data output from sequencing machine includes the information about the sequence fragment as well as a score corresponding to each base identification, we are considering ".fastq" format, widely used in many platforms, to explain the features. A single read is represented by four consecutive lines in .fastq format. The first and third line represent sequence identifiers and other optional information, such as machine version, flow cell information, etc., related to the specific run of the sample in the machine. The second line is the sequence bases, and fourth is the quality value for each base which is represented as ASCII characters.

This ASCII quality value or phred quality score gives the accurate measure of the base calling quality during sequencing. Phred quality score is mathematically defined as

$$Q = -10 \times \log_{10}(P) \text{ or } P = 10^{-Q/10} \quad (1)$$

Where Q is the phred quality score, and P is the probability of getting a faulty base.

In essence, a phred score of 30 is the probability of a base to be wrong is 1 in 1000. However, there are no standard methods to measure this exact quality; the phred score above 20–25 (**Figure 3a** and **b**) is considered as the average score to be acceptable for further analysis because phred quality assessments are probabilistically stable [13, 29].

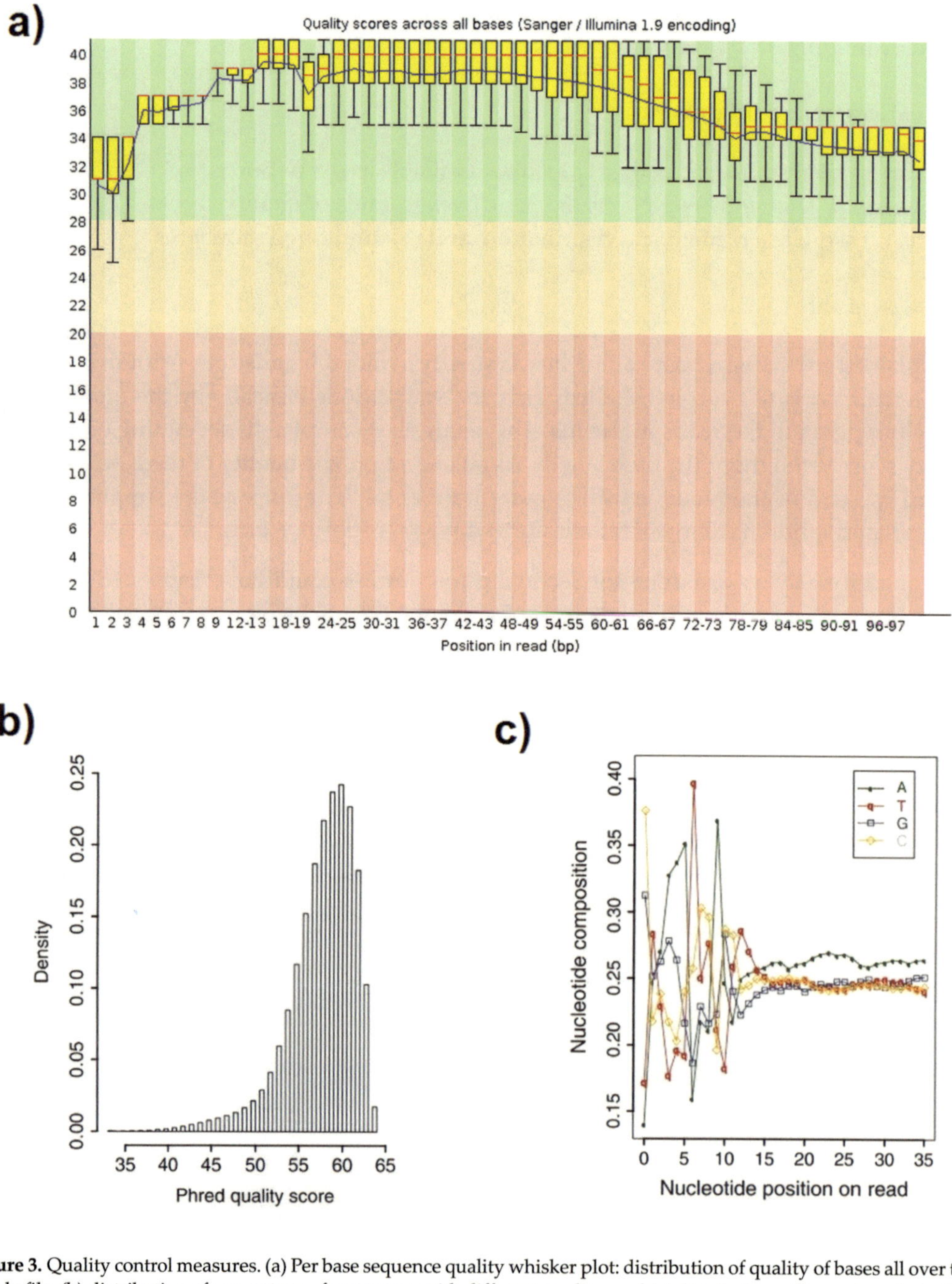

Figure 3. Quality control measures. (a) Per base sequence quality whisker plot: distribution of quality of bases all over the whole file, (b) distribution of percentage of sequences with different quality, and (c) distribution of bases in a .fastq file.

For each sequencer, they use different set of ASCII values to score each base calling and a maximum score of 41 which is almost 1 in 10,000 (99.99% accuracy) is the probability that a base is called incorrectly (**Table 1**). However, if the quality of any read falls to much lower scale, it is better to trim those regions off. There are many standard trimming tools available as open source. Few popular tools are FASTX-Toolkit [30], cutadapt [31], and trimgalore [32]. They cannot only be used for quality trimming but also has several other purposes, such as adapter trimming, demultiplexing, etc.

3.2. Evaluation of read quality

There are several statistical analysis pipelines available as open source to check the quality of the NGS data. This session explains the basic backgrounds of quality checks such as (1) base quality, (2) sequence content and distribution, and (3) duplicated sequences.

3.2.1. Base quality

As explained previously, base calling bias is strictly avoided because any error in base calling means the base is not correctly called. This analysis is done basically by the quality encoding values given to the reads in the file. This analysis is completely depending on the phred quality score throughout the base length. As an exception, the quality of reads will fall down toward the end of the reads, which is quite normal for long runs as the supplied base get reduced, and random calling of base leads to these false-positive errors.

Base quality analyzes are done for rectifying read errors could have happened during the run or library preparation. The data from the ".fastq" file can be plotted different ways based on the phred quality score of each bases, the proportion of reads being called wrong, N content distribution in the read, and finally, sequence length distribution. It is obvious that the sequence length would have uneven distribution in trimmed reads.

3.2.2. Sequence content and distribution

Evaluating GC content over the sequenced reads is as important as other modules because it leads to many biological reasoning. GC over AT is basically because of the stability of the

Phred quality score	Probability of incorrect base call	Base call accuracy
10	1 in 10	90%
20	1 in 100	99%
30	1 in 1000	99.9%
40	1 in 10,000	99.99%
50	1 in 100,000	99.999%
60	1 in 1,000,000	99.9999%

Table 1. Phred quality score.

bonds between them, and the annealing process of PCR is based on the melting temperature of GC bonding. DNA methylation happens at cytosine, and comparatively, exons are high in GC content than introns.

In an NGS run, the bases are provided with an equal ratio, and the average of each base as output is expected to be 25% of each base (**Figure 3c**). Any fluctuation from this composition is considered as bias which is due to overrepresented sequences like adapter dimers or rRNA in the sample. However, it is expected that a little bias at the first few bases from 5′ which is essentially produced by the random hexamer priming from PCR amplification.

Before starting any analysis, adapters are trimmed off from the reads because the presence of adapters in the sample will lead to the expression of overrepresented sequences. This is more like a final check to be done to make sure the overrepresented sequences or enrichment identified is not spurious.

3.2.3. *Duplicated sequences*

As discussed in the GC content, there are few other ways to check the overrepresented sequences. These methods are used to confirm the sample is not contaminated, unless there is some kind of enrichment in the reads. The enrichment analysis is done basically on different scales. The length of the read is considered as the scale here. Creating K-mers of different length can make sure that how often an enrichment or overrepresented sequence can occur in the read, and this can be calculated to double check the presence of contamination or enrichment study.

3.3. Genome alignment

This is the second major step in transcriptomic data analysis. If the reference genome is available for the organism, it can be referred to as resequencing analysis else should be referred to as de novo sequencing analysis. In resequencing data, the analysis pipeline is comparatively easier compared to de novo sequencing. If reference genome is available, all we need is to map the fragments to the genome and find out the genes showing expression in the experiment. Although the amount of data generated from the sequencer is huge, it is short in length compared to the actual size of the genome. However, an advanced computationally efficient algorithm is required to perform this time consuming and banal process [5].

Genome alignment is the most important step in transcriptome analysis as all the downstream analysis, and the result accuracy is based on the efficiency of the alignment algorithm. As the data are obtained from transcriptome, the algorithm cannot directly map the reads to reference genome. An efficient splice aligner algorithm is required to complete the task [12], and most of these algorithms use a technique called hashing or indexing either in raw data or the genome data or both.

Read alignment algorithm has a number of parameters such as input and index as mandatory, and many other optional parameters also based on the computational resources

available that can be set for the efficient mapping of reads. For example, we can set the number of multiple alignments for a single read and the maximum insertion or deletion length that can be allowed. A precise understanding of experimental conditions helps to set appropriate parameters according to a specific experiment. Moreover, default values provided to help and avoid confusions [7].

3.4. Gene quantification

Gene quantification is performed after alignment to a genome. The first step is to identify the amount of fragments or reads that could be mapped to each genomic location. Gene level or transcript level quantification can be performed according to user's choice. A number of software tools (coverageBED [33], htseq-count [34], and featureCounts [35]) are available for gene quantification. Quantification is performed against a reference annotation (GTF/GFF) file with coordinates for the gene, transcript, or exon. For example, htseq-count uses "--idattr=<id attribute>" that indicates GFF attribute to be used as feature ID from the ninth column where unique ids or accession numbers are available. Gene qualification has to be performed after normalization to avoid misleading measurements. Hence, gene level or sample level normalization of the data in terms of total number of reads mapped, read length, and coverage should be performed.

The reads per kilobase of exon model per million mapped reads (RPKM) measure normalizes with the sequencing depth that varies significantly between samples as well as the gene length. Fragments per kilobase of exon model per million mapped reads (FPKM) measure normalizes similar to RPKM but for the paired-end data and the transcripts per million (TPM) first normalizes by gene length, then by sequencing depth, preferably a better way of normalization [36].

3.5. Splice variation analysis

Transcriptome analysis can identify transcript sequence level features such as cassette exon, mutually exclusive exons, intron retentions, indels, alternative splice junctions, and hence, different possible isoforms all based on genome mapping (**Figure 1**). There are ~41,000 unique transcripts that are identified from a total of ~20,000 genes in human (NCBI RefSeq) [37].

Identification of transcripts from short and specific number of reads aligned across the gene, and the identification of splice junctions is a challenge in variation analysis. A number of algorithms such as Cufflinks [38], SLIDE [39], and StringTie [40] are available to analyze the alignment with user-provided existing annotations. Cufflinks [38] efficiently utilizes the advantage of paired-end sequencing data to annotate the splice variations (**Figure 4**).

3.6. Differential expression analysis

Once the genome assembly is completed, the downstream analysis can follow two routes—the variation analysis and the differential expression analysis. Differential expression analysis refers

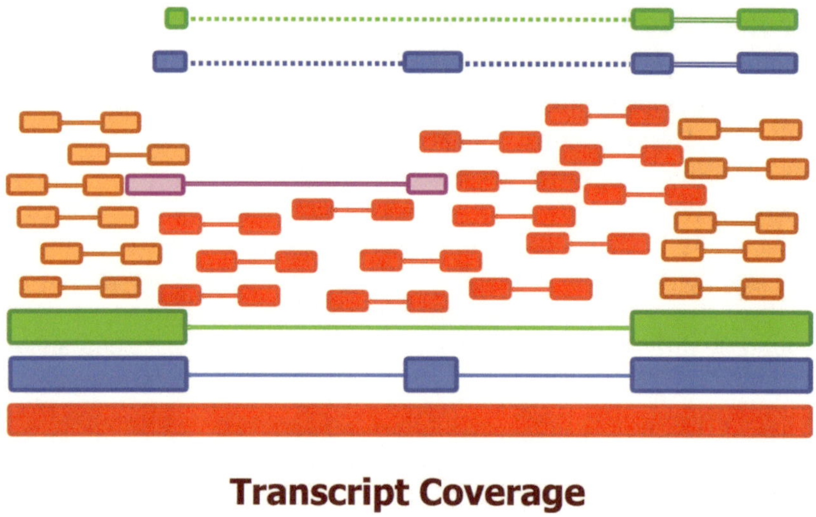

Figure 4. Transcript enrichment. Cufflinks identify three transcripts from reads mapped to the same genomic region.

the gene level expression difference between two or more samples. This can be performed using R packages like edgeR [9], DESeq [10] that can load gene quantification information from multiple samples and report the expression level difference for each transcript/gene. The above-mentioned R packages also can generate multiple figures such as heatmaps, histograms, dispersion plots, etc., which can be used for representing results as well as publications purposes. The comparison is performed after normalization of the data across samples that account the length of the fragments, sequencing depth, and the total number of reads mapped. RPKM, FPKM, and TPM are commonly used normalization values. Genes with at least 2-fold change are usually considered as differentially expressed, although a fold change of 1.5 is also considered in certain instances.

Types of graphical methods are available to visually represent the identified variations among experiments or samples used. Overview of gene expression studies can be represented by volcano plot, MA plot, heatmap, etc. Heatmap with hierarchical clustering clearly represents the trend of gene expression between samples.

Visualization is integral to NGS data from the evaluation of sequencing quality to the representation of the biologically significant results. Initially, the raw data have to undergo quality checking to assess the overall sequencing quality and decide quality measures (FastQC (**Figure 3a**) [28], NGSQC [41]). The next level of visualization is applicable to the alignment to the genome as perceived for the number of reads aligned to particular gene, exons, introns, and splice junctions with genome browsers such as UCSC browser [42], Integrative Genomics Viewer (IGV) [43], and Genome Maps [44]. Genome browsers load genome (.fasta), annotations (.gff, .gtf), variations (as bed files) to their interface to obtain clear visualization of collective data for a specified region along with the available annotation, identified evidence or mapped reads, and variations observed. They also host inbuilt tools to represent the data as plots and figures that can be used for publication [43].

4. TCGA: a genomic hub of cancer

The Cancer Genome Atlas well known as TCGA in short is a combined effort of National Cancer Institute (NCI) and National Human Genome Research Institute (NHGRI) investing $50 million each to increase the better understanding of molecular basis of cancer using advanced genome analysis technology. The overall aim of launching such a big project was to improve the ability to diagnose, treat, and prevent cancer. The first phase of the study started in the year 2005 focused on the brain, lung, and ovarian cancers was aimed to test and develop the infrastructure for further research. The second phase of the study comprises of around 30 different type of cancers started in the year 2009 and analyzed by the year 2014.

The first phase of the study proved that an atlas specific for cancer can be created with a worldwide network of research and teams working on different cancer and develop a single platform for making the data publically accessible pooling all the data. The publicly available data from TCGA would also enable researchers around the world to make validate important discoveries. TCGA is supported by Genomic Data Commons (GDC) as one among the several programs at the NCI's Center for Cancer Genomics along with another program Therapeutically Applicable Research to Generate Effective Treatments (TARGET). Now, GDCs host genomic alterations of exactly 39 projects combining the TCGA and TARGET.

Data availability has categorized based on primary site of study, and they are kidney, adrenal gland, brain, colorectal, lung, uterus, bile duct, bladder, bone marrow, breast, cervix, esophagus, eye, head and neck, liver, lymph nodes, ovary, pancreas, pleura, prostate, skin, soft tissue, stomach, testis, thymus, and thyroid. Some of the primary sites are again divided into different subdivions. For example, kidney again divided into three different projects: kidney renal clear cell carcinoma, kidney renal papillary cell carcinoma, and kidney chromophobe. So as the case with adrenal gland, brain, colorectal, lung, and uterus which all are divided again into two different sub categories as follows: pheochromocytoma & paraganglioma, adrenocortical carcinoma, glioblastoma multiforme, brain lower grade glioma, colon adenocarcinoma, rectum adenocarcinoma, lung adenocarcinoma, lung squamous cell carcinoma, uterine corpus endometrial carcinoma, uterine carcinosarcoma.

4.1. TCGA data and file formats

The main category of data available in TCGA are:

- Clinical
- Raw sequencing data
- Transcriptome profiling
- Simple nucleotide variation
- Biospecimen

- Copy number variation
- DNA methylation

Main categories of data type are:

- Aligned reads
- Gene expression quantification
- Annotated somatic mutation
- Raw simple somatic mutation
- Copy number segment
- Masked copy number segment
- Methylation beta value
- Isoform expression quantification
- miRNA expression quantification
- Biospecimen supplement
- Clinical supplement
- Aggregated somatic mutation
- Masked somatic mutation

These data that are generated from different experimental strategies such as WXS, RNA-Seq, and miRNA-Seq were studied under illumina platform, whereas Illumina Human Methylation 450 and Illumina Human Methylation 27 platforms were used for methylation array and genotyping array was carried out using Affymetrix SNP 6.0.

4.2. miRNA analysis

TCGA provides tissue-specific miRNA expression profiles, their isoforms, connection with diseases, and the discovery of unreported miRNAs. Alignment of the reads with BWA-aln is the very first step in the miRNA pipeline. Either the input can be FASTQ or BAM file format for alignment. The output after the alignment will be of BAM format. The alignment follows the expression workflow. The output from the expression workflow is raw read counts and normalized to reads per million mapped reads. There are two types of files, controlled and open. The aligned file which is having a controlled access, and the quantification files are open accessible (**Table 2**). The RPM comes in two separate files as "mirnas.quantification.txt" and "isoforms.quantification.txt." The mirna.quantification.txt data file describes the summed expression for each miRNA. The file contains the information:

- miRNA name
- raw read count

- reads per million miRNA reads
- cross-mapped to other miRNA forms (Y or N)

whereas the isoform.quantification.txt file contains every individual sequence isoform observed as follows:

- miRNA name
- alignment coordinates as <version>:<Chromosome>:<Start position>-<End position>:<Strand>
- raw read count
- reads per million miRNA reads
- cross-mapped to other miRNA forms (Y or N)
- region within miRNA

4.3. RNA-Seq analysis

TCGA uses an Illumina system as the basic platform. Information for nucleotide sequence and gene expression is found at TCGA. RNA sequence coverage, sequence variants (e.g., fusion genes), expression of genes, exon, or junction are different category of information available after the sequence alignment. The NCBI dbGaP database is the official repository for the actual sequence data [45]. After aligning the reads to reference genome, gene expression level is quantified in various forms such as HT-Seq raw mapping count, fragments per kilobase of transcript per million mapped reads (FPKM) and FPKM-UQ (upper quartile normalization) in TCGA mRNA quantification pipeline (**Table 3**). In case of mRNA analysis also the rules for data access are the same. Access for aligned reads file is controlled, whereas access for rest of the files is open.

4.4. DNA-Seq analysis

Genomic diversity across different cancer types has been characterized by utilizing DNA sequencing systems based on Sanger Sequencing at different Genome Sequencing Centers.

Type	Description	Format
Aligned reads	miRNA-Seq reads that have been aligned to the GRCh38 build. Reads that were not aligned are included to facilitate the availability of raw read sets	BAM
miRNA expression quantification	A table that associates miRNA IDs with read count and a normalized count in reads per million miRNA mapped	TXT
Isoform expression quantification	A table with the same information as the miRNA Expression Quantification files with the addition of isoform information such as the coordinates of the isoform and the type of region it constitutes within the full miRNA transcript	TXT

Table 2. Data types and file formats.

Type	Description	Format
RNA-Seq alignment	RNA-Seq reads that have been aligned to the GRCh38 build. Reads that were not aligned are included to facilitate the availability of raw read sets	BAM
Raw read counts	The number of reads aligned to each protein-coding gene, calculated by HT-Seq	TXT
FPKM	A normalized expression value that takes into account each protein-coding gene length and the number of reads mappable to all protein-coding genes	TXT
FPKM-UQ	A normalized raw read count in which gene expression values, in FPKM, are divided by the 75th percentile value	TXT

Table 3. Gene quantification data formats.

Somatic variants from whole-genome sequencing are identified using this pipeline. Somatic variants are identified by comparing the tumor samples with the normal samples allele frequency. After annotating each mutation, one project is created combining files from multiple cases. Identification of somatic mutation has achieved through four pipelines. Identified somatic variants are then annotated. Information from multiple files is combined into one single MAF for each pipeline. Mutations are listed in a tab delimited format as Mutation Annotation Format (MAF). Two types of MAF files are produced for each variant calling in a project, i.e., the protected and the somatic or public MAF files. These MAF files are produced on the basis of annotated Variant Call Format (VCF) file. This VCF file contains variants reported in multiple transcripts. Only the critical ones are reported in the protected MAF file, whereas Public MAF are processed to remove the low quality and potential germline variants restricting the confidential information.VCF files are of two type, raw unannotated simple somatic mutations and annotated somatic mutation VCF files.

4.5. Single-nucleotide polymorphism

TCGA utilized SNP-based technology to analyze genome-wide variations. It also includes platforms to define CNV and loss of LOH across multiple samples.

4.6. DNA methylation sequencing

TCGA utilizes the Illumina platform for the DNA methylation study ensures single-base-pair resolution, high accuracy, easy workflows, and low input of DNA requirements. DNA methylation data files (**Table 4**) contain information of signal intensities (raw and normalized), detection confidence, and calculated beta values for methylated (M) and unmethylated (U) probes.

4.7. Reverse-phase protein array (RPPA)

Is a high throughput, functional, and quantitative proteomic method for large-scale protein expression profiling which helps in biomarker discovery and cancer diagnostics eventually.

Protein arrays consist of data representing protein expression and concentration. These data archives are deposited to the TCGA DCC and include original images of protein arrays, calculated raw signals, relative concentrations of proteins and normalized protein signals (**Table 5**).

4.8. Data processing workflow

TCGA have a well-organized structure from sample collection to bioinformatics analysis with involvement of several centers (**Table 6**).

Platform code	File type	Description
IlluminaDNAMethylation_ OMA002_CPI	Tab-delimited, ASCII text (.txt)	Cy3 and Cy5 signals and detection confidence of methylated probes
IlluminaDNAMethylation_ OMA002_CPI	Tab-delimited, ASCII text (.txt)	Calculated beta values
IlluminaDNAMethylation_ OMA003_CPI	Tab-delimited, ASCII text (.txt)	Cy3 and Cy5 signals and detection confidence of methylated probes
IlluminaDNAMethylation_ OMA003_CPI	Tab-delimited, ASCII text (.txt)	Calculated beta values
HumanMethylation27	Binary (.idat)	Intensity data file with statistics for each bead type in terms of bead count, mean and standard deviation per dye
HumanMethylation27	Tab-delimited, ASCII text (.txt)	Calculated beta values and mean signal intensities for replicate methylated and unmethylated probes
HumanMethylation27	Tab-delimited, ASCII text (.txt)	Calculated beta values, gene symbols, chromosomes and genomic coordinates (build 36). Some data have been masked (including known SNPs)
HumanMethylation450	Binary (.idat)	Intensity data file with statistics for each bead type in terms of bead count, mean and standard deviation per dye
HumanMethylation450	Tab-delimited, ASCII text (.txt)	Background-corrected methylated (M) and unmethylated (U) summary intensities as extracted by the methylumi package
HumanMethylation450	Tab-delimited, ASCII text (.txt)	Calculated beta values, gene symbols, chromosomes and genomic coordinates (hg18). Some data have been masked (including known SNPs)

Table 4. DNA methylation data files format.

File type	Description
Array Slide Image (tiff)	Black and white, high-resolution image of protein array
RPPA Slide Image Measurements (txt)	Raw signals from a black and white, high-resolution image of protein array
Super Curve Results (tab-delimited, txt)	Supercurve results, use dilution to calculate relative concentration
Normalized Protein Expression (MAGE-TAB data matrix, txt)	Signals for genes

Table 5. Protein data file format.

http://dx.doi.org/10.5772/intechopen.70026

Project	Details	Source
Tissue Source Sites (TSSs)	Collection of the samples (blood and tissue from tumour and normal controls) and clinical metadata from patients (donors) Shipment of the annotated biospecimens to Biospecimen Core Resources (BCR) https://wiki.nci.nih.gov/display/TCGA/Tissue+Source+Site	https://tcga-data.nci.nih.gov/datareports/codeTablesReport.htm?codeTable=tissue%20source%20site
Biospecimen Core Resource (BCR)	Coordination of sample delivery and data collection, cataloguing, processing, and verifying the quality and quantity Isolation and distribution of RNA and DNA from biospecimens to other institutions for genomic characterization and high-throughput sequencing http://cancergenome.nih.gov/abouttcga/overview/howitworks/bcr http://www.nationwidechildrens.org/biospecimen-core-resource-about-us	Research Institute at Nationwide Children's Hospital in Columbus, Ohio
Genome Sequencing Centers (GSCS)	High-throughput sequencing (data are available in TCGA Data Portal or at NIH's database of Genotype and Phenotype) Identification of the DNA alterations http://cancergenome.nih.gov/abouttcga/overview/howitworks/sequencingcenters	Broad Institute Sequencing Platform in Cambridge Human Genome Sequencing Center, Baylor College of Medicine in Houston The Genome Institute at Washington University
Cancer Genome Characterization Centers (GCCs)	Utilization of novel technologies and multiple platforms Comprehensive description of the genomic changes: alterations in miRNA and gene expression, SNP, CNV, and others http://cancergenome.nih.gov/abouttcga/overview/howitworks/characterizationcenters	Copy Number Alteration (Brigham and Women's Hospital and Harvard Medical School in Boston, The Broad Institute in Cambridge) Epigenomics (University of Southern California in Los Angeles, Johns Hopkins University in Baltimore) Gene (mRNA) Expression (University of North California at Chapel Hill) miRNA Analysis (British Columbia Cancer Agency in Vancouver) Targeted Sequencing Center (Baylor College of Medicine in Houston) Functional Proteomics (MD Anderson Cancer Center)
Proteome Characterization Centers (PCCs)	Identification of cancer-specific proteins http://cancergenome.nih.gov/abouttcga/overview/howitworks/proteomecharacterization	Cancer Proteomic Center Center for Application of Advanced Clinical Proteomic Technologies for Cancer Proteo-Genomic Discovery Prioritization and Verification of Cancer Biomarkers Proteome Characterization Centre and Vanderbilt Proteome Characterization Center
Data Coordinating Center (DCC)	Management of all generated data and transfer them to public databases (TCGA Data Portal and Cancer Genomics Hub) http://cancergenome.nih.gov/abouttcga/overview/howitworks/datasharingmanagement	University of California Santa Cruz

Table 6. TCGA centers and data processing.

Eligible patient samples (blood and tissue) are collected by different Tissue Source Sites (TSSs) and delivered to the Biospecimen Core Resource (BCR). BCR catalogue, process, and verify the quality and quantity of these samples and then submit clinical data and metadata to the Data Coordinating Center (DCC). Genome Characterization Centers (GCCs) and Genome Sequencing Centers (GSCs) then do the genomic characterization and high-throughput sequencing once the DCC provide molecular analytes. After sequencing, DCC again receives the sequence-related data from GSS. Trace files, sequences, and alignment mappings from Genome Characterization Centers are also submitted to the NCI's secure repository Cancer Genomic Hub (CGHub). Access to research community for these data is made available along with Genome Data Analysis Centers (GDACs). Information managed by DCC that has stored into public free-access databases (TCGA portal, NCBI's Trace Archive, CGHub), allows researchers to access the data and hence helps to advance in cancer studies.

4.9. TCGA data identifiers

Barcodes were initially used as the primary identifier for biospecimen data in TCGA during the beginning of the data. Tissue source site delivers the patient sample and the metadata to Biospecimen Core Resource (BCR). Once the sample is received by BCR, a human readable TCGA barcode was assigned. TCGA barcode was assigned to keep the navigation of the various results produced by the different data-generating centers for one particular sample connected. Sections of barcode also provide metadata information about the sample. Nowadays, BCR is also assigning universally unique identifiers (UUIDs) along with TCGA barcode to samples keeping UUIDs as the primary identifier instead of barcodes.

4.9.1. Barcodes

BCR generates the barcode for each sample received from TSS. Barcode initial numbers after the program code are assigned according to the TSS and the participant from which the tissue sample was received. The barcodes TCGA-02 and TCGA-02-0001 are assigned, respectively. Types of tissue are also differentiated with codes (**Table 7**). Next number in the barcode stands for the sample followed by the vial number; the sample was split into TCGA-02-0001-01 and TCGA-02-0001-01B. This vial number is again divided into different portions—TCGA-02-0001-01B-02. Analytes represented with barcode, e.g., TCGA-02-0001-01B-02D was extracted and distributed across one or more than one plates TCGA-02-0001-01B-02D-0182. Each well represented as, e.g., TCGA-02-0001-01B-02D-0182-06 is identified as an aliquot. These plates are later given to various characterize and sequencing centers.

4.9.2. Universally unique identifier (UUID)

UUIDs are randomly generated 32-digit hexadecimal value. TCGA became more complex, and the barcode was not enough to handle the generated data because there was not enough barcode combinations to represent the data. Also, flexibility in altering the barcode was also less when the associated metadata changes with a barcode. Considering all these factors, TCGA changed from using barcode for biospecimen and clinical data.

Tissue code	Letter code	Definition
1	TP	Primary Solid Tumor
2	TR	Recurrent Solid Tumor
3	TB	Primary Blood Derived Cancer—Peripheral Blood
4	TRBM	Recurrent Blood Derived Cancer—Bone Marrow
5	TAP	Additional—New Primary
6	TM	Metastatic
7	TAM	Additional Metastatic
8	THOC	Human Tumor Original Cells
9	TBM	Primary Blood Derived Cancer—Bone Marrow
10	NB	Blood Derived Normal
11	NT	Solid Tissue Normal
12	NBC	Buccal Cell Normal
13	NEBV	EBV Immortalized Normal
14	NBM	Bone Marrow Normal
20	CELLC	Control Analyte
40	TRB	Recurrent Blood Derived Cancer—Peripheral Blood
50	CELL	Cell Lines
60	XP	Primary Xenograft Tissue
61	XCL	Cell Line Derived Xenograft Tissue

Table 7. Tissue code.

The generated data are not only categorized based on the type but also the level at which these data can be accessed. In addition to the analyzed tumor data, TCGA also collects non-tumor samples aimed to analyze every patients germ line DNA to identify which alteration found in tumor sample responsible for the oncogenic process. For most of the tumors, TCGA collects and analyzes normal blood samples. In the absence of a matching normal blood sample, a normal tissue sample from the same patient is used as the germ line control for DNA assays. But in the case of RNA assays, using a normal blood sample as a control is not logically correct. Because RNA profile of blood sample is expected to be different from the RNA profile of tissues from other organs such as brain, breast, and lungs or ovary. Because of this reason, TCGA attempts to collect normal tissue matched to the anatomic site of the tumor not matched to the patient.

4.10. Accessibility of data

Access to the data is strictly controlled. There are two levels of data access:

- Open access data tier [raw, non-normalized data (Level I), processed data (Level II)].
- Controlled access data tier [segmented/interpreted data (Level III) apply to individual samples, while summarized data (Level IV)].

4.10.1. Open access data tier

The open access data level is composed of public data not unique to a patient. The open access data tier does not require any user certification [45].

Type of data accessible at open tier:

- Biospecimen
- Transcriptomic profiling
- Copy number variations
- DNA methylation
- Clinical
- Single-nucleotide variation

4.10.2. Controlled access data tier

Patient's unique information falls into the controlled access tier. Each data type has unique identifiers. In order to get the access to the data, user needs the certification.

Type of data accessible at controlled level:

- BAM and FASTQ files
- Level 1 and level 2 SNP6 array data
- Level 1 and level 2 exon array data
- Variant Call Format files
- Peculiar data of MAFs

In order to attain the access to these data, the researchers must:

- Complete the Data Access Request (DAR) form which is available electronically through the Database of Genotypes and Phenotypes (dbGaP).

Once the submitted request is evaluated and approved, researchers must

- Agree to restrict their use of the information to biomedical research purposes only
- Agree with the statements within TCGA Data Use Certification (DUC)
- Have their institutions certifiably agree to the statements within TCGA DUC

All patient samples are sworn to use for TCGA and there is no provision of sharing the material with a third party. Even this is not the case because 95% of material used up in different characterization. Even there is chance left to get the samples from the TSS centers. One can directly contact the TSS center for samples, and the decision lays on them.

4.11. TCGA data: visualization and data analysis

A huge amount of data accumulation demanding for advanced visualization technology and number of tools are available (**Table 8**). Visualization is essential to understand the data at ease.

Tool	Application
The Cancer Imaging Archive, CIA (http://www.cancerimagingarchive.net)	TCIA hosts a large archive of medical images of cancer accessible for public download. Information regarding patients treatment details, outcomes, pathology and genomics are also provided as supporting information based on availability
Berkeley Morphometric Data (http://tcga.lbl.gov:9999/biosig/tcgadownload.do)	Characterize tumour histopathology, through the delineation of the nuclear regions, from hematoxylin and eosin (H&E) stained tissue sections. The advantages of such a database is that other samples can be cross-referenced for personalized therapy and precision medicine as it contains information regarding responses to therapies, molecular correlates and morphometric subtypes
The Cancer Digital Slide Archive, CDSA (http://cancer.digitalslidearchive.net/)	Is an integrated Web-based platform supporting whole-slide pathology image visualization and data integration of the TCGA data
The Broad GDAC Firehose (http://firebrowse.org/)	Is a powerful tool for exploring cancer data. FireBrowse helps researchers to easily find any of thousands of data archives generated by the same. A powerful RESTful API is provided, with bindings to the UNIX command line, Python and R for programmers. For easy access, graphical interface like viewGene to explore expression levels and iCoMut are provided to explore the mutation information of each TCGA disease study with an interactive figure
The MD Anderson GDAC's MBatch (http://bioinformatics.mdanderson.org/tcgabatcheffects)	Is designed to help researchers to assess, diagnose and correct for any batch effects in TCGA data. It first allows the user to assess and quantify the presence of any batch effects through Principal Component Analysis and Hierarchical Clustering algorithms. The results from these algorithms are presented graphically as diagrams
Cancer Genome Workbench, CGWB (https://cgwb.nci.nih.gov/)	NCI developed application which integrate and display genomic and transcription alterations across various cancers. Integrated tracks view, Heatmap view, Bambino are the major viewers
UCSC Cancer Genomics Browser (https://genome-cancer.soe.ucsc.edu/)	Is an open access suite integrate, visualize and cancer genomic data along with clinical data
Integrative Genomics Viewer, IGV (http://www.broadinstitute.org/igv)	Is a freely available visualization tool of the genome developed by Broad Institute
The cBioPortal for Cancer Genomics (http://cbioportal.org)	Is interactive open-access resource for the exploration of multidimensional cancer genomics data sets. The barriers between the genomic data and the researchers are reduced rapidly after the resources was established. This database stores DNA copy-number data (deep deletions or amplification), non-synonymous mutations, mRNA and microRNA expression data, protein level, phosphoprotein level (RPPA) data, limited de-identified clinical data and DNA methylation data
Regulome Explorer (http://explorer.cancerregulome.org/)	It explores the association between and molecular features of TCGA data. According to user-specified parameters the data can be filtered for the search and visualize

Table 8. Visualization and data analysis tools.

Author details

Bijesh George, Vivekanand Ashokachandran, Aswathy Mary Paul and Reshmi Girijadevi*

*Address all correspondence to: reshmisuresh@gmail.com

Cancer Research Program-9, Rajiv Gandhi Centre for Biotechnology, Thiruvananthapuram, Kerala, India

References

[1] Institute NHGR. Transcriptome The National Human Genome Research Institute: The National Human Genome Research Institute. 2015 [updated August 27, 2015; cited 2015 August 27, 2015]. Available from: https://www.genome.gov/13014330/transcriptome-fact-sheet/

[2] Tuffaha MSA. Phenotypic and Genotypic Diagnosis of Malignancies: An Immunohistochemical and Molecular Approach. 1st ed. Weinheim: Wiley-Blackwell, 2008. DOI: 10.1002/9783527621521

[3] Ramalho AS, Beck S, Farinha CM, Clarke LA, Heda GD, Steiner B, et al. Methods for RNA extraction, cDNA preparation and analysis of CFTR transcripts. Journal of Cystic Fibrosis: Official Journal of the European Cystic Fibrosis Society. 2004;**3**(Suppl 2):11-15

[4] Gilbert SF. Differential Gene Expression. Developmental Biology. 6th ed.; Sunderland (MA): Sinauer Associates; 2000

[5] Hoopes L. Introduction to the gene expression and regulation topic room. Nature Education. 2008;**1**(1):160

[6] Alberts B, Johnson A, Lewis J, et al. Studying Gene Expression and Function. Molecular Biology of the Cell. 4th ed.; New York: Garland Science; 2002

[7] Trapnell C, Pachter L, Salzberg SL. TopHat: Discovering splice junctions with RNA-Seq. Bioinformatics. 2009;**25**(9):1105-1111

[8] Zahler, A. M. Pre-mRNA splicing and its regulation in Caenorhabditis elegans The C. elegans Research Community WormBook. WormBook, 2012. 1551-8507. DOI:10.1895/wormbook.1.31.2

[9] Wang ET, Sandberg R, Luo S, Khrebtukova I, Zhang L, Mayr C, et al. Alternative isoform regulation in human tissue transcriptomes. Nature. 2008;**456**(7221):470-476

[10] Christie M. L. Linux: The glue that binds your next-generation sequencing analyses. The Molecular Ecologist. [Internet]. 2012. Available from: http://www.molecularecologist.com/2012/10/linux-the-glue-that-binds-your-next-generation-sequencing-analyses/ [Accessed:2017-07-18]

[11] Afgan E, Baker D, van den Beek M, Blankenberg D, Bouvier D, Cech M, et al. The Galaxy platform for accessible, reproducible and collaborative biomedical analyses: 2016 update. Nucleic Acids Research. 2016;**44**(W1):W3-W10

[12] Lindner R, Friedel CC. A comprehensive evaluation of alignment algorithms in the context of RNA-seq. PLoS One. 2012;**7**(12):e52403

[13] Ewing B, Green P. Base-calling of automated sequencer traces using phred. II. Error probabilities. Genome Research. 1998;**8**(3):186-194

[14] Guttman M, Garber M, Levin JZ, Donaghey J, Robinson J, Adiconis X, et al. Ab initio reconstruction of cell type-specific transcriptomes in mouse reveals the conserved multi-exonic structure of lincRNAs. Nature Biotechnology. 2010;**28**(5):503-510

[15] Marioni JC, Mason CE, Mane SM, Stephens M, Gilad Y. RNA-seq: An assessment of technical reproducibility and comparison with gene expression arrays. Genome Research. 2008;**18**(9):1509-1517

[16] Wang Z, Gerstein M, Snyder M. RNA-Seq: A revolutionary tool for transcriptomics. Nature Reviews Genetics. 2009;**10**(1):57-63

[17] Wilhelm BT, Landry JR. RNA-Seq-quantitative measurement of expression through massively parallel RNA-sequencing. Methods. 2009;**48**(3):249-257

[18] Katz Y, Wang ET, Airoldi EM, Burge CB. Analysis and design of RNA sequencing experiments for identifying isoform regulation. Nature Methods. 2010;**7**(12):1009-1015

[19] Trapnell C, Williams BA, Pertea G, Mortazavi A, Kwan G, van Baren MJ, et al. Transcript assembly and quantification by RNA-Seq reveals unannotated transcripts and isoform switching during cell differentiation. Nature Biotechnology. 2010;**28**(5):511-515

[20] Bahn JH, Lee JH, Li G, Greer C, Peng G, Xiao X. Accurate identification of A-to-I RNA editing in human by transcriptome sequencing. Genome Research. 2012;**22**(1):142-150

[21] Park E, Williams B, Wold BJ, Mortazavi A. RNA editing in the human ENCODE RNA-seq data. Genome Research. 2012;**22**(9):1626-1633

[22] Peng Z, Cheng Y, Tan BC, Kang L, Tian Z, Zhu Y, et al. Comprehensive analysis of RNA-Seq data reveals extensive RNA editing in a human transcriptome. Nature Biotechnology. 2012;**30**(3):253-260

[23] Ramaswami G, Zhang R, Piskol R, Keegan LP, Deng P, O'Connell MA, et al. Identifying RNA editing sites using RNA sequencing data alone. Nature Methods. 2013;**10**(2):128-132

[24] Cabili MN, Trapnell C, Goff L, Koziol M, Tazon-Vega B, Regev A, et al. Integrative annotation of human large intergenic noncoding RNAs reveals global properties and specific subclasses. Genes & Development. 2011;**25**(18):1915-1927

[25] Prensner JR, Iyer MK, Balbin OA, Dhanasekaran SM, Cao Q, Brenner JC, et al. Transcriptome sequencing across a prostate cancer cohort identifies PCAT-1, an unannotated lincRNA implicated in disease progression. Nature Biotechnology. 2011;**29**(8):742-749

[26] Benjamini Y, Speed TP. Summarizing and correcting the GC content bias in high-throughput sequencing. Nucleic Acids Research. 2012;**40**(10):e72

[27] Hansen KD, Brenner SE, Dudoit S. Biases in Illumina transcriptome sequencing caused by random hexamer priming. Nucleic Acids Research. 2010;**38**(12):e131

[28] Simon A. FastQC: A quality control tool for high throughput sequence data. [Internet]. 2016. Available from: https://www.bioinformatics.babraham.ac.uk/projects/fastqc/ [18 Jul. 2017]

[29] Ewing B, Hillier L, Wendl MC, Green P. Base-calling of automated sequencer traces using phred. I. Accuracy assessment. Genome Research. 1998;**8**(3):175-185

[30] FASTX-Toolkit

[31] Martin M. Cutadapt removes adapter sequences from high-throughput sequencing reads. EMBnet.journal, [S.l.], may. 2011;**17**(1):10-12. Available at: http://journal.embnet.org/index.php/embnetjournal/article/view/200. Date accessed: 18 Jul. 2017. doi:http://dx.doi.org/10.14806/ej.17.1.200

[32] Trimgalore

[33] Quinlan AR, Hall IM. BEDTools: A flexible suite of utilities for comparing genomic features. Bioinformatics. 2010;**26**(6):841-842

[34] Anders S, Pyl PT, Huber W. HTSeq—A Python framework to work with high-throughput sequencing data. Bioinformatics. 2015;**31**(2):166-169

[35] Liao Y, Smyth GK, Shi W. featureCounts: An efficient general purpose program for assigning sequence reads to genomic features. Bioinformatics. 2014;**30**(7):923-930

[36] Conesa A, Madrigal P, Tarazona S, Gomez-Cabrero D, Cervera A, McPherson A, et al. A survey of best practices for RNA-seq data analysis. Genome Biology. 2016;**17**:13

[37] O'Leary NA, Wright MW, Brister JR, Ciufo S, Haddad D, McVeigh R, et al. Reference sequence (RefSeq) database at NCBI: Current status, taxonomic expansion, and functional annotation. Nucleic Acids Research. 2016;**44**(D1):D733-D745

[38] Roberts A, Pimentel H, Trapnell C, Pachter L. Identification of novel transcripts in annotated genomes using RNA-Seq. Bioinformatics. 2011;**27**(17):2325-2329

[39] Li JJ, Jiang CR, Brown JB, Huang H, Bickel PJ. Sparse linear modeling of next-generation mRNA sequencing (RNA-Seq) data for isoform discovery and abundance estimation. Proceedings of the National Academy of Sciences of the United States of America. 2011;**108**(50):19867-19872

[40] Pertea M, Pertea GM, Antonescu CM, Chang TC, Mendell JT, Salzberg SL. StringTie enables improved reconstruction of a transcriptome from RNA-seq reads. Nature Biotechnology. 2015;**33**(3):290-295

[41] Dai M, Thompson RC, Maher C, Contreras-Galindo R, Kaplan MH, Markovitz DM, et al. NGSQC: Cross-platform quality analysis pipeline for deep sequencing data. BMC Genomics. 2010;**11**(Suppl 4):S7

[42] Speir ML, Zweig AS, Rosenbloom KR, Raney BJ, Paten B, Nejad P, et al. The UCSC Genome Browser database: 2016 update. Nucleic Acids Research. 2016;**44**(D1):D717-D725

[43] Thorvaldsdottir H, Robinson JT, Mesirov JP. Integrative Genomics Viewer (IGV): High-performance genomics data visualization and exploration. Briefings in Bioinformatics. 2013;**14**(2):178-192

[44] Medina I, Salavert F, Sanchez R, de Maria A, Alonso R, Escobar P, et al. Genome Maps, a new generation genome browser. Nucleic Acids Research. 2013;**41**(Web Server issue):W41-W46

[45] Health NIo. The Cancer Genome Atlas

Section 2

Omics: From Bioeconomy to Human Health

Chapter 7

Current Advances in Functional Genomics in Aquaculture

Hetron M. Munang'andu and Øystein Evensen

Additional information is available at the end of the chapter

http://dx.doi.org/10.5772/intechopen.69883

Abstract

Gene expression studies in aquaculture have slowly evolved from the traditional reductionist approach of single gene sequencing to high throughput sequencing (HTS) techniques able to sequence entire genomes of living organisms. The upcoming of HTS techniques has led to emergence of metagenomics, nutrigenomics, epigenetics and other omics technologies in aquaculture in the last decade. Metagenomics analyses have accelerated the speed at which emerging pathogens are being discovered, thereby contributing to the design of timely disease control strategies in aquaculture. Using metagenomics, it is easy to identify and monitor microbial communities found in different ecosystems. In vaccine production, genomic studies are being used to identify cross neutralizing antigens against variant strains of the same pathogens. In genetics and epigenetics, genomics traits have been identified that are beginning to gain commercial applications in aquaculture. Nutrigenomics have not only enhanced our understanding of the biological markers for nutrition-related diseases, but they have also enhanced our ability to formulate diets able to maintain a stable immune homeostasis in the gut. Overall, herein, we have shown that functional genomics provide multifaceted applications ranging from monitoring microbial communities in aquatic environments to optimizing production systems in aquaculture.

Keywords: genomics, aquaculture, metagenomics, nutrigenomics, epigenetics

1. Introduction

The ability to decipher the molecular composition of nucleic acids of living organisms is of prime importance in biological sciences. Although the traditional approaches of single gene expression analyses using polymerase chain reaction (PCR) tests [1, 2], quantitative real

time PCRs (qRT-PCRs) [3, 4], competitive PCRs [5] or nested PCRs [6] have been and are still widely used in biological sciences, they inherently lack the ability to provide a global overview of genomic transcripts found in living organisms. However, the recent advent of omics technologies such as metagenomics, nutrigenomics and epigenetics based on high throughput sequencing (HTS) is rapidly enhancing our ability to understand complex systems underlying different biological functions. These omics technologies have not only accelerated whole genome sequencing projects of different aquatic organisms [7, 8], but they also have the capacity to unravel the sequences of entire genomes without prior knowledge of the genes to be sequenced thereby enhancing the discovery and annotation of novel genes in non-model species. And as shown from recent studies, their applications in aquaculture have accelerated our ability to identify emerging pathogens [9], monitor the microbiomes of different aquatic environments [10], develop nutritional diets with less side effects [11, 12] and understand the cellular networks that regulate different biological processes in aquatic organisms [13–15]. It is evident from studies carried out this far that an integrated use of different omics technologies is bound to improve our production systems in aquaculture [10, 12, 16–18]. Hence, this chapter provides an overview of different omics technologies currently used in aquaculture mainly focusing on their overall contribution to transforming genomics studies into functional applications.

2. Application of metagenomics analyses

Studies carried out this far show that metagenomics can be used to identify novel pathogens as well as microbiota found on mucosal surfaces of cultured aquatic organisms.

2.1. Application of metagenomics in diagnostics and discovery of novel pathogens

The rapid expansion of aquaculture to become a leading source of proteins for human consumption in the world has brought with it a rapid increase in the number pathogens infecting farmed aquatic organisms [19]. To expedite the process of identifying emerging pathogens, there has been a shift in recent years from the use of traditional diagnostic tools based on isolation, culture and pathogen characterization to include metagenomics analyses in the identification of novel pathogens in aquaculture [10]. Metagenomics is a culture independent diagnostic tool that does not require prior knowledge of nucleic acids to be sequenced unlike conventional PCR that require prior knowledge of the nucleic acid to be sequenced for the design of primers [20]. Metagenomics analyses have the capacity to sequence all nucleic acids present in a sample at once thereby generating a vast array of data that requires computational analyses for interpretation [20, 21]. As pointed out in our previous studies [9, 10], it has the advantage of identifying co-infections and in the case of viral pathogens, it has the capacity to generate all variable proteins that form complete virions thereby permitting comparative phylogenetic analyses with other viruses present in public databases. Moreover, it is a proactive diagnostic tool able to identify novel pathogens before they cause outbreaks unlike the reactive traditional diagnostic tools in which etiological agents are only identified after

causing disease outbreaks reaching epidemic proportions [21]. Using metagenomics, several novel pathogens have been identified at a much faster rate than traditional approaches in which the duration from first observation of clinical signs to identification of the pathogens is long [10]. For example, infectious pancreatic necrosis (IPN) was first reported as an acute infectious enteritis [22] in salmonids in the 1940s while the etiological was later characterized as IPN virus after 20 years in 1960 [23]. Similarly, viral haemorrhagic septicaemia (VHS) was first reported in the early 1950s in salmonids while the causative agent was characterized later after 10 years in 1962 [24]. This trend was observed for several other diseases such as infectious hematopoietic necrosis virus (IHNV), nervous necrosis virus (NNV), heart and skeletal muscle inflammation (HSMI) and cardiac myopathy syndrome (CMS) in which identification of the etiological agents took long after clinical signs were first reported [25–33]. However, the upcoming of metagenomics has accelerated our discovery of novel pathogens in which the duration from observation of first clinical signs to identification of the etiological agent has been reduced. In fish, viruses discovered using metagenomics include circoviruses from common bream [34] and European eel [35], posavirus [36] and seadornavirus [37] from freshwater carp and totivirus from golden shiner. As shown in our recent study [9], more than 20 novel fish pathogenic viruses have been identified using metagenomics in the last 4 years, which is more than the number identified using traditional diagnostic tools in the last 5 decades, clearly showing the rapid rate at which metagenomics has accelerated our ability to identify novel pathogens compared with traditional diagnostic methods.

In crustaceans, mortalities due to white spot syndrome virus (WSSV) in shrimps were first reported in 1992 while the causative agent was identified in 2001 [38–40]. Mortalities due to taura syndrome virus (TSV) in shrimps were first reported in Ecuador in 1991 [41] and the virus was characterized in 1994 [42]. A similar trend was observed for Yellow heard disease virus (YTV) [43, 44], infectious hypodermal and hematopoietic necrosis virus (IHHNV) [45–47], shrimp infectious myonecrosis virus (SIMV) [48] and *Penaues vannamei* nodavirus (PvNV) [49, 50] in which the duration between the first report of the disease and identification of the etiological agent was long. Shrimps viruses discovered using metagenomics analyses include *Frafantepenaeus duorarum* nodavirus (FdNV) and shrimp hepatopancreas-associated circular nodavirus (ShrimpCDV) [51].

2.2. Monitoring of environmental microbiomes

A good understanding of microbial communities found in freshwater and marine environment used for aquaculture is a prerequisite to designing effective disease control strategies tailored for each ecosystem. Metagenomics analyses provide a unique opportunity to study infectious agents in water samples outside their susceptible hosts [10]. Its ability to sequence all nucleic acids present in a sample at once enables it to profile microbial communities found in different ecosystems. For example, Angly et al. [52] showed that microbial composition varies with latitude gradient with highest diversity being in warm climates around the equator and less diversity in the poles. After analysis of viromes from 32 different marine sites, Dinsdale et al. [53] noted that viral richness decreased from deep sea to surface waters and with distance from shore in surface waters and increased from winter to summer. Given that

over 40% of the global human population live within 100 km of coastlines, anthropogenic activities have been shown to influence the composition of microbial communities in coastal areas where aquaculture activities are mostly carried out [54]. These anthropogenic activities include host species composition changes introduced by aquaculture [55, 56], waste disposal [57], agriculture [58], recreation [59] and industrial activities [59]. As a result, metagenomics is currently being used to monitor the impact of anthropogenic activities on coastal microbial composition. Port et al. [60] found an increase in antibiotic resistance genes caused by coastal effluent discharges, while Morán et al. [61] showed significant changes in bacterial community structures caused by coastal copper disposal in La Lancha and Chañaral bay in the Pacific Ocean. Overall, these studies show that metagenomics is not only used to identify novel pathogens, but it is also used to monitor the impact of human activities on microbial composition in different aquatic environments.

2.3. Application of metagenomics in recirculation systems

In contrast to outdoor aquaculture systems that are dependent on natural water basins such as rivers and oceans, the recirculation aquaculture system (RAS) uses water that is filtered before it is recycled back into culture tanks in closed systems. Water used in RAS is subjected to several treatment processes such as biofiltration to reduce ammonium, removal of solids, oxygenation, pH control and pathogen denaturation using ozone and UV-light. Although a well-designed state-of-the-art RAS has the potential to reduce the presence of waterborne microorganisms, some pathogens are able to resist RAS disinfection. Bacteria phyla detected from RAS biofilters include Actinobacteria [62], Firmicutes, Bacteroides [63–65], Protobacteria [63, 65], Verrucomicrobia [65] and Sphingobacteria [62, 65]. Hence, some microorganisms are being used as biosafety indicators whose dominance points to increase in the proliferation of pathogenic microorganisms [66]. As a result, metagenomics analyses are being used to monitor the increase in proliferation of pathogens in RAS [67].

2.4. Metagenomics analyses of mucosa microbiota

Given that mucosal surfaces are the major portals of microbial invasion, there has been a growing interest to study mucosal microbiota of cultured aquatic organisms. Metagenomics studies show that different environmental factors influence the composition of mucosal microbiota on different fish species.

2.4.1. Skin mucosa microbiota

Larsen et al. [68] compared the skin microbiota of six different fish species (*Mugil cephalus, Lutjanus campechanus, Cynoscion nebulosus, Cynoscion arenarius, Micropogonias undulatus* and *Lagodon rhomboides*) from the Gulf of Mexico and showed that Proteobacteria was the predominant phylum followed by Firmicutes and Actinobacteria across all species. Although Aeribacillus was found in 19% of all fish species examined, genera such as Neorickettsia and Microbacterium were fish species-specific pointing to existence of phyla and genera associated

with particular fish species. Lokesh and Kiron [69] showed that the bacterial operational taxonomy unit (OTU) composition on the skin of Atlantic salmon (*Salmo salar* L.) changed significantly as a result of transfer from fresh to seawater. Proteobacteria was the dominant phylum both in fresh and seawater while Bacteroidetes, Actinobacteria, Firmicutes, Cyanobacteria and Verrucomicrobia were the most abundant in freshwater. The genus *Oleispira* was the most abundant in seawater. Similarly, Wilson et al. [70] showed that bacterial communities from the epidermal mucus of Atlantic cod (*Gadus morhua*) from the Baltic, Iceland and North seas collected over three seasons mainly comprised of Psychrobacter, Bacteroides and Photobacterium OTUs in all seasons although there were significant inter-site and seasonal variations in community composition.

Boutin et al. [71] combined 16S RNA metagenomics and QTL analyses to show that host genotype can regulate the microbiota composition on the skin surface of brook charr (*Salvelinus fontinalis*). They found a strong negative correlation between Flavobacterium and Methylobacterium, pointing to a mutually competitive relationship between pathogenic and non-pathogenic bacteria on the skin mucosa of brook charr. Flavobacterium is known to be pathogenic among different fish species, while Methylobacteria provide protection against pathogenic bacterial infections on skin surfaces suggesting that a shift from Methylobacteria to Flavobacterium dominance on the skin mucosal could point to increase in susceptibility to bacterial infection. Hence, by monitoring changes on mucosal bacteria composition, metagenomics can be used to determine the susceptibility of fish to microbial infections.

2.4.2. Gut mucosal microbiota

As pointed out by Lyons et al. [72] that to better understand the gut microbiome and its impact on the health status of aquatic organisms, it is vital to determine its structure, diversity and potential functional capacity. Gajardo et al. [12] analysed the microbiota profile of the digesta and gut mucosal of Atlantic salmon (*S. salar* L.) fed commercial diets and showed that microbiota richness and diversity differed significantly between the digesta and gut. The digesta had a higher and diverse richness than the gut mucosa. Proteobacteria was the dominant phyla in the mucosa whereas Proteobacteria and Firmicules were dominant in the digesta. In addition, there were significant differences in microbiota composition in different segments of the gut. Actinobacteria was dominant in the posterior intestinal (PI) than the mid-intestinal (MI) mucosa. Moreover, the PI showed presence of Spirochaetes that were not found in the MI showing that metagenomics can be used to identify microbial communities that inhabit different segments of the gut. In another study, Gajardo et al. [11] identified bacterial groups associated with diet-induced gut dysfunction that could serve as biological markers of the gut health status in Atlantic salmon. Mouchet et al. [73] compared the gut microbiota of 15 fish species from the Atlantic Ocean near Brazil and showed that the microbiota genetic diversity was highly influenced by the fish species, geographical location and diet. Put together, these studies show that metagenomics can be used to profile bacteria species on mucosal surfaces of different fish species and that different factors such as host species, geographical areas and diet influence mucosal microbiota in fish.

2.5. Metagenomics technologies and their limitations

Of the most widely used NGS technologies, both 454 pyrosequencing Roche and Illumina sequencers have been widely used in the metagenomics analyses of different aquatic organisms. For example, 454 pyrosequencing Roche has been used to study microbial communities of different fish species including rainbow trout (*Oncorhynchus mykiss*) [74], Atlantic cod (*G. morhua*) [75], Atlantic salmon [76], brook trout (*S. fontinalis*) [77], brown trout (*Salmo trutta*) [78], zebrafish (*Dario rerio*) [79], Gizzard shad (*Dorosoma cepedianum*) [80], silver carp (*Hypophthalmichthys molitrix*) [81], common carp (*Cyprinus carpio*) [82], grass carp (*Ctenopharyngodon idellus*) [83], orange spotted grouper (*Epinephelus coioides*) [84] and Senegalese sole (*Solea senegalensis*) [85]. On the other hand, Illumina sequencers have been used for the analyses of microbiota found in seabass (*Lates calcarifer*) [86], blunt snout bream (*Megalobrama amblycephala*) [87], grass carp (GC) [87], mandarin fish (*Siniperca chuatsi*) [87], topmouth culter (*Culter alburnus*), common carp [87] and Crucian carp (*Carassius auratus*) [87], silver carp [87] and bighead carp (*Hypophthalmichthys nobilis*) [87]. In terms of assembly, both whole genome shotgun and marker gene guided sequencing have been used on different aquatic organisms. The commonly used marker gene in metagenomics analyses is the 16S ribosomal RNA (16S rRNA), which has been widely used to characterize the microbiota of different aquatic organisms including rainbow trout [88, 89], Atlantic salmon [11, 12], turbot (*Scophthalmus maximus*) [90], lamprey (*Lampetra morii*) [91] and Baleen whale [92]. Whole genome shotgun sequencing has also been widely used in the study of environmental microbial communities and pathogens infecting different aquatic organisms. The major advantage with this approach is that it can be used to sequence whole genomes of known or unknown organisms using *de novo* assemblies unlike guided marker assemblies that are dependent on a reference gene [93–96].

Despite its positive contribution to the discovery of novel pathogens and environmental monitoring of microbial communities, metagenomics has significant limitations that require the support of other tools [95]. The immense metagenome data generated using NGS technologies require the support of other tools for clustering, classification and annotation of individual sequences [95]. For *de novo* assembled sequences, the most reliable annotation approach is by homology search using reference sequences available in public databases. However, the number of existing public databases for aquatic organisms is limited, which makes it difficult to identify novel pathogens [97]. In general, functional annotation lags behind the rate at which metagenome data is generated. Alternative methods used to identify novel pathogens include motif or pattern-based identification [98, 99], phylogenetic profiling [100] and neighbourhood tree alignments [101, 102].

3. Nutrigenomics in aquaculture

Nutrigenomics is the study of the role of nutrition on gene expression. Galduch-Giner et al. [103] showed that there was specialization in the functional properties of different components of the intestinal tract of the European seabass (*Dicentarchus labrax*). They observed that

molecular markers linked to nutrient digestion and absorption were high in the anterior (AI) and middle intestine (MI) while the posterior intestine (PI) predominantly expressed genes linked to immune defence mechanisms. These observations are in line with other scientists who showed that the AI and MI are mainly responsible for nutrient digestion and absorption [104, 105] while the PI is responsible for induction of innate immune responses linked to activation of adaptive immunity in teleosts fish [106–109].

Different scientists have studied the genomic changes induced by various nutrients in the guts of different fish species. Krol et al. [110] compared the differential response of the Atlantic salmon gut to soybean meal (SBM) and fish meal (FM) as positive and negative controls for enteritis, respectively. They noted that SBM altered the gut histology and induced extensive transcriptomic changes linked to underlying mechanisms of SBM-induced enteropathy. They found 18 enriched pathways linked to inflammation and immune responses induced by SBM enteropathy. Among these were the NF-kB and IL-8 signalling pathways known to induce the synthesis of various pro-inflammatory cytokines. Phagocytic pathways such as the Fcγ receptor mediated phagocytosis and monocyte pathways were highly enriched. In another study, Torrecillas et al. [111] showed downregulation of TCRβ, COX-2, TNFα, IL-8, IL-6, IL-10, TGFβ and IgM when MHC-II was upregulated in European seabass fed to Soya-bean oil (SBO). Expression of these genes corresponded with reduced lengths of intestinal folds and mucus density in the gut. Conversely, mannan oligosaccharides (MOS) diets increased the length of intestinal folds and mucus density and upregulated MHC-CD4, COX-2, TNFα and IgM expression. Combined MOS and SBO diets reduced the harmful effects of SBO diets by moderating the downregulation of GALT-related genes. Therefore, these observations show the importance of optimizing feed formulation in order to produce balanced diets able to preserve the GALT-immune homeostasis.

Apart from soyabean, nutrigenomics have also been used to evaluate the impact of other nutrients in fish diets. Azeredo et al. [112] showed that the immune status of the European seabass was impaired by arginine dietary supplements. They observed that different cell-mediated immune markers were downregulated in fish fed 1–2% arginine diets. Leukocytes obtained from fish fed arginine diets showed low respiratory burst compared to control fish. After challenge with *Vibrio aguillarum*, fish fed arginine diet supplements showed higher mortality than control fish. Interestingly, reducing arginine levels to 0.5% in the diet supplements significantly increased respiratory burst to levels comparable with control fish. In another study, Estensoro et al. [113] showed that butyrate (BP-70 ®NOREL) helped to restore the intestinal status of marine gilthead sea bream (*Sparus aurata*) fed extremely low diets of fish meal (FM) and fish oil (FO). They observed that extremely low FO and FM diet levels significantly altered the transcriptomic profiles linked to nutrient absorption in the AI and increased expression of inflammatory, antioxidant, permeability and mucus production genes that coincided with increased granulocyte and lymphocyte presence in the PI submucosa. Interestingly, expression of these genes was restored to control values by adding butyrate (BP-70) to the feed. As pointed out by Krol et al. [110], gut transcriptomic profiling is a useful tool for testing the adverse impacts of different feeds and that understanding gut-diet interactions is a prerequisite to designing diets able to prevent induction of diet-related diseases in the gut.

Omics technologies commonly used for nutrigenomics analyses in aquaculture mainly comprise of microarray and RNA-seq. RNA-seq has been widely used to study the impact of different diets in various fish species including Atlantic salmon [114], rainbow trout [115], channel catfish (*Iactalurus punctatus*) [116], blue catfish (*Ictalurus furcatus*) [117] and zebrafish [118]. On the other hand, microarray has also been widely used to study nutrigenomics in different fish species that include Atlantic salmon, rainbow trout, Atlantic cod (*G. morhua*) and Gilthead sea bream (*S. aurata*). However, the use of RNA-seq and microarray leads to several challenges that include the need for large data processing softwares as well as the need of bioinformatics tools required for differential gene expression, network pathway, alternative splicing and gene duplication analyses. To cope with these challenges, different bioinformatics tools have been developed and new innovations are being invented to cover different aspects of quality assessment of mapped genes, mapping for *de novo* assembled genes, expression quantification, differential expression analyses, alternative splicing and network pathway analyses [119–122]. Different reviews have been published providing in-depth comparative analyses of existing tools highlighting their strengths and weakness that could serve as a guide for end users to select the most appropriate tool suitable for nutrigenomics studies in different aquatic organisms [119, 123, 124].

4. Functional genomics in vaccine development

Given that most pathogens exist as multiple strains having different antigenic proteins, the challenge in vaccine design has been to find cross protective antigens against variant strains of the same pathogen. In the case of viruses, different approaches have been used aiming at finding the most neutralizing epitopes using methods such as epitope mapping, peptide-scan and reverse genetics [125–128]. However, the upcoming of next generation sequencing (NGS) supported with current advances of bioinformatics tools is expected to expedite our ability to identify the most immunogenic proteins for vaccine production against viral diseases. For example, Ou-yang et al. [129] used bioinformatics to identify the antigenic proteins for Singapore grouper iridovirus. They used the 162 open reading frames (ORFs) of SGIV for sequence similarity searches to identify motifs, cellular locations and other prediction domains to identify the most immunogenic epitopes required for vaccine production. They identified 13 genes that were cloned to produce DNA vaccines of which three vaccines produced relative percent survival (RPS) ranging from 58.3 to 66.7% in vaccinated grouper.

In the case of bacterial vaccines, identification of protective antigens can be a challenge given that they contain several antigenic proteins such as capsular antigens, fimbriae, pili and outer membrane proteins [130–132]. Some of these proteins lead to serotype, biovar or strain differences leading to antigenic diversity within bacterial species. Hence, the challenge is to identify broad neutralizing antigens able to confer cross protection against variant bacterial strains can be a difficult task. To overcome this problem, Handfield et al. [133] developed an *in vivo* induced antigen technology (IVIAT) that uses antibodies generated from individuals infected by the bacterial strain homologous to the vaccine strain to probe for immunogenic proteins using an *in vitro* expression system. To do this, a genomic library is generated using DNA fragments from the bacteria strain to be used for vaccine production. The DNA fragments are digested using

restriction enzymes and cloned into plasmid vectors. Induced colonies of the expression library are probed using pooled sera from bacterial infected individuals as shown in **Figure 1**. Reactive clones are purified and used as vaccine candidates [133]. This technology has been widely used to identify antigenic proteins for different bacteria species such as *Streptococcus iniae* [134], *Vibrio anguillarum* [135], *Aeromonas salmonicida* [136, 137], *Edwardsiella tarda* [138] and *Streptococcus parauberis* [139]. Jia et al. [138] used the IVIAT to identify a 510 aa peptidase protein, which they used to produce a subunit vaccine against *E. tarda* in Japanese flounder. Sun et al. [134] used the IVIAT technique to identify a secretory antigen, which they designated as Sia10, and cloned it to produce a DNA vaccine against *S. iniae*. In vaccinated turbot, the Sia10 protein was detected in the muscle, liver, kidney and spleen by 7 days post-vaccination (dpv) lasting until 49 dpv. Post-challenge RPS showed 73.9 and 92.3% in fish challenged with high- and low-challenge dose, respectively. In addition, the Sia10 protein produced protective antibodies in passively vaccinated fish. In another study, Sun et al. [140] used the IVIAT method to identify a surface

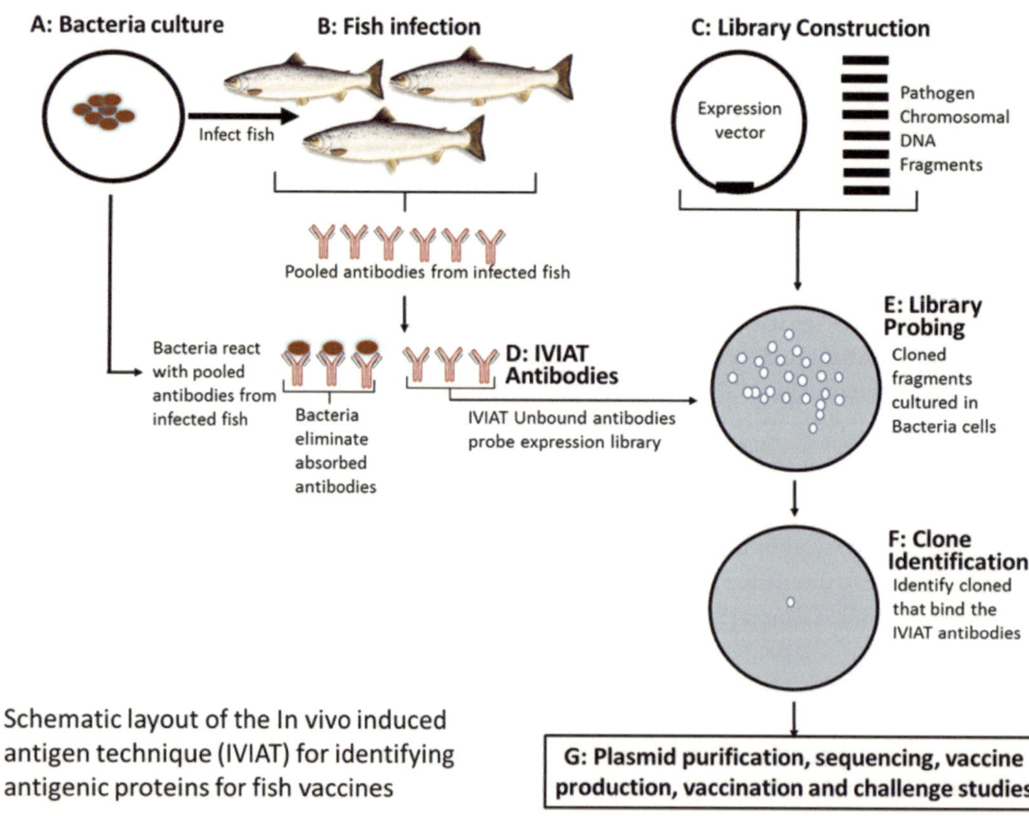

Figure 1. Schematic layout of the IVIAT technique for the identification of bacterial antigenic proteins essential for the production of fish vaccines: A: bacteria culture. B: bacteria infection in fish and the sera from infected fish is pooled. C: library construction using chromosomal DNA fragments of the bacteria cultured in (A). D: bacteria eliminate absorbed antibodies from sera while IVIAT unbound antibodies are used to probe the library constructed in (C). E: clones from fragments of bacterial chromosomal DNA are probed with IVIAT pooled sera. F: after probing with pooled sera from infected fish, clones depicting binding capacity to IVIAT sera are sub-cultured. G: the identified clones are purified, sequenced and used for subunit or DNA vaccine production followed by vaccination and challenge trials.

antigen designated as Esa1, which they used to produce a DNA vaccine against *E. tarda* in Japanese flounder. They showed that the pCEsa1 vaccine enhanced respiratory burst, acid phosphatase activity and bactericidal activity of headkidney macrophages. In addition, it produced RPS = 57% in passively vaccinated fish. Overall, these studies show that genomics approaches can be used to identify the most immunogenic proteins for different bacterial strains in order to produce the most protective vaccines for use in aquaculture.

5. Marker-assisted selection of growth and disease resistance traits

5.1. Growth traits

Genetic selection in which individuals with the best growth traits are selected as parent stock for the next generation is one of the major strategies used for improving production in aquaculture. And as such, several breeding programmes have been going on using natural selection approaches [141–143]. The major drawback with this approach is that it takes several generation cycles to identify individuals having positive growth traits. To expedite the process of identifying genetic traits for optimal growth performance, marker-assisted selection (MAS) processes such as single nucleotides polymorphism (SNP), microsatellite, amplified fragment length polymorphism (AFLP), random amplified polymorphism DNA (RAPD), restriction fragment length polymorphism (RFLP) and quantitative trait loci (QTL) are being used to scan chromosomal DNA of different farmed aquatic organisms. Among these, the most widely used is QTL analysis, which has been applied across most of the commercial fish and crustacean species used in aquaculture [144–147]. As defined by Geldermann [148], QTLs are chromosomal regions made of single genes or gene clusters determining a quantitative character of a given trait. Given their high heritability, mapped QTLs have proved to be a useful tool in selective breeding, which has played an important role in accelerating genetic improvement in aquaculture.

As shown in **Tables 1** and **2**, the most important genetic traits sought for in aquaculture are growth rate, body weight and length. These traits influence the commercial value of farmed aquatic organisms. Traits for body weight and length have been identified in several fish species such as Atlantic salmon [149], rainbow trout [150], Big heard carp (*H. nobilis*) [151], common carp [152, 153] and tilapia (*Oreochromis niloticus*) [154], nine spined stickleback (*Pungitius pungitius*) [155] and Arctic char (*Salvelinus alpinus*) [156]. In shrimps and prawns, body weight and length traits have been identified in kruma shrimp [157, 158], Chinese shrimp [159], Giant fresh water prawn [160], Ridge white prawn [161] and Oriental river prawns [162]. Another important trait, which has contributed to improved production in aquaculture is sexual maturation. It has been shown that in some some species, sex is closely related to growth. For example, Sun and Liang [163] showed that in common carp, females grow bigger than males at the same age, while in tilapia, the males grow faster than females [164]. Hence, the selection of males for aquaculture increases production in tilapia while the females increase production in carp. Important traits related to improving meat quality include muscle quality [154], muscle fibre [165], texture [165], colour [166, 167], fat percentage [166] and dressed weight percentage [166].

http://dx.doi.org/10.5772/intechopen.69883

Fish species	Trait	Method	References
Blue bream (*Ballerus ballerus*) (Cyprinidae	Thyroid hormones	Transcriptome	[241]
Blunt snout bream (*Megalobrama amblycephala*)	Growth trait	Transcriptome	[242]
Turbot (*Scophthalmus maximus*)	Growth trait	Transcriptome	[243]
Grouper hybrids (*Epinephelus fuscogutatus*)	Superiority in growth	Transcriptome	[244]
Mandarin fish (*Siniperca chuatsi*)	Growth traits	Microsatellite	[245]
Atlantic salmon (*Salmo salar* L.)	Growth traits	SNP/GWAS	[149]
Rainbow trout (*Oncorhynchus mykiss*)	Robustness	Transcriptome	[173]
Nile tilapia (*Oreochromis niloticus*)	Growth traits	Transcriptome	[154]
Nile tilapia (*Oreochromis niloticus*)	Skeletal muscle quality	Transcriptome	[154]
gilthead sea bream (*Sparus aurata*)	Skeletal muscle quality	Transcriptome	[246]
Rainbow trout (*Oncorhynchus mykiss*)	Growth traits	SNP	[150]
Rainbow trout (*Oncorhynchus mykiss*)	Stress factor traits	Transcriptome	[247]
Atlantic cod (*Gadus morhua*)	Growth/reproduction	Transcriptome	[248]
Lake whitefish pairs (*Coregonus* spp. *Salmonidae*)	Reproduction	Transcriptome	[249]
Lake whitefish pairs (*Coregonus* spp. *Salmonidae*)	Adaptation	QTL	[250]
Atlantic salmon (*Salmo salar* L.)	Smoltification	Transcriptome	[177]
Common carp (*Cyprinus carpio*)	Cold tolerance	QTL	[163]
Arctic char (*Salnelinus alpinus*)	Temperature tolerance	QTL	[176]
Arctic char (*Salnelinus alpinus*)	Growth rate	SNP	[251]
Tilapia (*Oreochromis niloticus*)	Cold tolerance	QTL	[175]
Tilapia (*Oreochromis niloticus*)	Fish size	QTL	[175]
Coho salmon (*Oncorhynchus kisutch*)	Flesh colour	QTL	[167]
Rainbow trout (*Oncorhynchus mykiss*)	Spawning time	QTL	[178]
Rainbow trout (*Oncorhynchus mykiss*)	Albinism	QTL	[170]
Rainbow trout (*Oncorhynchus mykiss*)	High temperature tolerance	QTL	[252]

Table 1. Growth and performance traits for different fish species.

Crustacean species	Trait	Method	References
Pandad shrimp (*Pandalus latirostris*)		Microsatellite	[253]
Giant freshwater prawn (*Macrobrachium rosenbergii*)	Growth traits	SNP	[160]
Ridgetail white prawn (*Exopalaemon carinicauda*)	Growth traits	Transcriptome	[161]
Kuruma shrimp (*Marsupenaeus japonicas*)	Growth traits	QTL	[157]
Kuruma shrimp (*Marsupenaeus japonicas*)	High temperature tolerance	QTL	[157]
Kuruma shrimp (*Marsupenaeus japonicas*)	Growth traits	AFLP	[158]
Pacific white shrimp (*Litopenaeus vannamei*)	Growth traits	QTL	[147]
Kuruma shrimp (*Marsupenaeus japonicas*)	Total and carapace length	ALFP	[254]
Indian black tiger shrimp (*Penaeus monodon*)	Sex determining loci	QTL	[255]
Pacific white shrimp (*Litopenaeus vannamei*)	Sex determining loci	Microsatellite	[256]
Chinese shrimp (*Fenneropenaeus chinensis*)	Body length	QTL	[159]
Pacific white shrimp (*Litopenaeus vannamei*)	Body weight and length	QTL	[257]
oriental river prawn (*Macrobrachium nipponense*)	Body length	QTL	[162]
Kuruma shrimp (*Marsupenaeus japonicas*)	Body length	QTL	[158]

Table 2. Growth and performance traits for different crustacean species.

Body appearance traits identified include the red body colour excluding normal black pigmentation in tilapia [168], silvery skin with few spots in rainbow trout [169], albinism in rainbow trout [170] and melanization in threespine sticklebacks (*Gasterosteus aculeatus*) [171]. Genetic traits essential for improving production in fish farming include traits for feed conversion ratio [172], robustness [173], maturation timing [174], cold tolerance [163, 175], high temperature tolerance [176] and salinity tolerance. In anadromous species such as Atlantic salmon, genetic traits for smoltification [177], migration and spawning timing [178] have been determined.

5.2. Disease resistance and susceptibility traits

The rapid expansion of aquaculture to become one of the leading sources of protein in the world has brought with it an increase in infectious diseases in aquaculture. To reduce the disease

burden and prevent the use of antibiotics, which have been shown to have adverse environmental effects, there has been a tremendous increase in genomics studies aimed at identifying disease resistance traits in different cultured organisms. And as such, different approaches such as SNP, MTLS, AFLP, RAPD, RFLP and QTL analyses have been used for the identification of disease resistance and susceptibility traits in different aquatic organisms. In the case of fish viral diseases, QTL resistance traits have been generated for grass cap reovirus (GCRV) infection in grass carp [179], nervous necrosis virus (NNV) in seabass [180], viral hemorrhagic septicemia (VHS) in turbot [181] and rainbow trout [182], infectious salmon anaemia (ISAV) virus in Atlantic salmon, lymphocytic disease virus in Japanese flounder [183] and infectious pancreatic necrosis virus (IPNV) in Atlantic salmon [184, 185]. Among these, the QTL for resistance against IPNV has contributed to significantly reducing the IPNV incidence by >80% from 2008 when IPNV resistance fish were introduced in the Norwegian Atlantic salmon industry to 2015 [186]. Bacteria disease for which QTL resistance traits have been identified include coldwater disease in rainbow trout [187], *Aeromonas hydrophila* in rohu (*Labeo rohita*) [188], *Vibrio anguillarum* in Japanese flounder [189], *Flavobacterium psychrophilum* in rainbow trout [190] and pastuerellosis in Gilhead seabream [191]. As for parasitic diseases, QTL resistance traits have been identified for *Gyrodactylus salaris* in Atlantic salmon [192] and Monohenean parasite (*Benedenia seriolae*) in Yellow tail (*Seriola quinqueradiata*) [193].

In shrimps, resistance traits have been identified for white spot syndrome virus (WSSV) in Indian black tiger shrimp (*Penaeus monodon*) [194, 195], Fenneropenaeus (*Penaeus chinensis*), infectious hypodermal and hematopoietic necrosis virus (IHHNV) resistance in shrimp (*Litopenaeus stylirostris*) [196] and taura syndrome resistance in Pacific white shrimp (*P. vannamei*) [197]. Among these, the QTL for resistance against TSV has contributed to significant reduction of the disease prevalence in shrimps by generating pathogen-specific free disease shrimps for us in breeding programmes in aquaculture.

6. Application of epigenetics in aquaculture

The term 'epigenetics' was first coined by Waddington in 1942 and was defined as changes in the phenotype without inducing changes in the genotype [198, 199]. Studies on chemical modification of DNA bases date as far back as 1948 [200] and by the 1970s, the role of DNA methylation in gene regulation was identified [201]. In subsequent years, the link between DNA methylation and gene expression was established [202] paving way to the discovery of therapeutic drugs such as 5-azacytidine used to block DNA methylation [203]. In principle, epigenetic changes are regulated by (i) chemical modifications on DNA cytosine residues resulting in DNA methylation and, (ii) histone protein modifications on DNA [204, 205]. Current advances in HTS have refined genomic analyses to base-pair resolution making it easier to map entire epigenomes of living organisms enabling us to identify biological markers predictive of the outcome of disease infections, reproduction, growth and adaptation to new environments [206]. As a result of these advances, epigenetics studies in aquaculture have tremendously increased in the last decades with the view to identifying biological markers relevant for improving the production of farmed aquatic organisms. Technologies used for epigenetics analyses in aquaculture include (i) RNA-seq in

Medaka [207] and Nile tilapia [208]; (ii) genome-wide methylated DNA immunoprecipitation sequencing (MeDIP-seq) in Nile tilapia [209] and Medaka [207]; (iii) bisulfite sequencing (BS-seq) in smooth tongue sole (*Cynoglossus semilaevis*) [210, 211], rainbow trout [212] and Nile tilapia [208]; (iv) genetic linkage map analysis using simple sequence length polymorphisms (SSLPs) in medaka [213, 214]; (v) methylation sensitivity amplified polymorphism (MSAP) in Atlantic salmon [18], grass carp [215], brown trout [17], sea urchin (*Glyptocidaris crenularis*) [216] and sea cucumber (*Apostichopus japonicas*) [217]; (vi) 5-methylcytosine immunolocation in sea lamprey (*Petromyzon marinus*) [218]; (vii) restriction endonuclease hydrolysis of DNA using methylation enzymes in Zebrafish [219] and (viii) bisulfite sequencing PCR in Pacific Oyster (*Crassostrea gigas*) [220] and grass carp [221]. As shown in **Table 3**, epigenetics studies carried out this far include studies on reproduction, growth and adaptation traits. In the case of Atlantic salmon, which is one of the most widely studied species, epigenetic studies have been carried out at different stages of the production cycle as shown in **Figure 2**.

6.1. Embryogenesis and reproduction traits

Embryogenesis and reproduction traits determined by epigenetic analyses in aquatic organisms include sexual dimorphism, embryo development, control of gonadal aromatase and male meiosis [208, 222, 223]. Mhanni and McGowan [219] examined the methylation patterns of the zebrafish genome during early embryogenesis and showed that parental genetic contributions to the zygote were differently methylated with the sperm being more hypermethylated than the oocyte genome. However, immediately after fertilization there was a significant decrease in the embryonic genome methylation, but increased rapidly as the embryo developed to normal levels by the gastrulation stage. These observations are consistent with those seen in mouse [224] suggesting that embryo demethylation/re-methylation is conserved across the vertebrate taxa as of part embryogenesis. As for reproduction traits, Wan et al. [208] found several differentially methylated regions (DMRs) on tilapia chromosomal DNA linked to sexual dimorphism in which the males had high methylation levels after prolonged exposure to high temperature conditions. Similarly, Navarro-Martín et al. [222, 223] showed that European seabass juvenile males had double DNA methylation levels than females in the promoter region of gonadal aromatase, the enzyme that converts androgens to estrogens suggesting that methylation levels on gonadal aromatase were predictive of sex determination. Other fish species for which DNA methylation of aromatase has been linked to sex determination include medaka [225] and Japanese flounder (*Paralichthys olivaceus*) [226]. In crustacean, Gómez et al. [227] analysed the post-translational histone modifications in the testis of *Daphnia magna* and identified cytological markers linked to meiosis progression and the silencing of unsynapsed chromatin. Put together, these studies show that DNA methylation and histone modification can induce reproduction and embryogenesis changes in different aquatic organisms.

6.2. Growth and productivity traits

Epigenetic factors associated with growth and productivity identified in aquatic organisms include early maturation, regulation of muscle growth and disease resistance. Early maturation in Atlantic salmon has emerged to be an interesting topic because prior to migration,

Aquatic organism	Epigenetic trait	References
Zebrafish (*Danio rerio*)	Carcinogenesis	[258]
Zebrafish (*Danio rerio*)	Embryo development	[219]
Zebrafish (*Danio rerio*)	Embryonic cardiogenesis	[259]
Medaka (*Oryzias latipes*)	Excision of ToL2 transposal	[260]
Medaka (*Oryzias latipes*)	Control of cardiomyocyte production in response to stress	[214]
Medaka (*Oryzias latipes*)	Hypoxia and transgenerational reproduction impairment	[207]
Nile tilapia (*Oreochromis niloticus*)	High temperature induced masculinization of skeletal muscles	[209]
Nile tilapia (*Oreochromis niloticus*)	Sexual dimorphism	[208]
Atlantic salmon (*Salmo salar* L.)	Early maturation	[18]
European seabass (*Dicentrarchus labrax*)	Temperature dependent sex ratio shift	[222, 223]
Tongue sole (Cynoglossidae)	Sex reversal	[210, 211]
Senegalese sole (*Solea senegalensis*)	Thermal epigenetic regulation of muscle growth	[261]
European eel (*Anguillarum anguillarum*)	Low cadmium exposure	[232]
European eel (*Anguillarum anguillarum*)	Abnormal ovarian DNA methylation-gonadal	[262]
Red eared slider turtle (*Trachemys scripta elegans*)	Control of gonadal aromatase	[263]
Daphnia magna	Male meiosis	[227]
Pacific oyster (*Crassostrea gigas*)	Growth	[220]
Rainbow trout (*Oncorhynchus mykiss*)	Glucose intolerance	[230]
Rainbow trout (*Oncorhynchus mykiss*)	Migration-related phenotypic divergence	[212]
Atlantic Cod (*Gadus morhua* L.)	Photoperiod influence	[228, 229]
Grass carp (*Ctenopharyngodon idella)*	Individual variations	[215]
Grass carp (*Ctenopharyngodon idella)*	Resistance against grass reovirus	[221]

Table 3. Epigenetics application in aquatic organisms.

parr can reach sexual maturity and successfully fertilize adult females. Up to 60% of total paternity in wild populations has been attributed to these precocious male parr or 'sneakers'. To determine the underlying causes of early sexual maturation in parr, Morán and Pérez-Figueroa [18] compared genetic and epigenetic differences of two populations of parr and mature fish originating from two different rivers and found no genetic difference between

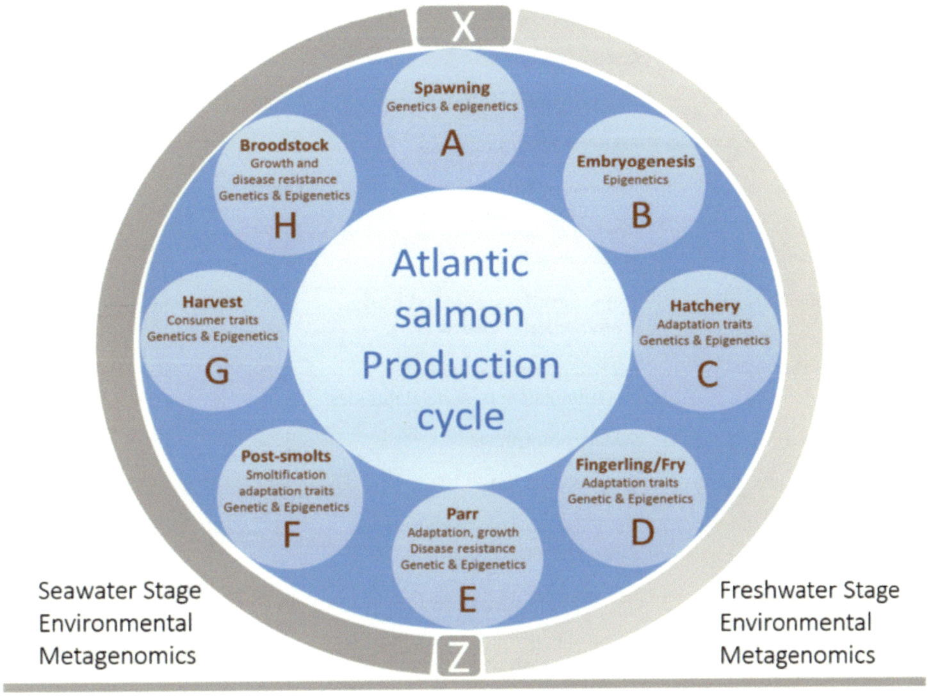

Figure 2. The cycle shows the use of different aspects of functional genomics to improve the production of Atlantic salmon at different stages of the production-cycle. Note that genetics and epigenetics studies are focused on identifying important traits in fish while metagenomics studies are mostly focused on environmental identification of infectious pathogens. Fish from different growth stages are also evaluated for the mucosal microbiota investigations using metagenomics analyses. Nutrigenomics is mostly applied at the outgrower stage. Growth stages are depicted from spawning (A), embryogenesis (B), hatching (C), fingerlings and fry stage (D), Parr stage (E), post-smolts (F), outgrower stage (G) and broodstock (H). Nutrigenomics are after through the feeding stages while the timing of most vaccinations is the parr (D) stage in order to enable fish develop protective antibodies by the post-smolt (E) stage and outgrower stage when they are most vulnerable to stress-related infectious diseases. (X): Depicts the migration of adult fish from seawater into freshwater for spawning. (Z): depicts migration from freshwater to seawater at the parr stage.

parr and mature fish. However, epigenetic analysis showed significant single-locus variations in the gonads followed by the brain and liver between parr and mature fish suggesting that early maturation in Atlantic salmon parr was mediated by epigenetic processes and not genetic differences. As for disease resistance, Shang et al. [221] showed that CpA/CpG methylation of grass carp *Ctenopharyngodon idella* melanoma differentiation associated gene 5 (MDA5) (CiMDA5) was tightly associated with resistance against GCRV. In their findings, they found CpA/CpG methylation sites in the CiMDA5 genome that consisted of putative densely methylated elements (DMEs) that were significantly higher in GCRV susceptible fish than in the resistant fish. In terms of muscle growth, Giannetto et al. [228] found a correlation between DNA (cytosine-5)-methyltransferases (DNMTs) increase in fast muscle with prolonged exposure to light indicating that photoperiod influence may be involved in the DNMTs regulation of muscle growth in Atlantic cod. Similarly, Nagasawa et al. [229] found high histone methyltransferases levels of the mixed-lineage leukaemia (MLL) gene in fast muscle of Atlantic cod subjected to prolonged light exposure, which corresponded with

increase in mRNA expression of myogenic regulatory factors (*Myog* and *Myf-5*) and *Pax7* in fast muscle. Overall, these studies show that DNA methylation and histone modification of chromosomal DNA play an important role in regulating muscle growth, disease resistance and sex maturation in fish.

6.3. Adaption epigenetic traits

Epigenetic factors shown to induce adaptation changes in cultured aquatic organisms include nutrition, migration, salinity and photoperiod exposure. Several nutritional studies have shown that rainbow trout displays persistent hyperglycaemia when fed high carbohydrate (HighCHO) diets. To underpin the underlying causes, Marandel et al. [230] examined the liver of rainbow trout fed HighCHO diets and found global DNA hypomethylation and hypoacetylation of histone H3K9 resembling hyperglycaemic and diabetes conditions in zebrafish and mammals. They also showed that *g6pcb2* ohnologs that encode the glucose-6-phosphatase (G6pc) enzyme involved in gluconeogenesis catalysis were hypomethylated at specific CpG sites indicating that the hepatic epigenetic landscape of rainbow trout can be affected by dietary carbohydrates. As for migration traits, Baerwald et al. [212] identified several DMRs between migratory smolts and resident rainbow trout juveniles in which most DMRs encoded proteins associated with migration showing that epigenetic variations were linked to migration traits in anadromous fish. Their findings were in concordance with Morán et al. [17] who found genome-wide methylation differences between hatchery reared and seawater brown trout. In addition, Morán et al. [17] showed that salt diets used during the seawater phase triggered genome-wide methylation changes when administered in freshwater reared trout indicating that DNA methylation could play a vital role in enabling anadromous fish acclimatize to seawater after transfer from freshwater. DNA methylation and histone modification have also been associated with adaptation changes induced by adverse environmental conditions as shown in Nile tilapia exposed to industrial pollutions [231], eels to cadmium exposure [232], sea urchin (*G. crenularis*) exposure to perfluoroctane sulfonate (PFOS) [216] and the three-spine stickleback (*G. aculeatus*) hexabromocyclododecane (HBCD) exposed to 17-β oestradiol (E_2) and 5-aza 2′ deoxycytidine (5AdC) pollutants [233]. In summary, these studies demonstrate that DNA methylation and histone modification contribute to nutritional, environmental and photoperiod adaptation in different aquatic organisms and that these factors could have an influence on improving production in aquaculture.

7. Whole genome sequencing of aquatic organisms

Although teleost fish are the largest known vertebrate group with more than 27,000 species [8], they account for a small proportion of vertebrate species whose whole genomes have been fully sequenced and characterized. The pufferfish genome is one of the earliest fish genome to be sequenced and characterized by 2002 [234], which raised interests to sequence the genomes of other fish species. The zebrafish (*Danio rerio*) whole genome sequencing project was started by Welcome Trust Sanger Institute in 2001 [235] while the Medaka genome was sequenced in 2007 [236]. Thus, Zebrafish and medaka are not only among the earliest

fish species to have their genomes sequenced and characterized, but they have attracted the highest research in genomic studies among teleost species. Their genomes have been widely used for comparative analyses as model species [235, 237–239]. Sequence analyses of the Atlantic cod genome in 2011 using the whole genome shotgun 454 pyrosequencing technology showed that this fish species lacks the major histocompatibility (MHC) II genes, which are compensated with expansion of the MHC-I and specific adaption of toll-like receptor genes demonstrating that whole genome sequencing can be used to elucidate evolutionary differences in the vertebrate taxa [240]. As shown in **Table 4**, there has been a spontaneous increase in the number of fish species whose genomes have characterized since the discovery of HTS technologies in recent years. Sequencing of other aquatic organism genomes is going on and it is anticipated that as HTS becomes cheaper, more sequences of aquatic organisms will become readily available for more advanced functional genomics research in aquaculture.

Common name	Scientific name	Year Published	Reference
Atlantic salmon	*Salmon salar* L.	2016	[264]
Atlantic cod	*Gadus morhua*	2011	[240]
Asian arowana	*Scleropages formosus*	2015	[8]
Medaka	*Oryzias latipes*	2007	[236]
Nile tilapia	*Oreochromis niloticus*	2015	[7]
Platyfish	*Xiphophorus maculatus*	2013	[265, 266]
Puffer fish	*Takifugu rubripes*	2002	[234]
Puffer fish	*Tetraodon nigroviridis*	2004	[267]
Three-spined stickleback	*Gasterosteus aculeatus*	2012	[268]
Rainbow trout	*Oncorhynchus mykiss*	2014/2016	[269, 270]
Killifish	*Nothobranchius furzeri*	2015	[271, 272]
Pearl oyster	*Pinctada fucata*	2012	[273]

Table 4. Whole genome sequencing of aquatic organisms.

8. Conclusions

In this chapter, we have shown that HTS has contributed to the rapid discovery of novel pathogens in aquaculture using metagenomics, which has significantly contributed in enhancing our ability to develop rationale disease control strategies unlike in the past when it took long from the first report of a clinical disease to identification of a novel pathogen. Moreover, metagenomics enable us to identify and monitor microbial communities found in different ecosystems

used in aquaculture. It has also proved to be an important tool able to map mucosal microbiota of different aquatic organisms. In vaccine production, genomics studies are being used to identify cross-neutralizing antigens able to confer protection across variant strains of the same pathogens. In genetics and epigenetics, several genomics traits have been identified that currently contributing to the improvement of production in aquaculture. Nutrigenomics have not only enhanced our understanding of the genetic markers for enteropathy and other nutritional diseases, but they have also highlighted our ability to formulate diets able to maintain stable GALT homeostasis in the gut. And as shown from the example of the Atlantic salmon production cycle in **Figure 2**, it is evident that functional genomics are used at different production stages of aquatic organisms to improve the overall production in aquaculture. Hence, genomics studies are not only useful at elucidating host-pathogen interactions [13-15], but they also serve as optimization tools for improving the quality and quantity of aquaculture products.

9. Future perspective

As HTS technologies become cheaper, it is anticipated that more genomes for different aquatic organisms will characterized and that this shall pave to a better understanding of the genome duplication seen in some fish species. The use of HTS technologies in pathogen discovery and microbiota inhabiting mucosal surfaces of different aquatic organisms is expected to pave way into timely design of rational disease control strategies. Hence, in future generations, we shall not only sequence whole genomes of all aquatic organisms, but we expect to provide a better understanding of the evolutionary aspects of the vertebrate taxa as well as providing new insight into host-pathogen interaction mechanisms at protein-protein level. It is our perception that current HTS studies are building a strong foundation for more advanced functional genomics developments in the future.

Author details

Hetron M. Munang'andu* and Øystein Evensen

*Address all correspondence to: hetroney.mweemba.munangandu@nmbu.no

Department of Basic Sciences and Aquatic Medicine, Section of Aquatic Medicine and Nutrition, Faculty of Veterinary Medicine and Biosciences, Norwegian University of Life Sciences, Ullevalsveien, Oslo, Norway

References

[1] Gibbs RA. DNA amplification by the polymerase chain reaction. Analytical Chemistry. 1990;**62**(13):1202-1214

[2] Mullis K, Faloona F, Scharf S, Saiki R, Horn G, Erlich H. Specific enzymatic amplification of DNA in vitro: The polymerase chain reaction. In: Cold Spring Harbor Symposia on Quantitative Biology. Edited by Michael A. Innis, David H. Gelfand, John J. Sninsky. Cold Spring Harbor Laboratory Press; Academic Press, San Dieago, USA. 1986. pp. 263-273

[3] Munang'andu HM, Fredriksen BN, Mutoloki S, Dalmo RA, Evensen Ø. The kinetics of CD4+ and CD8+ T-cell gene expression correlate with protection in Atlantic salmon (*Salmo salar* L.) vaccinated against infectious pancreatic necrosis. Vaccine. 2013;**31**(15):1956-1963

[4] Rhodes SD. Quantitative Real-time Polymerase Chain Reaction. In: Encyclopedia of Systems Biology. Dubitzky W., Wolkenhauer O., Yokota H., Cho K.-H. (Eds.) Springer, New York, USA; 2013. pp. 1807-1807

[5] Yamaguchi S, Kaji N, Munang'andu H, Kojima C, Mase M, Tsukamoto K. Quantification of chicken anaemia virus by competitive polymerase chain reaction. Avian Pathology. 2000;**29**(4):305-310

[6] Tsofack JEK, Zamostiano R, Watted S, Berkowitz A, Rosenbluth E, Mishra N, Briese T, Lipkin WI, Kabuusu RM, Ferguson H. Detection of Tilapia Lake virus in clinical samples by culturing and nested reverse Transcription-PCR. Journal of Clinical Microbiology. 2017;**55**(3):759-767

[7] Xia JH, Bai Z, Meng Z, Zhang Y, Wang L, Liu F, Jing W, Wan ZY, Li J, Lin H. Signatures of selection in tilapia revealed by whole genome resequencing. Scientific Reports. 2015;**5**:14168. doi: 10.1038/srep14168.

[8] Austin CM, Tan MH, Croft LJ, Hammer MP, Gan HM. Whole genome sequencing of the Asian arowana (Scleropages formosus) provides insights into the evolution of ray-finned fishes. Genome Biology and Evolution. 2015 Oct 6;**7**(10):2885-95. doi: 10.1093/gbe/evv186.

[9] Munang'andu HM, Mugimba KK, Byarugaba DK, Mutoloki S, Evensen Ø. Current advances on virus discovery and diagnostic role of viral metagenomics in aquatic organisms. Frontiers in Microbiology. 2017;**8**:406. doi: 10.3389/fmicb.2017.00406.

[10] Munang'andu HM. Environmental viral metagenomics analyses in aquaculture: Applications in epidemiology and disease control. Frontiers in Microbiology. 2016;7:1986

[11] Gajardo K, Jaramillo-Torres A, Kortner TM, Merrifield DL, Tinsley J, Bakke AM, Krogdahl Å. Alternative protein sources in the diet modulate microbiota and functionality in the distal intestine of Atlantic salmon (Salmo salar). Applied and Environmental Microbiology. 2016:02615-02616

[12] Gajardo K, Rodiles A, Kortner TM, Krogdahl Å, Bakke AM, Merrifield DL, Sørum H. A high-resolution map of the gut microbiota in Atlantic salmon (*Salmo salar*): A basis for comparative gut microbial research. Scientific Reports. 2016;**6**:30893. doi: 10.1038/srep30893.

[13] Xu C, Evensen O, Munang'andu HM. A de novo transcriptome analysis shows that modulation of the JAK-STAT signaling pathway by salmonid alphavirus subtype 3 favors virus replication in macrophage/dendritic-like TO-cells. BMC Genomics. 2016;**17**:390

[14] Xu C, Evensen O, Munang'andu HM. De Novo transcriptome analysis shows that SAV-3 infection upregulates pattern recognition receptors of the endosomal Toll-Like and RIG-I-Like receptor signaling pathways in Macrophage/Dendritic like TO-Cells. Viruses. 2016;**8**(4):114

[15] Xu C, Evensen Ø, Munang'andu HM. De novo assembly and transcriptome analysis of Atlantic salmon macrophage/dendritic-like TO cells following type I IFN treatment and Salmonid alphavirus subtype-3 infection. BMC Genomics. 2015;**16**(1):96

[16] Morais S, Silva T, Cordeiro O, Rodrigues P, Guy DR, Bron JE, Taggart JB, Bell JG, Tocher DR. Effects of genotype and dietary fish oil replacement with vegetable oil on the intestinal transcriptome and proteome of Atlantic salmon (*Salmo salar*). BMC Genomics. 2012;**13**(1):448

[17] Morán P, Marco-Rius F, Megías M, Covelo-Soto L, Pérez-Figueroa A. Environmental induced methylation changes associated with seawater adaptation in brown trout. Aquaculture. 2013;**392**:77-83

[18] Morán P, Pérez-Figueroa A. Methylation changes associated with early maturation stages in the Atlantic salmon. BMC Genetics. 2011;**12**(1):86

[19] Moffitt CM, Cajas-Cano L. Blue growth: The 2014 FAO state of world fisheries and aquaculture. Fisheries. 2014;**39**(11):552-553

[20] Bibby K. Metagenomic identification of viral pathogens. Trends in Biotechnology. 2013;**31**(5):275-279

[21] Alavandi S, Poornima M. Viral metagenomics: A tool for virus discovery and diversity in aquaculture. Indian Journal of Virology. 2012;**23**(2):88-98

[22] McGonigle R. Acute catarrhal enteritis of salmonid fingerling. Journal Transactions of the American Fisheries Society. 1941;**70**(7)

[23] Wolf K, Snieszko S, Dunbar C, Pyle E. Virus nature of infectious pancreatic necrosis in trout. Proceedings of the Society for Experimental Biology and Medicine. 1960;**104**(1):105-108

[24] Jensen MH. Research on the virus of Egtved disease. Annals of the New York Academy of Sciences. 1965;**126**:422-426

[25] Amin A, Trasti J. Endomyocarditis in Atlantic salmon in Norwegian seafarms. Bulletin-European Association of Fish Pathologists. 1988;**8**:70-71

[26] Boucher P, Castric J, Laurencin FB. Observation of virus-like particles in rainbow trout *Oncorhynchus mykiss* infected with sleeping disease virulent material. Bulletin of the European Association of Fish Pathologists (United Kingdom). 1995;**14**:215-216

[27] Castric J, Baudin Laurencin F, Bremont M, Jeffroy J, Ven Al, Bearzotti M. Isolation of the virus responsible for sleeping disease in experimentally infected rainbow trout

(*Oncorhynchus mykiss*). Bulletin of the European Association of Fish Pathologists. 1997;**17**(1):27-30

[28] Wingfield W, Fryer J, Pilcher K. Properties of the sockeye salmon virus (Oregon strain). Experimental Biology and Medicine. 1969;**130**(4):1055-1059

[29] Glazebrook J, Heasman M, Beer S. Picorna-like viral particles associated with mass mortalities in larval barramundi, Lates calcarifer Bloch. Journal of Fish Diseases. 1990;**13**(3):245-249

[30] Munday B, Kwang J, Moody N. Betanodavirus infections of teleost fish: A review. Journal of Fish Diseases. 2002;**25**(3):127-142

[31] Haugland Ø, Mikalsen AB, Nilsen P, Lindmo K, Thu BJ, Eliassen TM, Roos N, Rode M, Evensen Ø. Cardiomyopathy syndrome of Atlantic salmon (*Salmo salar* L.) is caused by a double-stranded RNA virus of the Totiviridae family. Journal of Virology. 2011;**85**(11):5275-5286

[32] Kongtorp R, Kjerstad A, Taksdal T, Guttvik A, Falk K. Heart and skeletal muscle inflammation in Atlantic salmon, *Salmo salar* L.: A new infectious disease. Journal of Fish Diseases. 2004;**27**(6):351-358

[33] Palacios G, Lovoll M, Tengs T, Hornig M, Hutchison S, Hui J, Kongtorp R-T, Savji N, Bussetti AV, Solovyov A. Heart and skeletal muscle inflammation of farmed salmon is associated with infection with a novel reovirus. PLoS one. 2010;**5**(7):e11487

[34] Tarján Z, Pénzes J, Tóth R, Benko M. First detection of circovirus-like sequences in amphibians and novel putative circoviruses in fishes. Acta Veterinaria Hungarica. 2013;**62**(1):134-144

[35] Fichtner D, Philipps A, Groth M, Schmidt-Posthaus H, Granzow H, Dauber M, Platzer M, Bergmann SM, Schrudde D, Sauerbrei A. Characterization of a novel picornavirus isolate from a diseased European eel (*Anguilla anguilla*). Journal of Virology. 2013;**87**(19):10895-10899

[36] Reuter G, Pankovics P, Delwart E, Boros Á. A novel posavirus-related single-stranded RNA virus from fish (*Cyprinus carpio*). Archives of Virology. 2015;**160**(2):565-568

[37] Reuter G, Boros Á, Delwart E, Pankovics P. Novel seadornavirus (family Reoviridae) related to Banna virus in Europe. Archives of Virology. 2013;**158**(10):2163-2167

[38] Lotz J. Viruses, biosecurity and specific pathogen-free stocks in shrimp aquaculture. World Journal of Microbiology and Biotechnology. 1997;**13**(4):405-413

[39] van Hulten MC, Witteveldt J, Peters S, Kloosterboer N, Tarchini R, Fiers M, Sandbrink H, Lankhorst RK, Vlak JM. The white spot syndrome virus DNA genome sequence. Virology. 2001;**286**(1):7-22

[40] Yang F, He J, Lin X, Li Q, Pan D, Zhang X, Xu X. Complete genome sequence of the shrimp white spot bacilliform virus. Journal of Virology. 2001;**75**(23):11811-11820

[41] Jimenez R. Sindrome de taura (Resumen). Acuacultura del Ecuador. 1992;**1**:1-16

[42] Hasson K, Lightner DV, Poulos B, Redman R, White B, Brock J, Bonami J. Taura syndrome in *Penaeus vannamei*: Demonstration of a viral etiology. Diseases of Aquatic Organisms. 1995;**23**(2):115-126

[43] Limsuwan C. Handbook for Cultivation of Black Tiger Prawns. Bangkok: Tansetakit Co Ltd; 1991

[44] Tang KF-J, Lightner DV. A yellow head virus gene probe: Nucleotide sequence and application for in situ hybridization. Diseases of Aquatic Organisms. 1999;**35**(3):165-173

[45] Brock J, Lightner D, Bell T. A review of four virus (BP, MBV, BMN and IHHNV) diseases of penaeid shrimp with particular reference to clinical significance, diagnosis and control in shrimp aquaculture. Proceedings of the 71st International Council for the Exploration of the Sea, CM. 1983:1-18.

[46] Lightner D, Pantoja C, Poulos B, Tang K, Redman R, Andreas T, Bonami J. Infectious myonecrosis (IMN): A new virus disease of Litopenaeus vannamei. Aquaculture. 2004;**242**:353

[47] Lightner DV, Redman R. A parvo-like virus disease of penaeid shrimp. Journal of Invertebrate Pathology. 1985;**45**(1):47-53

[48] Nunes AJ, Martins P, Gesteira TCV. Carcinicultura ameaçada. Rev Panoram Aquic. 2004;**83**:37-51

[49] Poulos BT, Tang KF, Pantoja CR, Bonami JR, Lightner DV. Purification and characterization of infectious myonecrosis virus of penaeid shrimp. Journal of General Virology. 2006;**87**(4):987-996

[50] Tang KF, Pantoja CR, Redman RM, Lightner DV. Development of in situ hybridization and RT-PCR assay for the detection of a nodavirus (PvNV) that causes muscle necrosis in *Penaeus vannamei*. Diseases of Aquatic Organisms. 2007;**75**(3):183-190

[51] Gadan K, Sandtro A, Marjara IS, Santi N, Munang'andu HM, Evensen O. Stress-induced reversion to virulence of infectious pancreatic necrosis virus in naive fry of Atlantic Salmon (*Salmo salar* L.). Plos One. 2013;**8**(2)

[52] Angly FE, Felts B, Breitbart M, Salamon P, Edwards RA, Carlson C, Chan AM, Haynes M, Kelley S, Liu H. The marine viromes of four oceanic regions. PLoS Biology. 2006;**4**(11):e368

[53] Dinsdale EA, Pantos O, Smriga S, Edwards RA, Angly F, Wegley L, Hatay M, Hall D, Brown E, Haynes M. Microbial ecology of four coral atolls in the Northern Line Islands. PloS One. 2008;**3**(2):e1584

[54] Programme UNE. Marine and coastal ecosystems and human well-being: A synthesis report based on the findings of the Millennium Ecosystem Assessment. UNEP. 2006:76

[55] Nogales B, Lanfranconi MP, Piña-Villalonga JM, Bosch R. Anthropogenic perturbations in marine microbial communities. FEMS Microbiology Reviews. 2011;**35**(2):275-298

[56] Roux S, Enault F, Robin A, Ravet V, Personnic S, Theil S, Colombet J, Sime-Ngando T, Debroas D. Assessing the diversity and specificity of two freshwater viral communities through metagenomics. PLoS One. 2012;7(3):e33641

[57] Tseng C-H, Chiang P-W, Shiah F-K, Chen Y-L, Liou J-R, Hsu T-C, Maheswararajah S, Saeed I, Halgamuge S, Tang S-L. Microbial and viral metagenomes of a subtropical freshwater reservoir subject to climatic disturbances. The ISME Journal. 2013;7(12):2374-2386

[58] Islam MS, Tanaka M. Impacts of pollution on coastal and marine ecosystems including coastal and marine fisheries and approach for management: A review and synthesis. Marine Pollution Bulletin. 2004;**48**(7):624-649

[59] Halpern BS, Walbridge S, Selkoe KA, Kappel CV, Micheli F, D'agrosa C, Bruno JF, Casey KS, Ebert C, Fox HE. A global map of human impact on marine ecosystems. Science. 2008;**319**(5865):948-952

[60] Port JA, Wallace JC, Griffith WC, Faustman EM. Metagenomic profiling of microbial composition and antibiotic resistance determinants in Puget Sound. PLoS One. 2012;7(10):e48000

[61] Morán AC, Hengst MB, De la Iglesia R, Andrade S, Correa JA, González B. Changes in bacterial community structure associated with coastal copper enrichment. Environmental Toxicology and Chemistry. 2008;**27**(11):2239-2245

[62] Sugita H, Nakamura H, Shimada T. Microbial communities associated with filter materials in recirculating aquaculture systems of freshwater fish. Aquaculture. 2005;**243**(1):403-409

[63] Itoi S, Niki A, Sugita H. Changes in microbial communities associated with the conditioning of filter material in recirculating aquaculture systems of the pufferfish *Takifugu rubripes*. Aquaculture. 2006;**256**(1):287-295

[64] Schneider O, Chabrillon-Popelka M, Smidt H, Haenen O, Sereti V, Eding EH, Verreth JA. HRT and nutrients affect bacterial communities grown on recirculation aquaculture system effluents. FEMS Microbiology Ecology. 2007;**60**(2):207-219

[65] Itoi S, Ebihara N, Washio S, Sugita H. Nitrite-oxidizing bacteria, Nitrospira, distribution in the outer layer of the biofilm from filter materials of a recirculating water system for the goldfish *Carassius auratus*. Aquaculture. 2007;**264**(1):297-308

[66] Fox BK, Tamaru CS, Hollyer J, Castro LF, Fonseca JM, Jay-Russell M, Low T. A preliminary study of microbial water quality related to food safety in recirculating aquaponic fish and vegetable production systems. College of Tropical Agriculture and Human Resources, University of Hawaii at Manoa Food Safety and Technology. 2012

[67] Munguia-Fragozo P, Alatorre-Jacome O, Rico-Garcia E, Torres-Pacheco I, Cruz-Hernandez A, Ocampo-Velazquez RV, Garcia-Trejo JF, Guevara-Gonzalez RG. Perspective for aquaponic systems: "Omic" technologies for microbial community analysis. BioMed Research International. 2015;**2015**:480386. doi: 10.1155/2015/480386.

[68] Larsen A, Tao Z, Bullard SA, Arias CR. Diversity of the skin microbiota of fishes: Evidence for host species specificity. FEMS Microbiology Ecology. 2013;**85**(3):483-494

[69] Lokesh J, Kiron V. Transition from freshwater to seawater reshapes the skin-associated microbiota of Atlantic salmon. Scientific Reports. 2016;**6**:19707. doi: 10.1038/srep19707.

[70] Wilson B, Danilowicz BS, Meijer WG. The diversity of bacterial communities associated with Atlantic cod Gadus morhua. Microbiology Ecology. 2008;**55**(3):425-434

[71] Boutin S, Sauvage C, Bernatchez L, Audet C, Derome N. Inter individual variations of the fish skin microbiota: Host genetics basis of mutualism? PLoS One. 2014;**9**(7):e102649

[72] Lyons PP, Turnbull JF, Dawson KA, Crumlish M. Phylogenetic and functional characterization of the distal intestinal microbiome of rainbow trout *Oncorhynchus mykiss* from both farm and aquarium settings. Journal of Applied Microbiology. 2016. **2017**;122(2):347-363. doi: 10.1111/jam.13347.

[73] Mouchet MA, Bouvier C, Bouvier T, Troussellier M, Escalas A, Mouillot D. Genetic difference but functional similarity among fish gut bacterial communities through molecular and biochemical fingerprints. FEMS Microbiology Ecology. 2012;**79**(3):568-580

[74] Desai AR, Links MG, Collins SA, Mansfield GS, Drew MD, Van Kessel AG, Hill JE. Effects of plant-based diets on the distal gut microbiome of rainbow trout (*Oncorhynchus mykiss*). Aquaculture. 2012;**350**:134-142

[75] Star B, Haverkamp TH, Jentoft S, Jakobsen KS. Next generation sequencing shows high variation of the intestinal microbial species composition in Atlantic cod caught at a single location. BMC Microbiology. 2013;**13**(1):248

[76] Navarrete P, Magne F, Araneda C, Fuentes P, Barros L, Opazo R, Espejo R, Romero J. PCR-TTGE analysis of 16S rRNA from rainbow trout (*Oncorhynchus mykiss*) gut microbiota reveals host-specific communities of active bacteria. PloS One. 2012;7(2):e31335

[77] Boutin S, Audet C, Derome N. Probiotic treatment by indigenous bacteria decreases mortality without disturbing the natural microbiota of Salvelinus fontinalis. Canadian Journal of Microbiology. 2013;**59**(10):662-670

[78] Skrodenyte-Arbaciauskiene V, Sruoga A, Butkauskas D. Assessment of microbial diversity in the river trout *Salmo trutta fario* L. intestinal tract identified by partial 16S rRNA gene sequence analysis. Fisheries Science. 2006;**72**(3):597-602

[79] Semova I, Carten JD, Stombaugh J, Mackey LC, Knight R, Farber SA, Rawls JF. Microbiota regulate intestinal absorption and metabolism of fatty acids in the zebrafish. Cell Host & Microbe. 2012;**12**(3):277-288

[80] Ye L, Amberg J, Chapman D, Gaikowski M, Liu W-T. Fish gut microbiota analysis differentiates physiology and behavior of invasive Asian carp and indigenous American fish. The ISME Journal. 2014;**8**(3):541-551

[81] Li X, Yu Y, Feng W, Yan Q, Gong Y. Host species as a strong determinant of the intestinal microbiota of fish larvae. The Journal of Microbiology. 2012;**50**(1):29-37

[82] Li X, Yan Q, Xie S, Hu W, Yu Y, Hu Z. Gut microbiota contributes to the growth of fast-growing transgenic common carp (*Cyprinus carpio* L.). PLoS One. 2013;**8**(5):e64577

[83] Wu S, Wang G, Angert ER, Wang W, Li W, Zou H. Composition, diversity, and origin of the bacterial community in grass carp intestine. PLoS One. 2012;**7**(2):e30440

[84] Sun Y, Yang H, Ling Z, Chang J, Ye J. Gut microbiota of fast and slow growing grouper *Epinephelus coioides*. African Journal of Microbiology Research. 2009;**3**(11):637-640

[85] Tapia-Paniagua ST, Chabrillón M, Díaz-Rosales P, de la Banda IG, Lobo C, Balebona MC, Moriñigo MA. Intestinal microbiota diversity of the flat fish *Solea senegalensis* (Kaup, 1858) following probiotic administration. Microbial Ecology. 2010;**60**(2):310-319

[86] Xia JH, Lin G, Fu GH, Wan ZY, Lee M, Wang L, Liu XJ, Yue GH. The intestinal microbiome of fish under starvation. BMC Genomics. 2014;**15**(1):266

[87] Liu H, Guo X, Gooneratne R, Lai R, Zeng C, Zhan F, Wang W. The gut microbiome and degradation enzyme activity of wild freshwater fishes influenced by their trophic levels. Scientific Reports. 2016;**6**:24340. doi: 10.1038/srep24340.

[88] Lyons PP, Turnbull JF, Dawson KA, Crumlish M. Phylogenetic and functional characterization of the distal intestinal microbiome of rainbow trout *Oncorhynchus mykiss* from both farm and aquarium settings. Journal of Applied Microbiology. 2017;**122**(2):347-363

[89] Wong S, Waldrop T, Summerfelt S, Davidson J, Barrows F, Kenney PB, Welch T, Wiens GD, Snekvik K, Rawls JF. Aquacultured rainbow trout (*Oncorhynchus mykiss*) possess a large core intestinal microbiota that is resistant to variation in diet and rearing density. Applied and Environmental Microbiology. 2013;**79**(16):4974-4984

[90] Xing M, Hou Z, Yuan J, Liu Y, Qu Y, Liu B. Taxonomic and functional metagenomic profiling of gastrointestinal tract microbiome of the farmed adult turbot (*Scophthalmus maximus*). FEMS Microbiology Ecology. 2013;**86**(3):432-443

[91] Li Y, Xie W, Li Q. Characterisation of the bacterial community structures in the intestine of *Lampetra morii*. Antonie van Leeuwenhoek. 2016;**109**(7):979-986

[92] Sanders JG, Beichman AC, Roman J, Scott JJ, Emerson D, McCarthy JJ, Girguis PR. Baleen whales host a unique gut microbiome with similarities to both carnivores and herbivores. Nature Communications. 2015;**6**:8285. doi: 10.1038/ncomms9285.

[93] Etyemez M, Balcázar JL. Bacterial community structure in the intestinal ecosystem of rainbow trout (*Oncorhynchus mykiss*) as revealed by pyrosequencing-based analysis of 16S rRNA genes. Research in Veterinary Science. 2015;**100**:8-11

[94] Jan C, Petersen JM, Werner J, Teeling H, Huang S, Glöckner FO, Golyshina OV, Dubilier N, Golyshin PN, Jebbar M. The gill chamber epibiosis of deep-sea shrimp Rimicaris exoculata: An in-depth metagenomic investigation and discovery of Zetaproteobacteria. Environmental Microbiology. 2014;**16**(9):2723-2738

[95] Prakash T, Taylor TD. Functional assignment of metagenomic data: Challenges and applications. Briefings in Bioinformatics. 2012;**13**(6):711-727

[96] Quinn NL, Levenkova N, Chow W, Bouffard P, Boroevich KA, Knight JR, Jarvie TP, Lubieniecki KP, Desany BA, Koop BF. Assessing the feasibility of GS FLX Pyrosequencing for sequencing the Atlantic salmon genome. BMC Genomics. 2008;**9**(1):404

[97] Edwards RA, Rohwer F. Viral metagenomics. Nature Reviews Microbiology. 2005;**3**(6): 504-510

[98] Hunter S, Jones P, Mitchell A, Apweiler R, Attwood TK, Bateman A, Bernard T, Binns D, Bork P, Burge S. InterPro in 2011: New developments in the family and domain prediction database. Nucleic Acids Research. 2011:(**Database** issue):D306-12. doi: 10.1093/nar/gkr948.

[99] Attwood TK, Bradley P, Flower DR, Gaulton A, Maudling N, Mitchell AL, Moulton G, Nordle A, Paine K, Taylor P. PRINTS and its automatic supplement, prePRINTS. Nucleic Acids Research. 2003;**31**(1):400-402

[100] Pellegrini M, Marcotte EM, Thompson MJ, Eisenberg D, Yeates TO. Assigning protein functions by comparative genome analysis: Protein phylogenetic profiles. Proceedings of the National Academy of Sciences. 1999;**96**(8):4285-4288

[101] Dandekar T, Snel B, Huynen M, Bork P. Conservation of gene order: A fingerprint of proteins that physically interact. Trends in Biochemical Sciences. 1998;**23**(9):324-328

[102] Overbeek R, Fonstein M, D'souza M, Pusch GD, Maltsev N. The use of gene clusters to infer functional coupling. Proceedings of the National Academy of Sciences. 1999;**96**(6):2896-2901

[103] Calduch-Giner JA, Sitjà-Bobadilla A, Pérez-Sánchez J. Gene expression profiling reveals functional specialization along the intestinal tract of a carnivorous teleostean fish (*Dicentrarchus labrax*). Frontiers in Physiology. 2016;**7**:359. doi: 10.3389/fphys.2016.00359.

[104] Ezeasor D, Stokoe W. Light and electron microscopic studies on the absorptive cells of the intestine, caeca and rectum of the adult rainbow trout, *Salmo gairdneri*, Rich. Journal of Fish Biology. 1981;**18**(5):527-544

[105] Nasruddin NS, Azmai MNA, Ismail A, Saad MZ, Daud HM, Zulkifli SZ. Histological features of the gastrointestinal tract of wild Indonesian shortfin eel, Anguilla bicolor bicolor (McClelland, 1844), captured in Peninsular Malaysia. The Scientific World Journal. 2014;**2014**:312670. doi: 10.1155/2014/312670.

[106] Munang'andu HM, Mutoloki S, Evensen Ø. A review of the immunological mechanisms following mucosal vaccination of finfish. Frontiers in Immunology. 2015;**6**:427

[107] Mutoloki S, Munang'andu HM, Evensen Ø. Oral vaccination of fish–antigen preparations, uptake, and immune induction. Frontiers in Immunology. 2015;**6**:519

[108] Salinas I. The mucosal immune system of teleost fish. Biology. 2015;**4**(3):525-539

[109] Munang'andu HM, Mutoloki S, Evensen Ø. An overview of challenges limiting the design of protective mucosal vaccines for finfish. Frontiers in Immunology. 2015;**6**:542

[110] Król E, Douglas A, Tocher DR, Crampton VO, Speakman JR, Secombes CJ, Martin SA. Differential responses of the gut transcriptome to plant protein diets in farmed Atlantic salmon. BMC Genomics. 2016;**17**(1):156

[111] Torrecillas S, Montero D, Caballero MJ, Pittman KA, Custódio M, Campo A, Sweetman J, Izquierdo M. Dietary mannan oligosaccharides: Counteracting the side effects of soybean meal oil inclusion on european sea bass (*Dicentrarchus labrax*) gut health and skin mucosa mucus production? Frontiers in Immunology. 2015;**6**:397. doi: 10.3389/fimmu.2015.00397.

[112] Azeredo R, Pérez-Sánchez J, Sitjà-Bobadilla A, Fouz B, Tort L, Aragão C, Oliva-Teles A, Costas B. European sea bass (*Dicentrarchus labrax*) immune status and disease resistance are impaired by arginine dietary supplementation. PLoS One. 2015;**10**(10):e0139967

[113] Estensoro I, Ballester-Lozano G, Benedito-Palos L, Grammes F, Martos-Sitcha JA, Mydland L-T, Calduch-Giner JA, Fuentes J, Karalazos V, Ortiz Á. Dietary butyrate helps to restore the intestinal status of a marine teleost (*Sparus aurata*) fed extreme diets low in fish meal and fish oil. PLoS One. 2016;**11**(11):e0166564

[114] Núñez-Acuña G, Gonçalves AT, Valenzuela-Muñoz V, Pino-Marambio J, Wadsworth S, Gallardo-Escárate C. Transcriptome immunomodulation of in-feed additives in Atlantic salmon *Salmo salar* infested with sea lice Caligus rogercresseyi. Fish & Shellfish Immunology. 2015;**47**(1):450-460

[115] Olsvik PA, Hemre G-I, Waagbø R. Correction: Exploring early micronutrient deficiencies in rainbow trout (*Oncorhynchus mykiss*) by Next-Generation sequencing Technology-From black box to functional genomics. PLoS One. 2016;**11**(5):e0156668

[116] Zhao H, Li C, Beck BH, Zhang R, Thongda W, Davis DA, Peatman E. Impact of feed additives on surface mucosal health and columnaris susceptibility in channel catfish fingerlings, *Ictalurus punctatus*. Fish & Shellfish Immunology. 2015;**46**(2):624-637

[117] Li C, Beck BH, Peatman E. Nutritional impacts on gene expression in the surface mucosa of blue catfish (*Ictalurus furcatus*). Developmental & Comparative Immunology. 2014;**44**(1):226-234

[118] Rurangwa E, Sipkema D, Kals J, ter Veld M, Forlenza M, Bacanu GM, Smidt H, Palstra AP. Impact of a novel protein meal on the gastrointestinal microbiota and the host transcriptome of larval zebrafish *Danio rerio*. Frontiers in Physiology. 2015;**6**:133. doi: 10.3389/fphys.2015.00133.

[119] Corthésy-Theulaz I, den Dunnen JT, Ferré P, Geurts JM, Müller M, van Belzen N, van Ommen B. Nutrigenomics: The impact of biomics technology on nutrition research. Annals of Nutrition and Metabolism. 2005;**49**(6):355-365

[120] Poirion OB, Zhu X, Ching T, Garmire L. Single-Cell transcriptomics bioinformatics and computational challenges. Frontiers in Genetics. 2016;**7**:163.

[121] Stegle O, Teichmann SA, Marioni JC. Computational and analytical challenges in single-cell transcriptomics. Nature Reviews Genetics. 2015;**16**(3):133-145

[122] Wang Z, Gerstein M, Snyder M. RNA-Seq: A revolutionary tool for transcriptomics. Nature Reviews Genetics. 2009;**10**(1):57-63

[123] Neeha V, Kinth P. Nutrigenomics research: A review. Journal of Food Science and Technology. 2013;**50**(3):415-428

[124] Müller M, Kersten S. Nutrigenomics: Goals and strategies. Nature Reviews Genetics. 2003;**4**(4):315-322

[125] Munang'andu HM, Mutoloki S, Evensen O. Acquired immunity and vaccination against infectious pancreatic necrosis virus of salmon. Developmental & Comparative Immunology. 2014;**43**(2):184-196

[126] Munang'andu HM, Sandtro A, Mutoloki S, Brudeseth BE, Santi N, Evensen O. Immunogenicity and cross protective ability of the central VP2 amino acids of infectious pancreatic necrosis virus in Atlantic salmon (*Salmo salar* L.). PLoS One;2013;**8**(1):e54263

[127] Christie K. Immunization with viral antigens: Infectious pancreatic necrosis. Developments in Biological Standardization. 1996;**90**:191-199

[128] Costa J, Adams A, Bron J, Thompson K, Starkey W, Richards R. Identification of B-cell epitopes on the betanodavirus capsid protein. Journal of Fish Diseases. 2007;**30**(7):419-426

[129] Ou-yang Z, Wang P, Huang Y, Huang X, Wan Q, Zhou S, Wei J, Zhou Y, Qin Q. Selection and identification of Singapore grouper iridovirus vaccine candidate antigens using bioinformatics and DNA vaccination. Veterinary Immunology and Immunopathology. 2012;**149**(1):38-45

[130] Munang'andu HM, Mutoloki S, Evensen Ø. Non-replicating Vaccines. Fish Vaccination. 22-32

[131] Munang'andu HM, Evensen Ø. A review of intra-and extracellular antigen delivery systems for virus vaccines of finfish. Journal of Immunology Research. 2015;**2015**

[132] Munang'andu HM, Paul J, Evensen Ø. An overview of vaccination strategies and antigen delivery systems for streptococcus agalactiae vaccines in Nile Tilapia (*Oreochromis niloticus*). Vaccines. 2016;**4**(4):48

[133] Handfield M, Brady LJ, Progulske-Fox A, Hillman JD. IVIAT: A novel method to identify microbial genes expressed specifically during human infections. Trends in Microbiology. 2000;**8**(7):336-339

[134] Sun Y, Hu Y-H, Liu C-S, Sun L. Construction and analysis of an experimental Streptococcus iniae DNA vaccine. Vaccine. 2010;**28**(23):3905-3912

[135] Zou YX, Mo ZL, Hao B, Ye XH, Guo DS, Zhang PJ. Screening of genes expressed in vivo after infection by *Vibrio anguillarum* M3. Letters in Applied Microbiology. 2010;**51**(5):564-569

[136] Menanteau-Ledouble S, El-Matbouli M. Antigens of *Aeromonas salmonicida* subsp. *salmonicida* specifically induced in vivo in Oncorhynchus mykiss. Journal of Fish Diseases. 2015;**39**(8):1015-9. doi: 10.1111/jfd.12430.

[137] Menanteau-Ledouble S, Soliman H, Kumar G, El-Matbouli M. Use of in vivo induced antigen technology to identify genes from *Aeromonas salmonicida* subsp. *salmonicida* that are specifically expressed during infection of the rainbow trout *Oncorhynchus mykiss*. BMC Veterinary Research. 2014;**10**(1):298

[138] Jiao X-D, Dang W, Hu Y-H, Sun L. Identification and immunoprotective analysis of an in vivo-induced *Edwardsiella tarda* antigen. Fish & Shellfish Immunology. 2009;**27**(5):633-638

[139] Nho SW, Hikima J-i, Cha IS, Park SB, Jang HB, del Castillo CS, Kondo H, Hirono I, Aoki T, Jung TS. Complete genome sequence and immunoproteomic analyses of the fish bacterial pathogen *Streptococcus parauberis*. Journal of Bacteriology. 2011: 00182-00111

[140] Sun Y, Liu C-S, Sun L. Construction and analysis of the immune effect of an *Edwardsiella tarda* DNA vaccine encoding a D15-like surface antigen. Fish & Shellfish Immunology. 2011;**30**(1):273-279

[141] Board BA. Norwegian breeding strategies—a success story of Long-term benefits

[142] Lester LJ. Developing a selective breeding program for penaeid shrimp mariculture. Aquaculture. 1983;**33**(1-4):41-50

[143] Argue BJ, Arce SM, Lotz JM, Moss SM. Selective breeding of Pacific white shrimp (*Litopenaeus vannamei*) for growth and resistance to Taura Syndrome Virus. Aquaculture. 2002;**204**(3):447-460

[144] López ME, Neira R, Yáñez JM. Applications in the search for genomic selection signatures in fish. Frontiers in Genetics. 2014;**5**

[145] McAndrew B, Napier J. Application of genetics and genomics to aquaculture development: Current and future directions. The Journal of Agricultural Science. 2011;**149**(S1):143-151

[146] Andriantahina F, Liu X, Huang H. Genetic map construction and quantitative trait locus (QTL) detection of growth-related traits in *Litopenaeus vannamei* for selective breeding applications. PloS One. 2013;**8**(9):e75206

[147] Li Y, Byrne K, Miggiano E, Whan V, Moore S, Keys S, Crocos P, Preston N, Lehnert S. Genetic mapping of the kuruma prawn *Penaeus japonicus* using AFLP markers. Aquaculture. 2003;**219**(1):143-156

[148] Geldermann, H. Investigations on inheritance of quantitative characters in animals by gene markers I. Methods. TAG Theoretical and Applied Genetics. 1975;**46**(7):319-330

[149] Tsai H-Y, Hamilton A, Tinch AE, Guy DR, Gharbi K, Stear MJ, Matika O, Bishop SC, Houston RD. Genome wide association and genomic prediction for growth traits in juvenile farmed Atlantic salmon using a high density SNP array. BMC Genomics. 2015;**16**(1):969

[150] Salem M, Vallejo RL, Leeds TD, Palti Y, Liu S, Sabbagh A, Rexroad III CE, Yao J. RNA-Seq identifies SNP markers for growth traits in rainbow trout. PLoS One. 2012;**7**(5):e36264

[151] Liu H, Fu B, Pang M, Feng X, Wang X, Yu X, Tong J. QTL fine mapping and identification of candidate genes for growth-related traits in bighead carp (*Hypophthalmichehys nobilis*). Aquaculture. 2016;**465**:134-143

[152] Lv W, Zheng X, Kuang Y, Cao D, Yan Y, Sun X. QTL variations for growth-related traits in eight distinct families of common carp (*Cyprinus carpio*). BMC Genetics. 2016;**17**(1):65

[153] Laghari M, Lashari P, Zhang X, Xu P, Xin B, Zhang Y, Narejo N, Sun X. Mapping quantitative trait loci (QTL) for body weight, length and condition factor traits in backcross (BC1) family of Common carp (*Cyprinus carpio* L.). Molecular Biology Reports. 2014;**41**(2):721-731

[154] Huang C, Li Y, Hu S, Chi J, Lin G, Lin C, Gong H, Chen J, Chen R, Chang S. Differential expression patterns of growth-related microRNAs in the skeletal muscle of Nile tilapia. Journal of Animal Science. 2012;**90**(12):4266-4279

[155] Laine VN, Shikano T, Herczeg G, Vilkki J, Merilä J. Quantitative trait loci for growth and body size in the nine-spined stickleback *Pungitius pungitius* L. Molecular Ecology. 2013;**22**(23):5861-5876

[156] Moghadam HK, Poissant J, Fotherby H, Haidle L, Ferguson MM, Danzmann RG. Quantitative trait loci for body weight, condition factor and age at sexual maturation in Arctic charr (*Salvelinus alpinus*): Comparative analysis with rainbow trout (*Oncorhynchus mykiss*) and Atlantic salmon (*Salmo salar*). Molecular Genetics and Genomics. 2007;**277**(6):647-661

[157] Lu X, Luan S, Hu LY, Mao Y, Tao Y, Zhong SP, Kong J. High-resolution genetic linkage mapping, high-temperature tolerance and growth-related quantitative trait locus (QTL) identification in *Marsupenaeus japonicus*. Molecular Genetics and Genomics. 2016;**291**(3):1391-1405

[158] Lyons R, Dierens L, Tan S, Preston N, Li Y. Characterization of AFLP markers associated with growth in the Kuruma prawn, *Marsupenaeus japonicus*, and identification of a candidate gene. Marine Biotechnology. 2007;**9**(6):712-721

[159] Wang W, Tian Y, Kong J, Li X, Liu X, Yang C. Integration genetic linkage map construction and several potential QTLs mapping of Chinese shrimp (*Fenneropenaeus chinensis*) based on three types of molecular markers. Russian Journal of Genetics. 2012;**48**(4):422-434

[160] Jung H, Lyons RE, Li Y, Thanh NM, Dinh H, Hurwood DA, Salin KR, Mather PB. A candidate gene association study for growth performance in an improved giant freshwater prawn (*Macrobrachium rosenbergii*) culture line. Marine Biotechnology. 2014;**16**(2):161-180

[161] Li J, Li J, Chen P, Liu P, He Y. Transcriptome analysis of eyestalk and hemocytes in the ridgetail white prawn Exopalaemon carinicauda: Assembly, Annotation and Marker Discovery. Molecular Biology Reports. 2015;**42**(1):135-147

[162] Ma K, Qiu G, Feng J, Li J. Transcriptome analysis of the oriental river prawn, *Macrobrachium nipponense* using 454 pyrosequencing for discovery of genes and markers. PloS One. 2012;7(6):e39727

[163] Sun X, Liang L. A genetic linkage map of common carp (*Cyprinus carpio* L.) and mapping of a locus associated with cold tolerance. Aquaculture. 2004;**238**(1):165-172

[164] Eshel O, Shirak A, Weller J, Hulata G, Ron M. Linkage and physical mapping of sex region on LG23 of Nile tilapia (*Oreochromis niloticus*). G3: Genes| Genomes| Genetics. 2012;**2**(1):35-42

[165] Zhang Y, Xu P, Lu C, Kuang Y, Zhang X, Cao D, Li C, Chang Y, Hou N, Li H. Genetic linkage mapping and analysis of muscle fiber-related QTLs in common carp (*Cyprinus carpio* L.). Marine Biotechnology. 2011;**13**(3):376-392

[166] Gjedrem T, Baranski M. Selective Breeding in Aquaculture: An Introduction. Vol. 10. Springer Science & Business Media; 2010

[167] Araneda C, Neira R, Iturra P. Identification of a dominant SCAR marker associated with colour traits in Coho salmon (*Oncorhynchus kisutch*). Aquaculture. 2005;**247**(1):67-73

[168] McAndrew B, Roubal FR, Roberts RJ, Bullock AM, McEwen I. The genetics and histology of red, blond and associated colour variants in *Oreochromis niloticus*. Genetica. 1988;**76**(2):127-137

[169] Kause A, Ritola O, Paananen T, Eskelinen U, Mäntysaari E. Big and beautiful? Quantitative genetic parameters for appearance of large rainbow trout. Journal of Fish Biology. 2003;**62**(3):610-622

[170] Nakamura K, Ozaki A, Akutsu T, Iwai K, Sakamoto T, Yoshizaki G, Okamoto N. Genetic mapping of the dominant albino locus in rainbow trout (*Oncorhynchus mykiss*). Molecular Genetics and Genomics. 2001;**265**(4):687-693

[171] Greenwood AK, Jones FC, Chan YF, Brady SD, Absher DM, Grimwood J, Schmutz J, Myers RM, Kingsley DM, Peichel CL. The genetic basis of divergent pigment patterns in juvenile threespine sticklebacks. Heredity. 2011;**107**(2):155-166

[172] Xuan-Peng W, Xiao-Feng Z, Wen-Sheng L, Tian-Qi Z, Xiao-Wen LCAS. Mapping and genetic effect analysis on quantitative trait loci related to feed conversion ratio of common carp (*Cyprinus carpio* L.). Acta Hydrobiologica Sinica. 2012;**2**:002

[173] Köbis JM, Rebl A, Kühn C, Goldammer T. Comparison of splenic transcriptome activity of two rainbow trout strains differing in robustness under regional aquaculture conditions. Molecular Biology Reports. 2013;**40**(2):1955-1966

[174] Shimada Y, Shikano T, Kuparinen A, Gonda A, Leinonen T, Merilä J. Quantitative genetics of body size and timing of maturation in two nine-spined stickleback (*Pungitius pungitius*) populations. PLoS One. 2011;**6**(12):e28859

[175] Cnaani A, Hallerman EM, Ron M, Weller JI, Indelman M, Kashi Y, Gall GA, Hulata G. Detection of a chromosomal region with two quantitative trait loci, affecting cold tolerance and fish size, in an F 2 tilapia hybrid. Aquaculture. 2003;**223**(1):117-128

[176] Somorjai IM, Danzmann RG, Ferguson MM. Distribution of temperature tolerance quantitative trait loci in Arctic charr (*Salvelinus alpinus*) and inferred homologies in rainbow trout (*Oncorhynchus mykiss*). Genetics. 2003;**165**(3):1443-1456

[177] Seear PJ, Carmichael SN, Talbot R, Taggart JB, Bron JE, Sweeney GE. Differential gene expression during smoltification of Atlantic salmon (*Salmo salar* L.): A first large-scale microarray study. Marine Biotechnology. 2010;**12**(2):126-140

[178] Sakamoto T, Danzmann RG, Okamoto N, Ferguson MM, Ihssen PE. Linkage analysis of quantitative trait loci associated with spawning time in rainbow trout (*Oncorhynchus mykiss*). Aquaculture. 1999;**173**(1):33-43

[179] Huang R, Sun J, Luo Q, He L, Liao L, Li Y, Guo F, Zhu Z, Wang Y. Genetic variations of body weight and GCRV resistance in a random mating population of grass carp. Oncotarget. 2015;**6**(34):35433

[180] Liu P, Wang L, Wan ZY, Ye BQ, Huang S, Wong S-M, Yue GH. Mapping QTL for resistance against viral nervous necrosis disease in Asian seabass. Marine Biotechnology. 2016;**18**(1):107-116

[181] Rodríguez-Ramilo ST, De La Herrán R, Ruiz-Rejón C, Hermida M, Fernández C, Pereiro P, Figueras A, Bouza C, Toro MA, Martínez P. Identification of quantitative trait loci associated with resistance to viral haemorrhagic septicaemia (VHS) in turbot (*Scophthalmus maximus*): A comparison between bacterium, parasite and virus diseases. Marine Biotechnology. 2014;**16**(3):265-276

[182] Verrier ER, Dorson M, Mauger S, Torhy C, Ciobotaru C, Hervet C, Dechamp N, Genet C, Boudinot P, Quillet E. Resistance to a rhabdovirus (VHSV) in rainbow trout: Identification of a major QTL related to innate mechanisms. PLoS One. 2013;**8**(2):e55302

[183] Fuji K, Kobayashi K, Hasegawa O, Coimbra MRM, Sakamoto T, Okamoto N. Identification of a single major genetic locus controlling the resistance to lymphocystis disease in Japanese flounder (*Paralichthys olivaceus*). Aquaculture. 2006;**254**(1):203-210

[184] Gheyas A, Houston R, Mota-Velasco J, Guy D, Tinch A, Haley C, Woolliams J. Segregation of infectious pancreatic necrosis resistance QTL in the early life cycle of Atlantic Salmon (*Salmo salar*). Animal Genetics. 2010;**41**(5):531-536

[185] Gheyas A, Haley C, Guy D, Hamilton A, Tinch A, Mota-Velasco J, Woolliams J. Effect of a major QTL affecting IPN resistance on production traits in Atlantic salmon. Animal Genetics. 2010;**41**(6):666-668

[186] Hjeltnes BWC, Bang Jensen B Haukaas A. A: Fish health report 3B—2016. Fiskehelserapporten, 2015. The Norwegian Veterinary Insititute; 2016

[187] Wiens GD, Vallejo RL, Leeds TD, Palti Y, Hadidi S, Liu S, Evenhuis JP, Welch TJ, Rexroad III CE. Assessment of genetic correlation between bacterial cold water disease resistance and spleen index in a domesticated population of rainbow trout: Identification of QTL on chromosome Omy19. PLoS One. 2013;**8**(10):e75749

[188] Robinson N, Baranski M, Mahapatra KD, Saha JN, Das S, Mishra J, Das P, Kent M, Arnyasi M, Sahoo PK. A linkage map of transcribed single nucleotide polymorphisms in rohu (*Labeo rohita*) and QTL associated with resistance to *Aeromonas hydrophila*. BMC Genomics. 2014;**15**(1):541

[189] Shao C, Niu Y, Rastas P, Liu Y, Xie Z, Li H, Wang L, Jiang Y, Tai S, Tian Y. Genome-wide SNP identification for the construction of a high-resolution genetic map of Japanese flounder (*Paralichthys olivaceus*): Applications to QTL mapping of *Vibrio anguillarum* disease resistance and comparative genomic analysis. DNA Research. 2015;**22**(2):161-70. doi: 10.1093/dnares/dsv001.

[190] Vallejo RL, Palti Y, Liu S, Evenhuis JP, Gao G, Rexroad III CE, Wiens GD. Detection of QTL in rainbow trout affecting survival when challenged with *Flavobacterium psychrophilum*. Marine Biotechnology. 2014;**16**(3):349-360

[191] Massault C, Franch R, Haley C, De Koning D, Bovenhuis H, Pellizzari C, Patarnello T, Bargelloni L. Quantitative trait loci for resistance to fish pasteurellosis in gilthead sea bream (*Sparus aurata*). Animal Genetics. 2011;**42**(2):191-203

[192] Gilbey J, Verspoor E, Mo TA, Sterud E, Olstad K, Hytterød S, Jones C, Noble L. Identification of genetic markers associated with *Gyrodactylus salaris* resistance in Atlantic salmon *Salmo salar*. Diseases of Aquatic Organisms. 2006;**71**(2):119-129

[193] Ozaki A, Yoshida K, Fuji K, Kubota S, Kai W, Aoki J-y, Kawabata Y, Suzuki J, Akita K, Koyama T. Quantitative trait loci (QTL) associated with resistance to a monogenean parasite (*Benedenia seriolae*) in yellowtail (*Seriola quinqueradiata*) through genome wide analysis. PloS One. 2013;**8**(6):e64987

[194] Wilson K, Li Y, Whan V, Lehnert S, Byrne K, Moore S, Pongsomboon S, Tassanakajon A, Rosenberg G, Ballment E. Genetic mapping of the black tiger shrimp *Penaeus monodon* with amplified fragment length polymorphism. Aquaculture. 2002;**204**(3):297-309

[195] Mukherjee K, Mandal N. A microsatellite DNA marker developed for identifying Disease-resistant population of Giant Black Tiger Shrimp, *Penaeus monodon*. Journal of the World Aquaculture Society. 2009;**40**(2):274-280

[196] Hizer SE, Dhar AK, Klimpel KR, Garcia DK. RAPD markers as predictors of infectious hypodermal and hematopoietic necrosis virus (IHHNV) resistance in shrimp (*Litopenaeus stylirostris*). Genome. 2002;**45**(1):1-7

[197] Ødegård J, Gitterle T, Madsen P, Meuwissen TH, Yazdi MH, Gjerde B, Pulgarin C, Rye M. Quantitative genetics of taura syndrome resistance in pacific white shrimp (*Penaeus vannamei*): A cure model approach. Genetics Selection Evolution. 2011;**43**(1):14

[198] Waddington CH. Canalization of development and the inheritance of acquired characters. Nature. 1942;**150**(3811):563-565

[199] Waddington CH. The epigenotype. Endeavour.1942;**1**:18-20

[200] Hotchkiss RD. The quantitative separation of purines, pyrimidines, and nucleosides by paper chromatography. Journal of Biological Chemistry. 1948;**175**(1):315-332

[201] Holliday R, Pugh JE. DNA modification mechanisms and gene activity during development. Cold Spring Harbor Monograph Series. 1996;**32**:639-645

[202] Razin A, Riggs AD. DNA methylation and gene function. Science. 1980;**210**(4470):604-610

[203] Taylor SM, Jones PA. Multiple new phenotypes induced in 10T12 and 3T3 cells treated with 5-azacytidine. Cell. 1979;**17**(4):771-779

[204] Goldberg AD, Allis CD, Bernstein E. Epigenetics: A landscape takes shape. Cell. 2007; **128**(4):635-638

[205] Bernstein BE, Meissner A, Lander ES. The mammalian epigenome. Cell. 2007;**128**(4): 669-681

[206] Martín-Subero J. How epigenomics brings phenotype into being. Pediatric Endocrinology Reviews: PER. 2011;**9**:506-510

[207] Wang Y, 王源. Hypoxia causes epigenetic changes and transgenerational reproductive impairments in marine medaka (*Oryzias melastigma*). HKU Theses Online (HKUTO). 2016

[208] Wan ZY, Xia JH, Lin G, Wang L, Lin VC, Yue GH. Genome-wide methylation analysis identified sexually dimorphic methylated regions in hybrid tilapia. Scientific Reports. 2016;**6**:35903. doi: 10.1038/srep35903.

[209] Sun L-X, Wang Y-Y, Zhao Y, Wang H, Li N, Ji XS. Global DNA methylation changes in Nile tilapia gonads during high temperature-induced masculinization. PLoS One. 2016;**11**(8):e0158483

[210] Shao C, Li Q, Chen S, Zhang P, Lian J, Hu Q, Sun B, Jin L, Liu S, Wang Z. Epigenetic modification and inheritance in sexual reversal of fish. Genome Research. 2014;**24**(4):604-615

[211] Zhang G. Epigenetic modification and inheritance in sexual reversal of tongue-sole fish. In: Proceeding of Plant and Animal Genome Asia (PAG), Grand Copthorn Waterfront Hotel. China, 2013.

[212] Baerwald MR, Meek MH, Stephens MR, Nagarajan RP, Goodbla AM, Tomalty KM, Thorgaard GH, May B, Nichols KM. Migration-related phenotypic divergence is associated with epigenetic modifications in rainbow trout. Molecular Ecology. 2015

[213] Kimura T, Yoshida K, Shimada A, Jindo T, Sakaizumi M, Mitani H, Naruse K, Takeda H, Inoko H, Tamiya G. Genetic linkage map of medaka with polymerase chain reaction length polymorphisms. Gene. 2005;**363**:24-31

[214] Taneda Y, Konno S, Makino S, Morioka M, Fukuda K, Imai Y, Kudo A, Kawakami A. Epigenetic control of cardiomyocyte production in response to a stress during the medaka heart development. Developmental Biology. 2010;**340**(1):30-40

[215] Cao Z, Ding W, Yu J, Cao L, Wu T. Differences in methylated loci among different grass carp individuals from one pair of parents. 2007: 1083-1088.

[216] Ding G, Wang L, Zhang J, Wei Y, Wei L, Li Y, Shao M, Xiong D. Toxicity and DNA methylation changes induced by perfluorooctane sulfonate (PFOS) in sea urchin *Glyptocidaris crenularis*. Chemosphere. 2015;**128**:225-230

[217] Zhao Y, Chen M, Storey KB, Sun L, Yang H. DNA methylation levels analysis in four tissues of sea cucumber *Apostichopus japonicus* based on fluorescence-labeled methylation-sensitive amplified polymorphism (F-MSAP) during aestivation. Comparative Biochemistry and Physiology Part B: Biochemistry and Molecular Biology. 2015;**181**:26-32

[218] Covelo-Soto L, Morán P, Pasantes JJ, Pérez-García C. Cytogenetic evidences of genome rearrangement and differential epigenetic chromatin modification in the sea lamprey (*Petromyzon marinus*). Genetica. 2014;**142**(6):545-554

[219] Mhanni A, McGowan R. Global changes in genomic methylation levels during early development of the zebrafish embryo. Development Genes and Evolution. 2004; **214**(8): 412-417

[220] Gavery MR, Roberts SB. DNA methylation patterns provide insight into epigenetic regulation in the Pacific oyster (*Crassostrea gigas*). BMC Genomics. 2010;**11**(1):483

[221] Shang X, Su J, Wan Q, Su J. CpA/CpG methylation of CiMDA5 possesses tight association with the resistance against GCRV and negatively regulates mRNA expression in grass carp, *Ctenopharyngodon idella*. Developmental & Comparative Immunology. 2015;**48**(1):86-94

[222] Navarro-Martín L, Viñas J, Ribas L, Díaz N, Gutiérrez A, Di Croce L, Piferrer F. Epigenetics and fish sex ratios: The case of the sea bass. II Jornada de Cromatina i Epigenètica. 2011. http://hdl.handle.net/10261/81182.

[223] Navarro-Martín L, Viñas J, Ribas L, Díaz N, Gutiérrez A, Di Croce L, Piferrer F. DNA methylation of the gonadal aromatase (cyp19a) promoter is involved in temperature-dependent sex ratio shifts in the European sea bass. PLoS Genetics. 2011;7(12):e1002447

[224] Santos F, Hendrich B, Reik W, Dean W. Dynamic reprogramming of DNA methylation in the early mouse embryo. Developmental Biology. 2002;**241**(1):172-182

[225] Contractor RG, Foran CM, Li S, Willett KL. Evidence of gender-and tissue-specific promoter methylation and the potential for ethinylestradiol-induced changes in Japanese medaka (*Oryzias latipes*) estrogen receptor and aromatase genes. Journal of Toxicology and Environmental Health, Part A. 2004;**67**(1):1-22

[226] Wen A, You F, Sun P, Li J, Xu D, Wu Z, Ma D, Zhang P. CpG methylation of dmrt1 and cyp19a promoters in relation to their sexual dimorphic expression in the Japanese flounder *Paralichthys olivaceus*. Journal of Fish Biology. 2014;**84**(1):193-205

[227] Gómez R, Van Damme K, Gosálvez J, Morán ES, Colbourne JK. Male meiosis in Crustacea: Synapsis, recombination, epigenetics and fertility in *Daphnia magna*. Chromosoma. 2016; **125**(4):769-787

[228] Giannetto A, Nagasawa K, Fasulo S, Fernandes JM. Influence of photoperiod on expression of DNA (cytosine-5) methyltransferases in Atlantic cod. Gene. 2013;**519**(2):222-230

[229] Nagasawa K, Giannetto A, Fernandes JM. Photoperiod influences growth and mll (mixed-lineage leukaemia) expression in Atlantic cod. PLoS One. 2012;7(5):e36908

[230] Marandel L, Lepais O, Arbenoits E, Véron V, Dias K, Zion M, Panserat S. Remodelling of the hepatic epigenetic landscape of glucose-intolerant rainbow trout (*Oncorhynchus mykiss*) by nutritional status and dietary carbohydrates. Scientific Reports. 2016;**6**

[231] Flohr L, Fuzinatto CF, Melegari SP, Matias WG. Effects of exposure to soluble fraction of industrial solid waste on lipid peroxidation and DNA methylation in erythrocytes of *Oreochromis niloticus*, as assessed by quantification of MDA and m 5 dC rates. Ecotoxicology and Environmental Safety. 2012;**76**:63-70

[232] Pierron F, Baillon L, Sow M, Gotreau S, Gonzalez P Effect of low-dose cadmium exposure on DNA methylation in the endangered European eel. Environmental Science & Technology. 2013;**48**(1):797-803

[233] Aniagu SO, Williams TD, Allen Y, Katsiadaki I, Chipman JK. Global genomic methylation levels in the liver and gonads of the three-spine stickleback (*Gasterosteus aculeatus*) after exposure to hexabromocyclododecane and 17-β oestradiol. Environment International. 2008;**34**(3):310-317

[234] Aparicio S, Chapman J, Stupka E, Putnam N, Chia J-m, Dehal P, Christoffels A, Rash S, Hoon S, Smit A. Whole-genome shotgun assembly and analysis of the genome of *Fugu rubripes*. Science. 2002;**297**(5585):1301-1310

[235] Howe K, Clark MD, Torroja CF, Torrance J, Berthelot C, Muffato M, Collins JE, Humphray S, McLaren K, Matthews L. The zebrafish reference genome sequence and its relationship to the human genome. Nature. 2013;**496**(7446):498-503

[236] Kasahara M, Naruse K, Sasaki S, Nakatani Y, Qu W, Ahsan B, Yamada T, Nagayasu Y, Doi K, Kasai Y. The medaka draft genome and insights into vertebrate genome evolution. Nature. 2007;**447**(7145):714-719

[237] Wittbrodt J, Shima A, Schartl M. Medaka—a model organism from the far East. Nature Reviews Genetics. 2002;**3**(1):53-64

[238] Hill AJ, Teraoka H, Heideman W, Peterson RE. Zebrafish as a model vertebrate for investigating chemical toxicity. Toxicological Sciences. 2005;**86**(1):6-19

[239] Chen X, Li L, Wong CKC, Cheng SH. Rapid adaptation of molecular resources from zebrafish and medaka to develop an estuarine/marine model. Comparative Biochemistry and Physiology Part C: Toxicology & Pharmacology. 2009;**149**(4):647-655

[240] Star B, Nederbragt AJ, Jentoft S, Grimholt U, Malmstrøm M, Gregers TF, Rounge TB, Paulsen J, Solbakken MH, Sharma A. The genome sequence of Atlantic cod reveals a unique immune system. Nature. 2011;**477**(7363):207-210

[241] Rastorguev S, Nedoluzhko A, Levina M, Prokhorchuk E, Skryabin K, Levin B. Pleiotropic effect of thyroid hormones on gene expression in fish as exemplified from the blue bream *Ballerus ballerus* (Cyprinidae): Results of transcriptomic analysis. In: Doklady Biochemistry and Biophysics: 2016. Springer; 2016. pp. 124-127

[242] Li F-G, Chen J, Jiang X-Y, Zou S-M. Transcriptome analysis of blunt snout bream (*Megalobrama amblycephala*) reveals putative differential expression genes related to growth and hypoxia. PloS One. 2015;**10**(11):e0142801

[243] Robledo D, Fernández C, Hermida M, Sciara A, Álvarez-Dios JA, Cabaleiro S, Caamaño R, Martínez P, Bouza C. Integrative transcriptome, genome and quantitative trait loci resources identify single nucleotide polymorphisms in candidate genes for growth traits in turbot. International Journal of Molecular Sciences. 2016;**17**(2):243

[244] Sun Y, Guo C-Y, Wang D-D, Li XF, Xiao L, Zhang X, You X, Shi Q, Hu G-J, Fang C. Transcriptome analysis reveals the molecular mechanisms underlying growth superiority in a novel grouper hybrid (*Epinephelus fuscogutatus*♀× *E. lanceolatus*♂). BMC Genetics. 2016;**17**(1):24

[245] Sun L, Li J, Liang X, Yi T, Fang L, Sun J, He Y, Luo X, Dou Y, Yang M. Microsatellite DNA markers and their correlation with growth traits in mandarin fish (*Siniperca chuatsi*). Genetics and Molecular Research. 2015;**14**(4):19128-19135

[246] Estévez A, Andree K, Johnston IA. Fast skeletal muscle transcriptome of the Gilthead sea bream (*Sparus aurata*) determined by next generation sequencing. BMC Genomics. 2012;**13**(1):181

[247] Sánchez CC, Weber GM, Gao G, Cleveland BM, Yao J, Rexroad CE. Generation of a reference transcriptome for evaluating rainbow trout responses to various stressors. BMC Genomics. 2011;**12**(1):626

[248] Hemmer-Hansen J, Nielsen EE, Meldrup D, Mittelholzer C. Identification of single nucleotide polymorphisms in candidate genes for growth and reproduction in a nonmodel organism; the Atlantic cod, *Gadus morhua*. Molecular Ecology Resources. 2011;**11**(s1):71-80

[249] Renaut S, Bernatchez L. Transcriptome-wide signature of hybrid breakdown associated with intrinsic reproductive isolation in lake whitefish species pairs (Coregonus spp. Salmonidae). Heredity. 2011;**106**(6):1003-1011

[250] Whiteley AR, Derome N, Rogers SM, St-Cyr J, Laroche J, Labbe A, Nolte A, Renaut S, Jeukens J, Bernatchez L. The phenomics and expression quantitative trait locus mapping of brain transcriptomes regulating adaptive divergence in lake whitefish species pairs (Coregonus sp.). Genetics. 2008;**180**(1):147-164

[251] Tao W, Boulding E. Associations between single nucleotide polymorphisms in candidate genes and growth rate in Arctic charr (*Salvelinus alpinus* L.). Heredity. 2003;**91**(1):60-69

[252] Perry GM, Danzmann RG, Ferguson MM, Gibson JP. Quantitative trait loci for upper thermal tolerance inoutbred strains of rainbow trout (*Oncorhynchus mykiss*). Heredity. 2001;**86**(3):333-341

[253] Kawahara-Miki R, Wada K, Azuma N, Chiba S. Expression profiling without genome sequence information in a non-model species, Pandalid shrimp (*Pandalus latirostris*), by next-generation sequencing. PLoS One. 2011;**6**(10):e26043

[254] Li Y, Dierens L, Byrne K, Miggiano E, Lehnert S, Preston N, Lyons R. QTL detection of production traits for the Kuruma prawn *Penaeus japonicus* (Bate) using AFLP markers. Aquaculture. 2006;**258**(1):198-210

[255] Robinson NA, Gopikrishna G, Baranski M, Katneni VK, Shekhar MS, Shanmugakarthik J, Jothivel S, Gopal C, Ravichandran P, Gitterle T. QTL for white spot syndrome virus resistance and the sex-determining locus in the Indian black tiger shrimp (*Penaeus monodon*). BMC Genomics. 2014;**15**(1):731

[256] Zhang L, Yang C, Zhang Y, Li L, Zhang X, Zhang Q, Xiang J. A genetic linkage map of Pacific white shrimp (*Litopenaeus vannamei*): Sex-linked microsatellite markers and high recombination rates. Genetica. 2007;**131**(1):37-49

[257] Yu Y, Zhang X, Yuan J, Li F, Chen X, Zhao Y, Huang L, Zheng H, Xiang J. Genome survey and high-density genetic map construction provide genomic and genetic resources for the Pacific White Shrimp *Litopenaeus vannamei*. Scientific Reports. 2015;**5**:15612

[258] Anelli V, Santoriello C, Distel M, Köster RW, Ciccarelli FD, Mione M. Global repression of cancer gene expression in a zebrafish model of melanoma is linked to epigenetic regulation. Zebrafish. 2009;**6**(4):417-424

[259] Hove JR, Köster RW, Forouhar AS, Acevedo-Bolton G, Fraser SE, Gharib M. Intracardiac fluid forces are an essential epigenetic factor for embryonic cardiogenesis. Nature. 2003;**421**(6919):172-177

[260] Bhandari RK. Medaka as a model for studying environmentally induced epigenetic transgenerational inheritance of phenotypes. Environmental Epigenetics. 2016;**2**(1):dvv010

[261] Dos Santos Campos MCM. Thermal epigenetic regulation of muscle growth and development in the Senegalese sole (Solea senegalensis Kaup, 1858) [thesis]. Instituto de Ciências Biomédicas, Abel Salazar da Universidade do Porto; 2013

[262] Pierron F, Bureau du Colombier S, Moffett A, Caron A, Peluhet L, Daffe G, Lambert P, Elie P, Labadie P, Budzinski Hln. Abnormal ovarian DNA methylation programming during gonad maturation in wild contaminated fish. Environmental Science & Technology. 2014;**48**(19):11688-11695

[263] Matsumoto Y, Buemio A, Chu R, Vafaee M, Crews D. Epigenetic control of gonadal aromatase (cyp19a1) in temperature-dependent sex determination of red-eared slider turtles. PLoS One. 2013;**8**(6):e63599

[264] Lien S, Koop BF, Sandve SR, Miller JR, Kent MP, Nome T, Hvidsten TR, Leong JS, Minkley DR, Zimin A. The Atlantic salmon genome provides insights into rediploidization. Nature. 2016;**533**(7602):200-5. doi: 10.1038/nature17164.

[265] Schartl M, Walter RB, Shen Y, Garcia T, Catchen J, Amores A, Braasch I, Chalopin D, Volff J-N, Lesch K-P. The genome of the platyfish, *Xiphophorus maculatus*, provides insights into evolutionary adaptation and several complex traits. Nature Genetics. 2013;**45**(5):567-572

[266] Walter RB, Shen Y, Garcia T, Catchen J, Amores A, Braasch I, Chalopin D, Volff J-N, Lesch K-P, Bisazza A. The Genome of the Platyfish, *Xiphophorus Maculatus*, Provides Insights into Evolutionary Adaptation and Several Complex Traits [Internet]. 2013. Available from: http://www nature com/ng/index.html.

[267] Jaillon O, Aury J-M, Brunet F, Petit J-L, Stange-Thomann N, Mauceli E, Bouneau L, Fischer C, Ozouf-Costaz C, Bernot A. Genome duplication in the teleost fish Tetraodon nigroviridis reveals the early vertebrate proto-karyotype. Nature. 2004;**431**(7011):946-957

[268] Jones FC, Grabherr MG, Chan YF, Russell P, Mauceli E, Johnson J, Swofford R, Pirun M, Zody MC, White S. The genomic basis of adaptive evolution in threespine sticklebacks. Nature. 2012;**484**(7392):55-61

[269] Berthelot C, Brunet F, Chalopin D, Juanchich A, Bernard M, Noël B, Bento P, Da Silva C, Labadie K, Alberti A. The rainbow trout genome provides novel insights into evolution after whole-genome duplication in vertebrates. Nature Communications. 2014;**5**:3657. doi: 10.1038/ncomms4657.

[270] Guiguen Y. The rainbow trout genome provides novel insights into evolution after Whole-Genome duplication in vertebrates. In: Plant and Animal Genome XXIV Conference: 2016: Plant and Animal Genome; 2016

[271] Harel I, Benayoun BA, Machado B, Singh PP, Hu C-K, Pech MF, Valenzano DR, Zhang E, Sharp SC, Artandi SE. A platform for rapid exploration of aging and diseases in a naturally short-lived vertebrate. Cell. 2015;**160**(5):1013-1026

[272] Valenzano DR, Benayoun BA, Singh PP, Zhang E, Etter PD, Hu C-K, Clément-Ziza M, Willemsen D, Cui R, Harel I. The African turquoise killifish genome provides insights into evolution and genetic architecture of lifespan. Cell. 2015;**163**(6):1539-1554

[273] Takeuchi T, Kawashima T, Koyanagi R, Gyoja F, Tanaka M, Ikuta T, Shoguchi E, Fujiwara M, Shinzato C, Hisata K. Draft genome of the pearl oyster Pinctada fucata: A platform for understanding bivalve biology. DNA Research. 2012;dss005

Chapter 8

Transcriptome Analysis and Genetic Engineering

Uzma Qaisar, Samina Yousaf, Tanzeela Rehman,
Anila Zainab and Asima Tayyeb

Additional information is available at the end of the chapter

http://dx.doi.org/10.5772/intechopen.69372

Abstract

Genetic engineering is the most powerful technology of this century which is dramatically revolutionizing the agriculture, health, pharmaceutical, and food industries all over the world. Transcriptomics and genetic engineering go hand in hand from the development of a genetically modified organism (GMO) to its utilization by the humans. Transcriptome analysis is the analysis of messenger RNAs (mRNAs), which are produced by transcription of deoxyribonucleic acid (DNA) in an organism in response to a specific internal/external environment. Transcriptome analysis is not only useful to dig out the potential target genes for genetic modifications but also utilized to study the proper functioning of a genetically engineered gene, evaluation of the GMO for biosafety risks and for monitoring the presence and movement of GMO. Despite huge scope of genetic engineering, these manipulations can upset the natural balance of a genome by insertional, soma clonal, and pleiotropic effects of a foreign gene resulting in unintended alterations along with the targeted changes. The untargeted alterations pose risks to environment and health of animals and plants. In this chapter, the key advancements in the field of biotechnology and the relevant biosafety issues are reviewed. The advantages and limitations of the current methods used for the evaluation, monitoring, and regulation of GMOs are discussed.

Keywords: genetic engineering, gene silencing, genetically modified organisms, unintended modifications, pleiotropic effects, enzyme-linked immunosorbent assay, soma clonal effects, next-generation sequencing

1. Introduction

Genetic engineering is an advanced field of biology that deals with modification of genomic deoxyribonucleic acid (DNA) in the living organisms to introduce desired traits to benefit mankind. Through genetic engineering, a DNA fragment (gene) is isolated from the donor organism

and transferred to the recipient where it can be transcribed into messenger RNA (mRNA) and translated to proteins by utilizing the recipient machinery. The donor protein in the recipient system performs its targeted function to modify the desired character of recipient plant, animal, or microorganism. Genomic DNA manipulations may involve addition of a foreign gene from another genome, deletion of an existing gene, or enhancing the expression of an indigenous gene. RNA interfering (RNAi) technology is used to silence the expression of an unwanted gene by inhibiting the mRNA availability for protein synthesis [1]. The genome-level genetic engineering approaches require an insight in the genome, transcriptome, and metabolome [2] of the organisms under study. Like all other applied fields, genetic engineering requires comprehensive information about the genome structure of the donor and recipient before genetic modification. Decision about the morphological character that needs to be improved, the choice of a particular donor and recipient species, genetic networks, and metabolic pathways involved in the expression of a specific trait need to be explored.

Transcriptome analysis is a robust and cost-efficient method which provides information about the internal biological processes, cellular biosynthesis, and metabolic functions of a cell, tissue, or living organism [3]. This technique can be utilized by the genetic engineering scientists for the identification and quantification of genetic factors which positively or negatively regulate a particular trait of interest [4]. Comparison of gene expression profiles of an organism exhibiting the desired traits with the genetically similar organism lacking that trait can help in the identification of genetic factors involved in the development of that trait [5, 6]. These genetic factors might affect that trait positively or negatively. Enhanced accumulation of a particular transcript in the organism with desired phenotype as compared to the reference organism indicates that overexpression of that transcript is required for the exhibition of that trait. This phenomenon is called as positive regulation. In negative regulation, reduced expression of a gene is responsible for the exhibition of a desired trait [7, 8].

Positively regulated genes serve as genetic engineering tools for overexpression of a gene regulating a particular trait resulting in the introduction of that trait in genetically modified organism (GMO). For example, in transgenic cotton, expression of crystal protein (Cry10Aa) is responsible for resistance against boll weevil [9]. Advances in gene silencing technology through RNAi have led to utilization of genes which are negatively correlated with the desired traits. In cotton plant, seed-oil content increased by 16.7% by silencing GhPEPC1 gene through RNAi technology [8].

Transcriptome analysis and genetic engineering go hand in hand in the modern era of genetic improvements. Comparative transcriptional studies using single gene approaches or high-throughput approaches are used to identify the differentially expressed genes in a specific condition/organism as compared to reference. In single gene approaches, the expression of a gene of interest is quantified in different sets of conditions/tissues using northern blotting or reverse transcriptase polymerase chain reaction (RT-PCR). Northern blotting technique utilizes the gene-specific probes for comparative quantification of mRNAs of the target gene, whereas RT-PCR uses gene-specific primers to amplify and subsequently quantify the mRNA molecules. High-throughput technologies have the power to measure and analyze the expression of all the genes in a set of conditions. Differential display reverse

transcriptase PCR (DDRT-PCR), gene expression microarray, and next-generation sequencing (NGS) techniques are high-throughput techniques which are currently used. DDRT-PCR can study the expression of hundreds of genes at the same time, whereas microarray and NGS can study the whole transcriptome in a single experiment. Expression microarrays can give insight of the comparative transcriptomics, whereas NGS can provide absolute quantification of each transcript. All these techniques help in the identification of genes which give differential expression under different conditions.

These identified genes serve as targets to be used in different genetic engineering events. These genes are manipulated in the living organisms to produce GMOs. The modified organism is tested for the proper functioning of the transgene by single gene transcriptional analysis. Then the GMO is tested for the potential risks to the environment and human/animal health using targeted approaches which are biased and require preexisting knowledge of the risk. The comprehensive and unbiased assessment of the GMO should be done using global transcriptome analysis of the GMO with the commercial safe variety. After biosafety testing, GMO is released for commercialization and human/animal utilization. There is great deal of resentment and resistance against utilization of genetically altered organisms. Many governments have designed policies to properly monitor the presence and movement of GMOs. Transcriptional analysis is widely being utilized for the monitoring of various newly developed organisms.

2. Genetic engineering for human benefit

Genetic engineering is the field of science which is revolutionizing the world by manipulating the genome and transcriptome of living organisms to introduce desired traits in them. Since the commercialization of "Flavr Savr" tomato in 1994 [10], 357 GM crops belonging to 27 species all over the world have been commercialized [11], and this number is increasing day by day. Genetic engineering is widely being used for the improvement of crops, animals, fungi [12], bacteria [13], and other organisms to benefit mankind. Insect resistance, herbicide resistance, disease resistance, and abiotic resistance are being incorporated in the industrially important crops to make them tolerant to stresses. Yield and nutritional content of food crops are being modified to improve the feed for humans and animals. Scientists [14] produced transgenic maize with overexpressing *Oryza sativa* myeloblastosis 55 (OsMYB55) gene and found that the transgenic maize became more tolerant to heat and drought stress through activating the expression of stress-responsive genes. Microorganisms (bacteria and fungi) are being genetically engineered for the production of useful enzymes [13], secondary metabolites, beneficial oils [12], and antibiotics on commercial scale to be utilized in the pharmaceutical, food, and medical industry.

In 2010, 29 countries were growing genetically modified crops, and 31 countries had the approval to import GM crops. In USA, more than 94% of the cultivated soybean and cotton while 92% of corn is genetically modified [15]. The commercialization of the first genetically modified animal "AquAdvantage Salmon" for food was approved recently in 2015 [16].

RNA-based genetic engineering technology is becoming more attractive after the approval of white button mushroom for commercialization without stringent testing by the USDA, as this technology does not involve the introduction of foreign DNA [17].

3. GMOs and biosafety issues

Due to the advancements in the field of biotechnology and genetic engineering, new varieties are extensively prevailing in the society. Despite their huge potential for human welfare, their commercialization is controversial. Many people perceive all the GMOs to be bad for their health and environment. People who are aware of the mechanism of genetic engineering are concerned about the unintended modifications and their effect on the soil microorganisms [18], plant-microbe interaction [19], and imbalances in the natural biosystems. GMO's controversy mainly revolves around environmental safety [20], human and animal health [21], concerns over interfering with nature [22], and patent issues [23].

Genetically modified organisms produced by genetic engineering or conventional plant breeding are targeted to enhance the desired commercial traits, but GMOs might exhibit unintended traits as well. In the international meeting on "Genetic Basis of Unintended Effects in Modified Plants," biotechnology industry, government, and academia emphasized that no genetic modification is without unintended effects whether conventional breeding or genetic engineering [24]. The source of unintended modifications could be attributed to gene insertions or deletions involving deletion or disruption of endogenous genes and chimeric protein production which perform abnormal function. Genetic engineering approaches involving tissue culturing and in vitro culturing pose the risk of soma clonal modifications arising from the genetic and epigenetic effects of in vitro cultures [25]. Pleiotropic effects may contribute to the unintended modifications if the transgene plays multiple roles or is the part of multiple pathways in an organism leading to the production of potentially harmful secondary metabolites [26].

Biosafety policies involve principles, procedures, and rules devised and adapted for protecting the environment and health of the individuals against potentially harmful metabolites and toxins. Biosafety involves containment of harmful material to avoid unintentional exposure to toxic agents produced by genetically modified organisms [27].

4. Monitoring of GMOs

Due to the resentment of the consumers in utilizing GMOs for food and animal feed purposes, many governments have devised policies to give its people freedom over utilization of GMOs. Policies mainly revolve around detection, proper labeling, isolation of propagation area, and tracking of GMOs. International trading requires standardization of procedures and policies related to GMO monitoring and marketing among trading countries. Moreover, in order to

limit the entry of approved varieties across the borders of a country, proper monitoring of GMOs is required.

The first step in the monitoring of GMO is the detection of transgene in an organism under question. Many methods are being used to detect the genetically modified varieties. GMOs produced by insertion of DNA fragments can be detected by protein-based assays [Enzyme-linked immunosorbent assay (ELISA), Western blotting, etc.] or nucleotide-based assays including PCR. PCR-based detection is the most sensitive method which makes use of sequence-specific primers [28]. Due to the abundance of GMOs in the market, it has become very difficult to keep the sequence information of all the transgenes. The advanced high-throughput technologies for GMO detection/monitoring are developed to detect multiple transgenes or related nucleotide components (promoter, enhancer, and terminator) of the cassette [29, 30] in a single experiment. For rapid PCR at atmospheric temperature, various methods have been developed [31]. DNA microarray chips are being developed which contain the probes against all the transgenes present in the commercial varieties [32]. Sampling and hybridization of DNA of a variety under question can detect the presence of any transgene. More efficient, sensitive, and robust methods are required for proper monitoring.

All the above methods are used for the detection of DNA insertion in the transgenic organisms. However, in the RNA-based GMOs, the detection of transgene requires transcriptomic approaches. Transcriptional methods including RT-PCR, gene expression microarray, and RNA-seq can detect all types of GMOs produced through RNA- or DNA-based methods. In transcriptomic approaches, RNA is isolated from the sample and reverse transcribed to produce complementary DNA (cDNA). Due to resemblance in the biochemical properties of RNA and DNA, DNA is often present in the RNA preparations which is eliminated by treating the sample with DNase enzyme. By avoiding this step of DNase treatment, we get both RNA and DNA in the sample. This crude RNA is transcribed and RT-PCR is used for the detection of RNA or DNA of the transgene.

5. Validation of genetically modified organisms

The developers of GMOs are required to assess the phenotypic and molecular characteristics of modified organisms. Many countries have adopted regulations for commercialization of GMOs which mainly include the comprehensive risk assessment of the new organism before field trials, to be used as feed/food or before release to the environment. These risk assessment methods mainly involve the comparison of the agronomic traits, composition, animal nutrition, and production of toxins of the new product with commercially available for multiple years and at multiple sites. But these assessments are targeted and require the prior information about the risk. The untargeted risks can be left without evaluation with the potential to harm the environment and health.

During the screening and selection of a GMO, the emphasis is given to the insertion of the transgene as a single copy without disruption of an endogenous gene, preserving the gene

cassette and the absence of vector backbone. Safety of the GMO is tested on a very limited scale only when the GMO is ready to be commercialized. The main focus of the biosafety studies is limited to the assessment of the effect of the GMO on the consumer health and safety. The phenotypic and agronomic traits of the newly produced plant and a genetically similar organism are compared [33], but thorough profiling of the genetically modified organism is lacking.

Newly produced plants by genetic engineering and other genetic methods should not only be assessed by target-based approaches as these assessments are biased and cannot recognize the unintended risks thoroughly [34]. Genome-wide approaches like transcriptome analysis, proteome analysis, or metabolome analysis have the advantage of being unbiased and robust [35–37] and provide a lot of information about the new plant variety. Scientists compare the protein profiles of genetically modified organisms with their wild types to identify the aberrant proteins. Proteome of a commercial variety of maize was compared with the isogenic transgenic line which was resistant to European corn borer by expressing Cry1Ab gene [38]. The results spotted unwanted/unintended protein expression in the transgenic lines and suggested for the untargeted evaluation of the new transgenic organisms. Other studies using proteomic or transcriptomic approaches to compare the GMO with the wild type found only intended alterations [7], while no unintended changes were found.

Unintended changes arising as a result of pleiotropic effects of genetic modification are not always harmful. A group of scientists has performed transcriptome analysis in GMO lines developed for enhanced insect attraction in *Arabidopsis* and compared it with naturally occurring non-GMO lines to identify transcriptional distance between the two groups [39]. They identified that the pleiotropic effects of gene insertion are equivalent to the gene expression changes naturally occurring in *Arabidopsis* indicating that the specific modified lines of *Arabidopsis* were equally safe as naturally occurring lines. Thus unbiased and untargeted risk assessment of GMOs through newly developed "omic" techniques is necessary [40] before its release in the environment or trials for human and animal use.

6. Transcriptome analysis for GMO validation

Unbiased detection of unintended effects of transgene in a genetically modified organism requires comparison of transcriptome [41], proteome [38] and metabolome [40] of the modified organism with the isogenic unmodified organism. The thorough profiling helps in the identification of genes, proteins, and metabolites modified in the newly developed organism. By digging the gene networks, protein functions, and metabolic processes of the altered biomolecule, scientists can depict the effects of GMO on the environment, health, and nutrition of the consumer. The absence of unintended aberrations in the biomolecules declares the new variety as safe, whereas the presence of unintended aberrations does not declare it to be unsafe but indicates that the variety requires more targeted validation before commercialization [7].

Transcriptome analysis stands out of the other omic-based approaches due to its comparative simplicity and cost efficiency. Latest technologies of gene expression microarray and NGS are commonly used for global transcriptional profiling of GMO and wild-type ecotype for transcriptional equivalence. Gene expression microarray involves the use of chips containing probes which represent the complete genome of an organism under study. Hybridization of these chips with fluorescently labeled cDNA can identify the genes which are differentially expressed between GMO and wild type. NGS technologies involve sequencing and quantification of nucleotides at the same time. RNA-seq is the type of NGS which specifically deals with the transcriptional studies. Gene expression microarray and RNA-seq have proved themselves equally for the detection of intended and unintended effects. However, both approaches have some advantages and disadvantages. Microarray experiments are comparatively cheaper and easier than RNA-seq. But the chips are commercially available only for a limited number of organisms, and custom printed chips require the genome sequence information of the specific organism. The full power of this technology can only be utilized for sequenced genomes. While RNA-seq is the only technology which can sequence as well as quantify the mRNA libraries of unsequenced genomes. Moreover, RNA-seq provides us the absolute quantification as compared to microarray which give comparative quantification. **Table 1** shows some examples where scientists have utilized these transcriptomic approaches for GMO validation.

Gene expression microarray and RNA-seq methods not only identify the unintended effects of genetic engineering but are also useful in elucidating the mechanism of action of a transgene. Pathway analysis and gene ontology analysis of modified genes lead to the evaluation of molecular basis of phenotypic changes in the newly produced organisms [48]. Transgenic variety of papaya (*Carica papaya* L.) fruit which was resistant to papaya ring spot virus (PRSV) was evaluated against its progenitor variety through RNA-seq analysis. The transcriptional profiles revealed the transcription factors, signaling pathways which were responsible for the stress tolerance and pathogen resistance [43].

Biotic and abiotic stress tolerance is a complex mechanism involving many gene networks and pathways causing changes in the morphology and physiology. Stress-related transcription factors which can bind to the promoters of multiple genes are largely used as transgenes to produce stress-tolerant GMOs. Genetically engineered crops for tolerance against stresses are difficult to get approval for commercialization due to increased risk of pleiotropic effects. Global transcriptome analysis can identify all the pathways affected by any kind of genetic modification and targets for risk assessment.

Transcriptomic approaches have an added benefit of detection of gene silencing in the GMOs produced by gene silencing technology. RNAi-based technologies where double-stranded RNA targeting a specific gene is introduced in an organism. This RNA after being processed in the recipient organism is converted into smaller piece of nearly 21–22 nucleotides. These RNAs reach their targets and inhibit the translation of specific messenger RNA into respective proteins, thus functionally silencing the genes post-transcriptionally. The increasing popularity of this technology is due to its ability to not affect the genome of the GMO [49].

Organism	Altered trait	Gene	Method of evaluation	References
Wheat	Drought and salt tolerance	Glycine max drought-responsive element-binding factor (GmDREB1)	RNA-seq	Jiang et al. [7]
Arabidopsis	Drought tolerance	Abscisic acid-responsive element binding factor 3 (ABF3)	Expression microarray	Abdeen et al. [42]
Arabidopsis	Insect attraction	Farnesyl diphosphate synthase 1 long isoform (FPS1L), nerolidol synthase 1 from Fragaria ananassa (FaNES1), short (cytosolic) isoform of 3-hydroxy-3-methylglutaryl coenzyme A reductase 1 (HMGRIS)	Expression microarray	Houshyani et al. [39]
Papaya	Resistance against papaya ring spot virus	Coat protein (CP) of PRSV	RNA-seq	Fang et al. [43]
Maize	Insect resistance	Cry1Ab	Expression microarray	Coll et al. [44]
Rice	Antifungal protein	Antifungal protein (AFP)	Expression microarray	Montero [45]
Barley	Defense against stresses	Endochitinase	Expression microarray	Kogela [46]
Soybean	Human and viral protein production in plants	Human myelin basic protein (hMBP), human thyroglobulin protein (hTG), mutant nontoxic staphylococcal enterotoxin B gene (mSEB)	RNA-seq	Lambirth et al. [47]

Table 1. Evaluation of GMOs by transcriptome analysis.

7. Conclusion

The newly produced GMOs could be very harmful for the environment, microbial life, and human and animal health, but they are not always harmful. The producers of genetically modified organisms should analyze the global transcriptional profiles of the GMO in comparison with the safe commercial variety to assess the presence or absence of unintended modifications. This data would also provide comprehensive and unbiased information about the metabolic pathways altered in the new organism that can be helpful in designing the strategy for biosafety risk assessment of GMOs.

Transcriptome analysis is very useful for detection and evaluation of transgenics produced by RNAi technology or transcription factor transformations. However, evaluation of gene expression is a very sensitive phenomenon and variable in different tissues and changing conditions. So, for transcriptional analysis, the selection of suitable sample and experimental conditions is critical for reliable results.

Author details

Uzma Qaisar[1]*, Samina Yousaf[2], Tanzeela Rehman[1], Anila Zainab[3] and Asima Tayyeb[1]

*Address all correspondence to: uzma67@hotmail.com

1 School of Biological Sciences, University of the Punjab, Lahore, Pakistan

2 Botany Department, University of the Punjab, Lahore, Pakistan

3 Institute of Agriculture Sciences, University of the Punjab, Lahore, Pakistan

References

[1] Scacheri PC, Rozenblatt-Rosen O, Caplen NJ, Wolfsberg TG, Umayam L, Lee JC, Hughes CM, Shanmuqam KS, Bhattacharjee A, Meyerson M, Collins FS. Short interfering RNAs can induce unexpected and divergent changes in the levels of untargeted proteins in mammalian cells. Proceedings of the National Academy of Sciences of the United States of America 2004;**101**:1892-1897

[2] Enot DP, Beckmann M, Draper J. Detecting a difference – assessing generalisability when modelling metabolome fingerprint data in longer term studies of genetically modified plants. Metabolomics. 2007;**3**(3):335-347. DOI: 10.1007/s11306-007-0064-4

[3] Riesgo A, Peterson K, Richardson C, Heist T, Strehlow B, McCauley M, Cotman C, Hill M, Hill A. Transcriptomic analysis of differential host gene expression upon uptake of symbionts: A case study with Symbiodinium and the major bioeroding sponge Cliona varians. BMC Genomics 2014;**15**:376

[4] Wang S, Qaisar U, Yin X, Grammas P. Gene expression profiling in Alzheimer's disease brain microvessels. Journal of Alzheimer's Disease 2012;**30**:1-13. DOI: 10.3233/JAD-2012-120454

[5] Qaisar U, Irfan M, Meqbool A, Zahoor M, Khan MY, Rashid B, Riazuddin S, Husnain T. Identification, sequencing and characterization of a stress induced homologue of fructose bisphosphate aldolase from cotton. Canadian Journal of Plant Science 2010;**90**(1):41-48

[6] Maqbool A, Zahur M, Irfan M, Qaisar U, Rashid B, Husnain T, Riazuddin S. Identification, characterization and expression of drought related alpha-crystalline heat shock protein gene (GHSP26) from Desi cotton. Crop Science 2007;**47**:2437-2444

[7] Jiang Q, Niu F, Sun X, Hu Z, Li X, Ma Y, Zhang H. RNA-seq analysis of unintended effects in transgenic wheat overexpressing the transcription factor GmDREB1, The Crop Journal 2016;**5**:207-218. DOI: 10.1016/j.cj.2016.12.001

[8] Xu Z, Li J, Guo X, Jin S, Zhang X. Metabolic engineering of cottonseed oil biosynthesis pathway via RNA interference. Scientific Reports 2016;**6**:33342. DOI: 10.1038/srep33342

[9] Ribeiro TP, Arraes FBM, Lourenço-Tessutti IT, Silva MS, Lisei-de-Sá ME, Lucena WA, Macedo LLP, Lima JM, Amorim RMS, Artico S, Alves-Ferreira M, Silva MCM, Sa MFG. Transgenic cotton expressing Cry10Aa toxin confers high resistance to the cotton boll weevil. Plant Biotechnology Journal 2017:1-13. DOI: 10.1111/pbi.12694

[10] James C. Global review of the field testing and commercialization of transgenic plants: 1986-1995. The International Service for the Acquisition of Agri-biotech Applications. 1996

[11] James C. 2014. Global status of commercialized biotech/GM crops. ISAAA Brief 49

[12] Ren L, Zhou P, Zhu Y, Ran RZ, Yu L. Improved eicosapentaenoic acid production in *Pythium splendens* RBB-5 based on metabolic regulation analysis. Applied Microbiology and Biotechnology. 2017;**101**(9):3769-3780. DOI 10.1007/s00253-016-8044-0

[13] Campbell-Platt G. 2011. Food Science and Technology. Ames, IA: John Wiley & Sons; ISBN 978-1-4443-5782-0

[14] Casaretto JA, El-kereamy A, Zeng B, Stiegelmeyer SM, Chen X, Bi Y-M, Rothstein SJ. Expression of OsMYB55 in maize activates stress-responsive genes and enhances heat and drought tolerance. BMC Genomics 2016;**17**:312. DOI: 10.1186/s12864-016-2659-5

[15] Adoption of Genetically Engineered Crops in the USA. Economic Research Service USDA; 2015

[16] Bodnar A. 2010. Risk assessment and mitigation of AquAdvantage Salmon. ISB News Report

[17] Waltz E. Gene-edited CRISPR mushroom escapes US regulation. Nature 2016;**532**:293. DOI: 10.1038/nature.2016.19754

[18] Guana Z-J, Luc S-B, Huod Y-L, Guane Z-P, Liuf B, Weib W. Do genetically modified plants affect adversely on soil microbial communities? Agriculture, Ecosystems and Environment 2016;**235**:289-305

[19] Icoz I, Stotzky G. Fate and effects of insect-resistant Bt crops in soil ecosystems. Soil Biology and Biochemistry 2008;**3**:559-586

[20] Thomson J. Genetically modified food crops for improving agricultural practice and their effects on human health. Trends in Food Science and Technology 2003;**14**:210-228

[21] Craig W, Tepfer M, Degrassi G, Ripandelli D. An overview of general features of risk assessments of genetically modified crops. Euphytica 2008;**164**:853-880

[22] Frewer L, Lassen J, Kettlitz B, Scholderer J, Beekman V, Berdal KG. Societal aspects of genetically modified foods. Food and Chemical Toxicology 2004;**42**:1181-1193

[23] Vergragt PJ, Brown HS. Genetic engineering in agriculture: New approaches for risk management through sustainability reporting. Technological Forecasting and Social Change. 2008;**75**:783-798

[24] Ladics GS, Bartholomaeus A, Bregitzer P, Doerrer NG, Gray A, Holzhauser T, Jordan M, Keese P, Kok E, Macdonald P, Parrott W, Privalle L, Raybould A, Rhee SY, Rice E,

Romeis J, Vaughn J, Wal J-M, Glenn K. Genetic basis and detection of unintended effects in genetically modified crop plants. Transgenic Research 2015;**24**:587-603

[25] Latham JR, Wilson AK, Steinbrecher RA. The mutational consequences of plant transformation. Journal of Biomedicine and Biotechnology. 2006;**253**(76):1-7

[26] Ioset J-R, Urbaniak B, Ndjoko-Ioset K, Wirth J, Martin F, Gruissem W, Hostettmann K, Sautter C. Flavonoid profiling among wild type and related GM wheat varieties. Plant Molecular Biology. 2007;**65**:645-654. DOI: 10.1007/s11103-007-9229-9

[27] Kumar S. Biosafety issues in laboratory research. Biosafety. 2012;**1**:e116

[28] Gachet E, Martin GG, Vigneau F, Meyer, G. Detection of genetically modified organisms (GMOs) by PCR: A brief review of methodologies available. Trends in Food Science & Technology 1999;**9**:380-388

[29] Singh M, Bhoge RK, Randhawa G. Crop-specific GMO matrix-multiplex PCR: A cost-efficient screening strategy for genetically modified maize and cotton events approved globally. Food Control 2016;**70**:271-280

[30] Zhang D, Guo J. The development and standardization of testing methods for genetically modified organisms and their derived products. Journal of Integrative Plant Biology 2011;**53**:539-551

[31] Ha MN, Lee NY. Miniaturized polymerase chain reaction device for rapid identification of genetically modified organisms. Food Control 2015;**57**:238-245. DOI: 10.1016/j.foodcont.2015.04.014

[32] Turkec A, Lucas SJ, Karacanli B, Baykut A, Yuksel H. Assessment of a direct hybridization microarray strategy for comprehensive monitoring of genetically modified organisms (GMOs). Food Chemistry. 2016;**194**:399-409

[33] Preeti R, Kumar A, Ray K, Chaudhary B, Kumar S, Gautam T, Kanoria S, Kaur G, Kumar P, Pental D, Burma PK. Detrimental effect of expression of Bt endotoxin Cry1Ac on in vitro regeneration, in vivo growth and development of tobacco and cotton transgenics. Journal of Biosciences. 2011;**36**(2):363-376

[34] Holst-Jensen A, Spilsberg B, Arulandhu AJ, Kok E, Shi J, Zel J. Application of whole genome shotgun sequencing for detection and characterization of genetically modified organisms and derived products. Analytical and Bioanalytical Chemistry 2016;**408**:4595-4614. DOI: 10.1007/s00216-016-9549-1

[35] Tanaka H. Omics-based medicine and systems pathology: A new perspective for personalized and predictive medicine. Methods of Information in Medicine 2010;**49**:173-185

[36] de Ligt J, Willemsen MH, van Bon BW, Kleefstra T, Yntema HG, Kroes T, Vulto-van Silfhout AT, Koolen DA, de Vries P, Gilissen C, del Rosario M, Hoischen A, Scheffer H, de Vries BB, Brunner HG, Veltman JA, Vissers LE. Diagnostic exome sequencing in persons with severe intellectual disability. The New England Journal of Medicine 2012;**367**:1921-1929

[37] Rauch A, Wieczorek D, Graf E, Wieland T, Endele S, Schwarzmayr T, Albrecht B, Bartholdi D, Beygo J, Di Donato N, Dufke A, Cremer K, Hempel M, Horn D, Hoyer J, Joset P, Röpke A, Moog U, Riess A, Thiel CT, Tzschach A, Wiesener A, Wohlleber E, Zweier C, Ekici AB, Zink AM, Rump A, Meisinger C, Grallert H, Sticht H, Schenck A, Engels H, Rappold G, Schröck E, Wieacker P, Riess O, Meitinger T, Reis A, Strom TM. Range of genetic mutations associated with severe non-syndromic sporadic intellectual disability: An exome sequencing study. Lancet. 2012;**380**:1674-1682

[38] Albo G, Mila S, Digilio G, Motto M, Aime S, Corpillo D. 2007. Proteomic analysis of a genetically modified maize flour carrying cry1ab gene and comparison to the corresponding wild-type. Maydica. 2007;**52**:443-455

[39] Houshyani B, Krol AR, Bino RJ, Bouwmeester HJ. Assessment of pleiotropic transcriptome perturbations in Arabidopsis engineered for indirect insect defence. BMC Plant Biology 2014;**14**:170

[40] Metzdorff SB, Kok EJ, Knuthsen P, Pedersen J. 2006. Evaluation of a nontargeted "omic" approach in the safety assessment of genetically modified plants. Plant Biology (Stuttgart, Germany). 2006;**8**:662-672

[41] Wang L, Wang X, Jin X, Jia R, Huang Q, Tan Y, Guo A. 2015. Comparative proteomics of Bt-transgenic and non-transgenic cotton leaves. Proteome Science. 2015;**13**:15. DOI: 10.1186/s12953-015-0071-8

[42] Abdeen A, Schnell J, Miki B. Transcriptome analysis reveals absence of unintended effects in drought-tolerant transgenic plants overexpressing the transcription factor ABF3. BMC Genomics 2010;**11**:69

[43] Fang F, Lin A, Qiu W, Cai H, Umar M, Chen R, Ming R. Transcriptome profiling revealed stress-induced and disease resistance genes up-regulated in PRSV resistant transgenic papaya. Frontiers in Plant Science. 2016;7:855. DOI: 10.3389/fpls.2016.00855

[44] Coll A, Nadal A, Collado R, Capellades G, Kubista M, Messeguer J, Pla M. Natural variation explains most transcriptomic changes among maize plants of MON810 and comparable non-GM varieties subjected to two N-fertilization farming practices. Plant Molecular Biology 2010;**73**:349-362. DOI: 10.1007/s11103-010-9624-5

[45] Montero M, Coll A, Nadal A, Messeguer J and Pla M. Only half the transcriptomic differences between resistant genetically modified and conventional rice are associated with the transgene. Plant Biotechnology Journal 2011;**9**:693-702

[46] Kogel KH, Voll LM, Schäfer P, Jansen C, Wu Y, Langen G, Imani J, Hofmann J, Schmiedl A, Sonnewald S, Wettstein D, Cook RJ, Sonnewald U. 2009. Transcriptome and metabolome profiling of field grown transgenic barley lack induced differences but show cultivar-specific variances. Proceedings of the National Academy of Sciences. 2009;**107**(14):6198-6203. DOI: 10.1073/pnas.1001945107

[47] Lambirth KC, Whaley AM, Blakley IC, Schlueter JA, Bost KL, Loraine AE, Piller KJ. A comparison of transgenic and wild type soybean seeds: Analysis of transcriptome profiles using RNA-Seq. BMC Biotechnology 2015;**15**:89. DOI: 10.1186/s12896-015-0207-z

[48] Jiang Y, Guo L, Liu R, Jiao B, Zhao X, Ling Z. Overexpression of poplar PtrWRKY89 in transgenic arabidopsis leads to a reduction of disease resistance by regulating defense-related genes in salicylate- and jasmonate-dependent signaling. PloS One. 2016;**11**(3):e0149137. DOI: 10.1371/journal.pone.0149137

[49] Aelbrecht T, Vuylsteke M, Bauwens M, Houdt HV, Depicker A. Introduction of silencing-inducing transgenes does not affect expression of known transcripts. FEBS Letters 2006;**580**:4154-4159

Chapter 9

Transcriptomic Studies in Non-Model Plants: Case of *Pisum sativum* L. and *Medicago lupulina* L.

Olga A. Kulaeva, Alexey M. Afonin,
Aleksandr I. Zhernakov, Igor A. Tikhonovich and
Vladimir A. Zhukov

Additional information is available at the end of the chapter

http://dx.doi.org/10.5772/intechopen.69057

Abstract

Transcriptomics is a dynamically developing branch of biology highly important for geneticists and molecular ecologists alike. A large number of studies concerning differential gene expression, mapping of genes and quantitative trait loci (QTL), analysis of genotyping variations and so on has been conducted recently on several non-model plants using next-generation sequencing techniques. One example of non-model legumes is garden pea (*Pisum sativum* L.), a valuable pulse crop capable of forming nitrogen-fixing nodules and arbuscular mycorrhiza. Adaptation of standardised RNA-seq approaches and data analysis developed for model plants to *P. sativum* should facilitate both studying of pea molecular genetics and breeding of new cultivars possessing agriculturally important traits. Another non-model legume is black medick *Medicago lupulina* L. (a close relative of model legume plant barrel medick, *Medicago truncatula* Gaertn.), for which unique genetic lines almost obligatory dependent on arbuscular mycorrhiza symbiosis formation have been obtained. Such lines show promise as the perfect model for studying the genetic bases of arbuscular mycorrhiza development. In this chapter, we give a brief description of the current developments in the field of garden pea and black medick transcriptomics. Our aim is to provide a quick start guide to the non-expert researchers for next-generation sequencing (NGS)-based transcriptome analysis.

Keywords: transcriptomics, RNA-seq, non-model legume plants, nitrogen-fixing symbiosis, arbuscular mycorrhiza, *Pisum sativum* L., *Medicago lupulina* L.

1. Introduction

Transcriptome is defined as the sum of all the messenger RNA molecules expressed from the genes of an organism, tissue, or a cell. Transcriptome analysis is a powerful method for

plant biology research since studying expressed genes facilitates investigation into plant development, responses to environmental stresses, plant-microbe interactions and so on. Transcriptomic analysis of model organisms, such as the classical object of plant genetics, *Arabidopsis thaliana* (L.) Heyhn., with available full-genome sequence enables researchers to conduct more precise measurements of gene expression level, including alternative splicing and epigenetic modifications studies, in order to reveal the molecular mechanisms involved in specific biological processes [1]. Undoubtedly, many aspects of plant biology, for example, economically important traits such as specific immunity, pathogen resistance and symbiotic efficiency contributing to high crop productivity, cannot be studied with the use of model plants only, making the investigation of non-model plants a necessity.

The rapid decrease of per-base sequencing cost coupled with unprecedented development rates of computational biology practices opened the field of transcriptomics for in-depth investigation of non-model plants [1]. In the last few years, a large number of studies concerning differential gene expression, mapping of genes and quantitative trait loci (QTLs), analysis of genotyping variations and so on using next-generation sequencing (NGS) techniques has been conducted on several non-model plants including legumes (members of family Fabaceae) [2–4].

The leguminous plants (chickpea (*Cicer arietinum* L.), pea (*Pisum sativum* L.) and lentil (*Lens culinaris* Medik.)) were among the earliest domesticated plant species [5] and are to this day an integral part of agricultural systems [6]. These and other members of the Fabaceae family are essential for economics as a food, fodder and oil source [3]. A significant feature of most legume species is their capability of forming mutualistic symbioses with soil microorganisms. Root-nodule symbiosis, the association of the legumes with nodule bacteria collectively called rhizobia, provides the plant with fixed atmospheric nitrogen [7]. This fact makes the legume-rhizobial inter-organismal system an essential component of natural and agricultural ecosystems [8]. Arbuscular-mycorrhizal (AM) symbiosis (association with arbuscular mycorrhizal fungi), inherent to over 80% of land plants including most of legumes [9], facilitates water and mineral (especially phosphorous) uptake of the plant and consequently the nutritional value of the crop. Legumes are also capable of forming symbioses with endophytic plant growth promoting bacteria also contributing to plant productivity [10, 11].

In the early 1990s, two legume species—*Medicago truncatula* Gaertn. and *Lotus japonicus* (Regel.) K. Larsen—were introduced as model objects for studying plant genetics of symbiotic nitrogen fixation and AM development [12–14]. Both species have small diploid genomes (approx. 500 Mb) [15] and are self-pollinators with short generation time able to produce hundreds to thousands of seeds per plant. Intensive studies of genetics resulted in high-quality annotated genomes for both *L. japonicus* and *M. truncatula*, accumulation of gene expression microarray datasets and development of several tools and repositories combining the diverse genetic, genomic and transcriptomic data in these model species (the *Medicago* Gene Expression Atlas [16, 17], the *Medicago* genome database [18], the *Lotus* Base information portal [19], etc.).

During the last decade, rapid development of sequencing and bioinformatics technologies significantly improved the state of genomics in non-model legumes. In the past few years, genomes of important legumes, such as *Glycine max* (L.) Merr. [20], *Phaseolus vulgaris* L. and *Trifolium*

pratense L. [21], were sequenced and are currently available at Phytozome website (https://phytozome.jgi.doe.gov/pz/portal.html) and in the integrative bioinformatic platform Legume IP providing information about gene and protein sequences, gene models and annotations, syntenic regions, protein families and phylogenetic trees [22].

Despite all the recent research progress, most of the agriculturally important legumes were considered 'orphan' crops for a long time as separated from the intense genomic studies due to large genomes, and their agricultural significance mainly in developing countries lacking funds for large-scale 'omics' studies [3]. Most genome and transcriptome analysis tools were developed for particular model objects [23] and can generally be used for studying 'orphan' species [24, 25], although careful fine-tuning may be necessary for successful deployment of said tools in non-model organisms (see **Figure 1**). With the cost of genome assemblies remaining prohibitively high, researchers are forced to work with only transcriptome data, making the analysis strategy all the more important.

It is worth noting that one of the most challenging steps of transcriptome analysis pipelines is correct transcript annotation. The simplest approach giving a sufficiently accurate result is BLAST search against annotated sequences of other species. The development of transcriptome annotation pipelines, for example, Trinotate [26], has more or less taken the burden of transcriptome

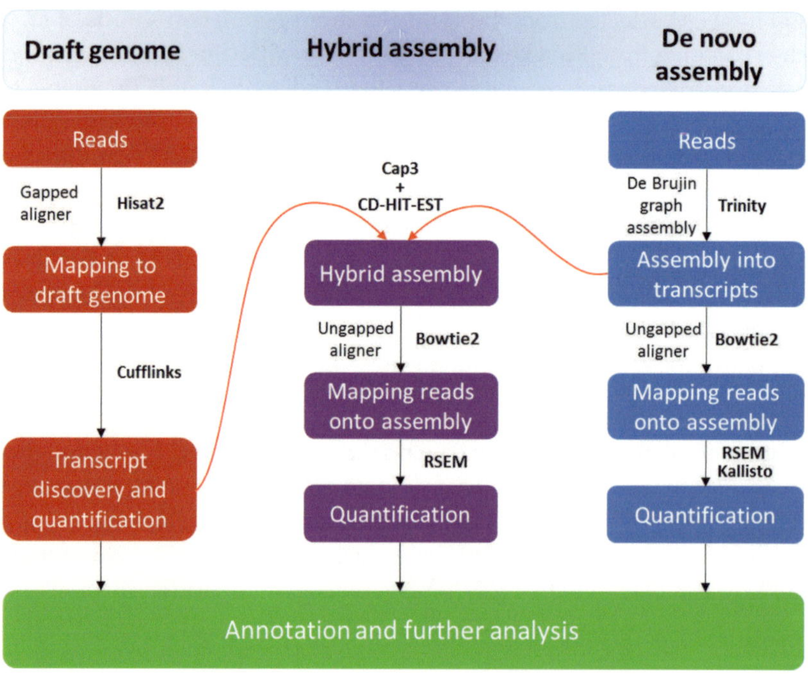

Figure 1. Pipelines of transcriptome assembly in non-model plants (based on the information from Refs. [23, 24].) Three strategies for RNA-seq analysis. (A) Using a draft genome. Novel transcript discovery, quantification and functional annotation. (B) De novo transcriptome assembly with no reference. For quantification, reads are mapped back to the novel reference transcriptome followed by the functional annotation of the novel transcripts as in (A). (C) Combination of the two methods. Transcriptomes are first assembled using methods (A) and (B) then merged using CD-HIT-EST and cap3. Transcripts are then annotated as in (B).

annotation off of the researcher. Trinotate combines the output of a number of annotation tools into an integrated database simplifying the following deeper analysis of acquired data.

One example of an 'orphan' legume is garden pea (*Pisum sativum* L.), a valuable pulse crop capable of forming both nitrogen-fixing symbiosis and arbuscular mycorrhiza. Global production of green pea in 2014 was 17.4 million tons, harvested from 2.3 million hectares, with an additional 11.2 million tons of dried pea from 6.9 million hectares [6]. The genome of the species is considered to be about 4300 Mb with high percentage of repetitive sequences [27]. Adaptation of RNA-seq data analysis approaches standardised for model plants to *P. sativum* should facilitate both studying of pea molecular genetics and breeding of new cultivars possessing agriculturally important traits.

Black medick (*Medicago lupulina* L.), a close relative of a model legume plant barrel medick (*M. truncatula* Gaertn.), is another example of an important (but almost not studied in terms of genetics) non-model legume. It is valuable as a pasture legume component in complex grass mixtures and can also be used as an intermediate culture in crop rotation and as green manure. Black medick is characterised by high protein, vitamin and mineral content, long growing season and ability for improving soil fertility due to nitrogen fixation, therefore being a perfect lawn plant [28]. Black medick is a very promising object for studying AM functioning and development, since a unique genetic line of *M. lupulina* obligatory dependent on arbuscular mycorrhiza symbiosis formation has been selected from the spring landrace population VIK-32 of *M. lupulina* var. *vulgaris* Koch originating from Kazakhstan [28, 29]. Plants of the line MlS-1 (for *Medicago lupulina* Spring) [28] demonstrate dwarfism when grown in the soil with low Pi (inorganic phosphorus) level in the absence of the AM fungi inoculation but can grow normally when inoculated with AM fungus. Therefore, MlS-1 line is considered highly effective in AM symbiosis formation (as inoculation by fungi dramatically heightens the plant biomass). Apparently, MlS-1 line is only capable of using the symbiotrophic way of phosphorus uptake from the soil, supposedly due to yet unidentified mutation(s) and, consequently, can serve as a model object for the investigation of arbuscular-mycorrhizal symbiosis. For instance, this line is suitable for mutagenesis aimed at selection of mutants with defects in arbuscular mycorrhiza development, since plants carrying mutations in genes related to AM formation can be easily identified by visual examination as demonstrating dwarfism under inoculation with AM fungi [29].

High level of genome synteny, similarity of gene sequences and developmental processes provide the opportunity to use the vast amounts of data accumulated on *M. truncatula* in genetics, genomic and transcriptomics of these non-model legumes *M. lupulina* and *P. sativum*. In this chapter, we give a brief description of the current achievements in the field of transcriptomics of non-model legumes black medick (*M. lupulina*) and garden pea (*P. sativum*).

2. Transcriptome assembly studies

2.1. *P. sativum* transcriptomics

The genome of *P. sativum* is as of yet not assembled due to its comparatively large size and numerous repeats, greatly reducing the number of research methods available. Pea transcriptome,

unlike genome, is closer in size to transcriptomes of other legumes, including model plant *M. truncatula*, making it more susceptible to analysis. Due to the existence of tissue-specific gene expression, different plant tissues possess unique sets of transcripts, making the choice of tissue samples important for further research. Furthermore, transcriptome assemblies from distinct plant organs should be used as reference for analysis of tissue-specific processes. A high-quality transcriptome assembly with full tissue representation is therefore crucial for studies associated with gene interactions (differential gene expression, see section 3), gene polymorphism studies and proteome analysis.

In the last 5 years, several pea transcriptome assemblies of distinct organs and tissues were presented by different workgroups. The first publication of pea transcriptome sequencing and assembly was made by Franssen et al. [30]. Total of 20 libraries from flowers, leaves, cotyledons, epicotyls and hypocotyls and etiolated and light-treated etiolated seedlings were sequenced using the Roche 454 sequencing platform. Several iterations of de novo assembly and merging yielded 81,449 unigenes. Sudheesh et al. [31] sequenced transcriptomes from different parts (leaf, stipule, stem, tendril tissues from multiple nodes, root-tip tissues, flowers, stamens, pistils, immature pods, immature seeds and nodules) of two pea cultivars (Parafield and Kaspa) differing in both seed and plant morphological characteristics. Read assembly for separate cultivars yielded 126,335 and 145,730 contigs, respectively, with 87% showing significant expression levels in both cultivars. Later on, Liu et al. sequenced samples from pea seeds harvested at the stage of 10 and 25 days after pollination and assembled 77,273 unigenes [32].

Several transcriptome assembly sets were generated for Single Nucleotide Polymorphism (SNP) marker development and genetic mapping in pea (see section 4). Duarte et al. [33] sequenced libraries from eight pea cultivars (six spring sown, one winter sown field pea, one fodder pea cultivar) with Roche 454 technology. A total of 3,826,797 reads were assembled into 68,850 contigs by MIRA transcriptome assembler [34]. Sindhu et al. sequenced 3′-anchored libraries of eight diverse pea accessions (six *P. sativum* cultivars (CDC Bronco, Alfetta, Cooper, CDC Striker, Nitouche and Orb) and two wild accessions P651 (*P. fulvum*), PI 358610 (*P. sativum* ssp. *abyssinicum*)) with Roche 454 technology, generating 4,008,648 reads in total. De novo assembly was performed for 520,797 reads from the CDC Bronco by MIRA, resulting in a set of 29,725 reference contigs representing a significant proportion of the 3′ end of genes in pea [35].

Since analysis of inter organismal genetic network between pea and rhizobia is a poorly developed field, assembly of a high-quality transcriptome provided researchers with the much-needed data on nodule-specific transcripts. Transcriptomes of pea nodules and root tips were obtained by Zhukov et al. [36]. Transcriptome sequencing using the Illumina Genome Analyzer IIx platform (Illumina Inc.) generated 52,021,865 reads from the 'Nodules' library and 17,684,604 reads from the 'Root Tips' library, yielding 58,397 and 37,287 contigs assembled de novo by Trinity, respectively [37]. A total of 13,000 nodule-specific contigs were annotated by alignment to known plant protein-coding sequences and by Gene Ontology search. Of these, 581 sequences were found to possess full Coding DNA Sequence (CDSs) and could thus be considered novel nodule-specific transcripts of pea. Further investigation of those transcripts can potentially lead to the discovery of key regulators of nodule symbiosis, such as identification of pea gene homologous to *Nodulation signaling pathway 1 (NSP1)* gene of *M. truncatula* [38]. In this study, pea gene *Sym34* was shown to be homologous to the *M. truncatula NSP1* gene,

based on preliminary stop codons detected in an open reading frame of *NSP1* homologous sequence in two *sym34* allelic mutants (RisNod1 and RisNod23) and full co-segregation of the alleles of the hypothetical pea *Nsp1* gene with the nodulation phenotype in F_2 generation.

Alves-Carvalho et al. [39] sequenced transcriptomes of roots, nodules, shoots, leaves, flowers, seeds, tendrils and pods harvested at different developmental stages of pea cultivar 'Caméor'. Sequencing of 20 cDNA libraries produced one billion reads. After de novo assembly and several steps of redundancy reduction, 46,099 contigs were obtained. The main objective of their study was to obtain the most complete transcriptome and to filter out all the artefacts and chimeric contigs so a rigorous filtration pipeline was developed and implemented. The accumulated transcriptome data was used for the development of the Pea RNA-Seq gene atlas containing expression profiles of thousands of genes in several organs, including symbiotic nodules. It is worth noting that the pipeline used in this work filtered out a large proportion of short protein-coding transcripts, including a number of NCR peptide-coding transcripts [40], making the Pea RNA-Seq gene atlas less useful than tissue-specific transcriptomes in some cases.

Pea RNA-Seq gene atlas is also lacking information regarding mycorrhiza-specific transcripts. Genetic framework of mycorrhizal symbiosis is as of yet not fully understood in either model or non-model legumes [38]. In order to discover symbiotically active genes both in plant roots and arbuscular-mycorrhizal fungus, a transcriptome of Frisson pea cultivar roots colonised by *Rhizophagus irregularis* isolate BEG144 was assembled by our workgroup. Sequencing was performed on an Illumina HiSeq2000 sequencing platform yielding 120 million pair end reads. In order to separate the transcriptomes of two organisms present in the samples, all the reads were mapped using the HISAT2 mapper [41] to the genome of *R. irregularis* [42]. Over 5 million successfully mapped reads were assembled by Trinity with default parameters yielding 30,000 transcripts, in good correlation with 28,000 of known genes for the fungus [42, 43].

All the transcripts not mapped to the *R. irregularis* genome were then assembled with the Trinity pipeline with standard assembly parameters and quality trimming parameters. This resulted in more than 200,000 contigs, of which more than 100,000 were similar to genes of pea and other plants of the Fabaceae family.

An assessment of transcriptome assembly and annotation completeness with single-copy orthologs for all available pea transcriptomes was carried out using BUSCO V.2 software with OrthoDB v9.1 'embryophyta' base as a reference [44]. The lowest number of present groups in the transcriptome published by Franssen et al. [30] named 'Franssen' is due to low transcriptome coverage. High number of missing groups in 'Kaspa', 'Parafield' and 'SGE' assemblies are most likely the result of limited tissue representation (see **Figure 2**). Deep sequencing of mycorrhized roots yielded similar results in regard to transcriptome completeness as a combined transcriptome from 20 tissues, indicative of assembly of low-copy transcripts due to high transcriptome coverage.

2.2. *M. lupulina* transcriptomics

M. lupulina is a plant of the Fabaceae family, a close relative to the *M. truncatula*, for which a unique genetic line MlS-1 characterised by obligate mycotrophic lifestyle was obtained [28].

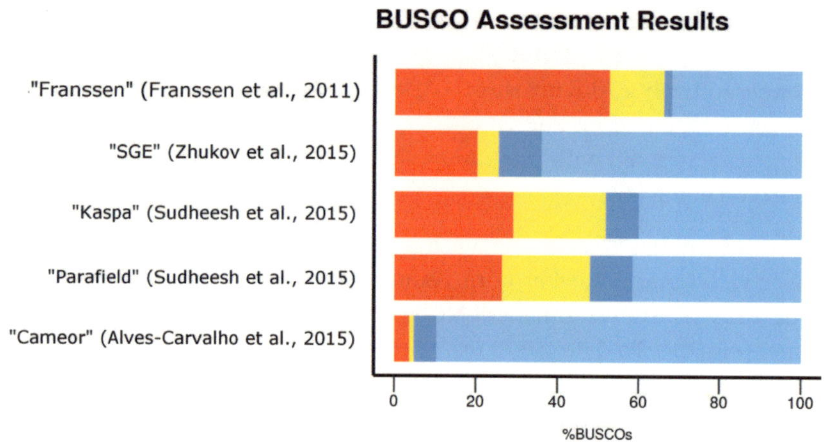

Figure 2. The results of BUSCO analysis of pea transcriptomes. Light-blue: complete and single-copy genes; dark-blue: complete and duplicated genes; yellow: fragmented genes; red: missing genes.

This line may potentially be extremely useful as a model for investigation of genetic foundations of mycorrhizal symbiosis. *M. lupulina* is a novel object for genomic studies, so to kick-start its analysis the transcriptome of the mycorrhized roots of *M. lupulina* was sequenced using the Illumina 2500 platform. Plants of MlS-1 line were grown in soil under inoculation with *R. irregularis* strain RCAM00320, followed by total RNA extraction from the mycorrhized root system and appropriate preparation of cDNA libraries for Illumina sequencing. Using Trinity assembly pipeline, 41 million paired reads were assembled yielding over 138,000 contigs, of which 19,022 showed resemblance to genes of *R. irregularis*. Further analysis revealed over 70,000 contigs similar to known genes of *M. truncatula*. The assembled transcriptome can be used as reference for differential gene expression analysis.

3. Differential gene expression (DGE)

Analysis of alterations in gene expression between conditions or genotypes is the most significant part of transcriptomic data analysis. The differences in expression levels can help determine the important genes and elucidate the processes taking place in the investigated samples.

Extensive analysis of gene expression can be carried out by microarray analysis or RNA sequencing technology. Microarray technology requires prior knowledge of gene sequences and is more suitable for objects with available genome sequence. In the case of model object *M. truncatula,* combination of microarray data resulted in development of atlas of gene expression profiles (*Medicago truncatula* Gene Expression Atlas (MtGEA)) (https://mtgea.noble.org/v3/). MtGEA contains information about gene expression in roots, nodules, stems, petioles, leaves, vegetative buds, flowers, seeds, pods and is potentially helpful for studying other legumes. Despite the fact that pea genome is not sequenced yet, several studies of pea gene expression have been carried

out by microarray technology. Analysis of gene expression during *Mycosphaerella pinodes* infection was carried out using a microarray [45] containing 16,470 different 70-mer oligonucleotides from *M. truncatula* and only 25 did not show a detectable signal [46]. In another study, microarray transcriptome profiling based on known pea Expressed Sequence Tags (ESTs) revealed altered expression of genes associated with programmed cell death, oxidative stress and protein ubiquitylation during seed aging [47].

In spite of many advantages of microarrays, this technique is not effective for quantification of transcript splice variants and, furthermore, cannot provide information about novel genes not included in the array. The development of NGS technology made analysis of full transcriptome gene expression possible. To date, there were several studies of pea gene expression based on RNA-seq technology. Comparative analysis of transcriptional control of pea seed development conducted by RNA-seq revealed significant differences in gene expression between vegetable and grain pea. Genes associated with sugar and starch biosynthesis were significantly activated during seed maturation. Analysis of differential expression of these genes revealed a negative correlation between soluble sugar and starch flux in vegetable and grain pea seeds [32]. Alves-Carvalho et al. [39] developed the Pea RNA-Seq gene atlas containing expression profiles of thousands of genes in different pea tissues harvested at distinct developmental stages [48].

Although RNA-seq technology is indispensable for exhaustive transcriptome studies, it is not the most cost-efficient tool for gene expression analysis due to substantial sequencing depth required for rare transcript detection. There are RNA-seq modifications, for example, Massive Analysis of cDNA Ends (MACE) developed by GenXPro GmbH (Frankfurt am Main, Germany) (http://genxpro.net/) that increase the sequencing depth (number of reads per-transcript) by sequencing only a 50–500 bp fragment (adjacent to the 5′ or 3′-end of the transcript, dependent on the version) [49]. As each read originates from a distinct copy of mRNA, MACE technology is free of duplications and similar artefacts, leading to much more accurate transcript quantification. Even though MACE data cannot be used to distinguish expression of splice-variants of genes, it can be successfully applied in a number of scenarios even with species not possessing a high-quality transcriptome.

In our opinion, 5′MACE is a technology possessing potential for simultaneous analysis of gene expression in prokaryotic and eukaryotic organisms; therefore, this technology is practically tailor-made for the analysis of plant-microbe interaction, particularly for studying the process of root nodule development in the plants of the Fabaceae family.

One of the many challenges in analysing the onset of nodule symbiosis is the small amounts of tissue available. Enclosed environments of symbiotic compartments complicate direct measurements. Implementation of 5′MACE technology made it possible to analyse the gene expression patterns of both organisms simultaneously in a developing nodule and at a fraction of the cost of a full RNA-seq study.

In our group, 5′MACE was implemented in a study investigating the expression changes in pea nodules caused by a mutation in the *Sym31* gene with unknown function. This gene is responsible for the unique fix$^-$ mutant phenotype (non-nitrogen-fixing nodules) with halted bacteroid development [50]. Two plant genotypes Sprint-2Fix$^-$ (carrying a mutation in the

Sym31 gene) and parental wild-type line Sprint-2 were inoculated with an efficient *Rhizobium leguminosarum* bv. *viciae* RCAM1026 [51]. All the obtained reads were sequentially mapped to the RCAM1026 genome (about 8% mapped reads), then to the pea transcriptome assembly from Alves-Carvalho et al. [39] (about 60% mapped reads) resulting in two sets of differential transcriptome data. The transcript quantification was carried out using the edgeR package [52]. Differentially expressed genes were then visualised on a metabolic map using KOBAS 2.0 annotation server [53]. Analysis resulted in the discovery of a coordinated shift in sulphur metabolism in both organisms. These preliminary data show the great potential of the 5′MACE technology in furthering our understanding of inter-organismal gene regulatory networks in plant-microbe interactions.

4. Transcript-based markers and their usage

The application of NGS for massive genetic polymorphism discovery is widely used due to being much more labour and time efficient than previously used methods such as microarray hybridisation [54] or denaturing high-performance liquid chromatography (HPLC) [55]. Originally, the main challenge in using NGS methods for massive polymorphism screening was obtaining sequences of a particular genomic locus for multiple lines due to complexity of plant genomes and the relatively low productivity of the first-generation NGS-sequencing platforms, leading to the development of several methods for sequencing optimisation.

For example, Restriction site Associated DNA-sequencing method (RAD-Seq) consists of genome cleavage and selection of fragments of appropriate size flanked by specific restriction sites (as with RFLP and AFLP analyses) [56]. RAD-Seq yields fragments distributed randomly over a genome and is suitable for discovering indels (insertion-deletion polymorphisms), SNVs (single nucleotide variations) and microsatellites simple sequence repeats (SSR). Using RAD-Seq, Boutet et al. [57] discovered a total of 419,024 SNVs between at least two of the four pea lines analysed in their work. Pea genetic map constructed by genotyping a subset of 64,754 SNVs on a subpopulation of 48 RILs (recombinant inbred lines) was collinear with previous pea consensus maps and therefore with the *M. truncatula* genome. Yang et al. [58] using Illumina HiSeq 2500 platform uncovered 8899 putative SSR-containing sequences. Reliable amplifications of detectable polymorphic fragments among 24 genotypes of pea were obtained for about a half of randomly selected SSR, 820 in total.

Another way of data complexity reduction is transcriptome sequencing. It makes the discovery of polymorphic sites in open reading frames (ORFs) and 5′- and 3′-untranslated regions (UTR) of a gene possible. Moreover, polymorphic sites associated with individual genes may have special meaning for evolutionary studies and QTL analyses. Even though the transcriptome sequencing omits introns and intergenic regions, it can successfully be used for SSR site detection.

Several polymorphism-screening studies aimed on SNVs and SSR sites discovering in transcriptomic data were performed on pea (see **Table 1**). SNVs detection may be executed by mapping NGS reads to an existing reference transcriptome assembly [59] or by de novo assembly of those reads [33, 35, 60]. In the case of existing assembly, the additional data complexity

Year	Plant material	Platform, technique	Number of putative discovered SNVs	Number of putative discovered SSR-sites	Number of created and mapped markers	References
2013	Parafield, Yarrum, Kaspa, 96–286	454 Roche, GS-FLX	36,188	2932	705	Leonforte et al. [60]
2014	*Six spring sown*: Lumina, Hardy, Panache, Rocket, Kayanne, Terese *One winter sown*: Cherokee *One fodder*: Champagne	Roche 454, GS-FLX	35,455	2397	1340	Duarte et al. [33]
2014	*Pisum sativum*: CDC Bronco, Alfetta, Cooper, CDC Striker, Nitouche, Orb. *P. fulvum*: P651 *P. sativum* ssp. *abyssinicum*: PI 358610	Roche 454, Titanium	over 20,000	406	1536	Sindhu et al. [35]
2017	SGE = JI3023 Finale = JI2678 Frisson = JI2491 NGB1238 = JI0073 Sparkle = JI0427 Sprint-2 = JI2612	Illumina HiSeq 2000, MACE	34,711	-	-	Zhernakov et al. [59]

Table 1. Studies aimed at gene polymorphism detection in pea (*Pisum sativum* L.) using transcriptome NGS-sequencing.

reduction is achievable by limiting sequenced mRNA regions. Since UTRs are generally more polymorphic than ORFs using sequences from the 3′ and 5′ mRNA, ends in SNV analysis should yield comparable results to those obtained with RNA-seq. 3′MACE protocol for cDNA-libraries preparation was used by Zhernakov et al. [59] to discover SNVs distinguishing six pea lines. Mapping MACE reads to the reference nodule transcriptome assembly of the pea line SGE [36] resulted in characterisation of over 34,000 polymorphic sites in more than 9700 contigs. Several of these SNVs were located within recognition sites of restriction endonucleases which allowed the design of co-dominant Cleaved Amplified Polymorphic Sequences (CAPS) markers for the particular transcript.

SNVs are markers of choice now due to their abundance and the availability of high-throughput screening techniques. SNV genotyping systems are now available, varying in the number of samples and markers to be genotyped, such as GoldenGate® and Infinium from Illumina Inc., SNPStream from Beckman Coulter and GeneChip from Affymetrix [61]. Illumina GoldenGate® oligonucleotide pool assay (OPA) designed for transcriptome-discovered SNVs was used for pea salinity tolerance QTLs search [60].

As the pea genome is not sequenced yet, the genetic linkage maps are still relevant, since determination of loci responsible for target traits requires their fine mapping and subsequent

search for candidate genes in the already sequenced genome of the model legume plant *M. truncatula*. Transcriptome-discovered SNVs and high-throughput genotyping systems made the construction of several highly saturated genetic maps of pea possible (see **Table 1**) [33, 35, 60].

5. Conclusion

Next-generation sequencing techniques make the analysis of differential gene expression and molecular marker development by transcriptome sequencing possible even in species lacking genomic information. Further development of sequencing and bioinformatics should substantially promote the investigation into genetics of non-model plants. It is worth noting that numerous traits like effectiveness of symbioses development [62] or specific resistance to pathogens can only be studied in each particular cultivated plant species, most having limited genomic data available. In addition, the decline in biodiversity makes the investigation of unique secondary metabolites inherent to non-model medicinal plants a pressing matter.

Leguminous plants capable of improving the soil quality due to the formation of the mutualistic symbioses with nodule bacteria and arbuscular mycorrhizal fungi are an integral part of agricultural systems. The genetics of most crop legumes lags behind that of model plants, and some are even considered 'orphan' crops, separated from the intense genomic studies due to a number of factors. Fortunately, the similarity of genome organisation, or 'genome synteny', characteristic for most related species, can help 'translate' the genomic data from the model legumes to their pulse crop relatives [63].

Using RNA-seq technologies for de novo transcriptome assembly provides opportunities for finding novel genes and isoforms in non-model species and investigation of their differential expression. Comparison to genomes and transcriptomes of closely related species can help determine the level of evolutionary distance between the two species and discover possible evolutionary pressures shaping contemporary species. Technologies for determining gene expression levels using transcript ends (like 3′ and 5′ MACE) can be used to conduct large-scale gene expression studies on a smaller budget. 5′ MACE, a technology for simultaneous analysis of prokaryotic and eukaryotic transcript abundancies, is particularly useful for studying plant-bacteria interactions. Using transcriptome-sequencing data in genetic marker development streamlines the construction of high-quality genomic maps, crucial for routine gene identification tasks as well as potentially for refining genome assemblies for non-model organisms. All the methods are useful in investigation of the unique phenotypes not present in the model plants, for example, *M. lupulina* MlS-1 genetic line, uniquely dependent on the AM formation. Adaptation of standardised RNA-seq approaches and data analysis developed for model plants to an important crop culture *P. sativum* should facilitate the breeding of new cultivars that meet the requirements of the present-day agriculture and possess the complex of beneficial traits, including increased efficiency of interactions with nodule bacteria and arbuscular-mycorrhizal fungi.

Acknowledgements

The work was supported by Russian Foundation for Basic Research (grant # 16-34-60132 for O.A. Kulaeva), by grant of the President of the Russian Federation (project NSh-6759.2016.4 for A.M. Afonin), by Russian Science Foundation (grant # 14-24-00135 for I.A. Tikhonovich and grant # 16-16-00118 for A.I. Zhernakov and V.A. Zhukov). The authors thank Dr A.P. Yurkov (ARRIAM, St. Petersburg, Russia) for providing the *Medicago lupulina* L. MlS-1 line and A.S. Sulima (ARRIAM, St. Petersburg, Russia) for critical reading of the manuscript.

Author details

Olga A. Kulaeva[1], Alexey M. Afonin[1], Aleksandr I. Zhernakov[1], Igor A. Tikhonovich[1,2] and Vladimir A. Zhukov[1]*

*Address all correspondence to: zhukoff01@yahoo.com

1 All-Russia Research Institute for Agricultural Microbiology, Saint Petersburg, Russia

2 Saint Petersburg State University, Saint Petersburg, Russia

References

[1] Dong Z, Chen Y. Transcriptomics: Advances and approaches. Science China Life Sciences. 2013;**56**:960-967. DOI: 10.1007/s11427-013-4557-2

[2] Kumawat G, Gupta S, Ratnaparkhe MB, Maranna S, Satpute GK. QTLomics in soybean: A way forward for translational genomics and breeding. Frontiers in Plant Science. 2016;**7**:1852. DOI: 10.3389/fpls.2016.01852

[3] Varshney RK, Close TJ, Singh NK, Hoisington DA, Cook DR. Orphan legume crops enter the genomics era! Current Opinion in Plant Biology. 2009;**12**:202-210. DOI: 10.1016/j.pbi.2008.12.004

[4] Xiao M, Zhang Y, Chen X, Lee EJ, Barber CJ, Chakrabarty R, et al. Transcriptome analysis based on next-generation sequencing of non-model plants producing specialized metabolites of biotechnological interest. Journal of Biotechnology. 2013;**166**:122-134. DOI: 10.1016/j.jbiotec.2013.04.004

[5] Zohary D, Hopf M, Weiss E. Domestication of Plants in the Old World: The origin and spread of domesticated plants in Southwest Asia, Europe, and the Mediterranean Basin. Oxford University Press Inc., New York; 2012

[6] Food and Agriculture Organization of the United Nations (FAOSTAT) [Internet]. 2017. Available from: http://www.fao.org/faostat/en/

[7] Sprent JI, Nodulation in legumes. Royal Botanic Gardens. Kew: Royal Botanic Gardens; 2001.

[8] Provorov N, Tikhonovich I. Genetic resources for improving nitrogen fixation in legume-rhizobia symbiosis. Genetic Resources and Crop Evolution. 2003;**50**:89-99. DOI: 10.1023/A:1022957429160

[9] Smith SE, Read DJ. Mycorrhizal symbiosis. Academic press; 2008

[10] Elvira-Recuenco M, Van Vuurde J. Natural incidence of endophytic bacteria in pea cultivars under field conditions. Canadian Journal of Microbiology. 2000;**46**:1036-1041

[11] Mishra PK, Mishra S, Selvakumar G, Bisht J, Kundu S, Gupta HS. Coinoculation of Bacillus thuringeinsis-KR1 with Rhizobium leguminosarum enhances plant growth and nodulation of pea (*Pisum sativum* L.) and lentil (*Lens culinaris* L.). World Journal of Microbiology and Biotechnology. 2009;**25**:753-761. DOI: 10.1186/1471-2164-8-427

[12] Barker DG, Bianchi S, Blondon F, Dattée Y, Duc G, Essad S, et al. *Medicago truncatula*, a model plant for studying the molecular genetics of theRhizobium-legume symbiosis. Plant Molecular Biology Reporter. 1990;**8**:40-49

[13] Cook DR. *Medicago truncatula*—a model in the making!: Commentary. Current Opinion in Plant Biology. 1999;**2**:301-304

[14] Stougaard J. Genetics and genomics of root symbiosis. Current Opinion in Plant Biology. 2001;**4**:328-335

[15] Young ND, Cannon SB, Sato S, Kim D, Cook DR, Town CD, et al. Sequencing the genespaces of *Medicago truncatula* and *Lotus japonicus*. Plant Physiology. 2005;**137**:1174-1181. DOI: 10.1104/pp.104.057034

[16] Benedito VA, Torres-Jerez I, Murray JD, Andriankaja A, Allen S, Kakar K, et al. A gene expression atlas of the model legume *Medicago truncatula*. The Plant Journal. 2008;**55**:504-513. DOI: 10.1111/j.1365-313X.2008.03519.x

[17] He J, Benedito VA, Wang M, Murray JD, Zhao PX, Tang Y, et al. The *Medicago truncatula* gene expression atlas web server. BMC Bioinformatics. 2009;**10**:441. DOI: 10.1186/1471-2105-10-441

[18] Krishnakumar V, Kim M, Rosen BD, Karamycheva S, Bidwell SL, Tang H, et al. MTGD: The *Medicago truncatula* genome database. Plant and Cell Physiology. 2014;**56**:pcu179. DOI: 10.1093/pcp/pcu179

[19] Mun T, Bachmann A, Gupta V, Stougaard J, Andersen SU. Lotus base: An integrated information portal for the model legume *Lotus japonicus*. Scientific Reports. 2016;**6**:39447. DOI: 10.1038/srep39447

[20] Schmutz J, Cannon SB, Schlueter J, Ma J, Mitros T, Nelson W, et al. Genome sequence of the palaeopolyploid soybean. Nature. 2010;**463**:178-183. DOI: 10.1038/nature08670

[21] De Vega JJ, Ayling S, Hegarty M, Kudrna D, Goicoechea JL, Ergon Å, et al. Red clover (*Trifolium pratense* L.) draft genome provides a platform for trait improvement. Scientific Reports. 2015;**5**:17394. DOI: 10.1038/srep17394

[22] Li J, Dai X, Zhuang Z, Zhao PX. LegumeIP 2.0—a platform for the study of gene function and genome evolution in legumes. Nucleic Acids Research. 2016;**44**:D1189-D1194. DOI: 10.1093/nar/gkv1237

[23] Conesa A, Madrigal P, Tarazona S, Gomez-Cabrero D, Cervera A, Mcpherson A, et al. A survey of best practices for RNA-seq data analysis. Genome Biology. 2016;**17**:13. DOI: 10.1186/s13059-016-0881-8

[24] Marchant A, Mougel F, Almeida C, Jacquin-Joly E, Costa J, Harry M. De novo transcriptome assembly for a non-model species, the blood-sucking bug *Triatoma brasiliensis*, a vector of Chagas disease. Genetica. 2015;**143**:225-239. DOI: 10.1007/s10709-014-9790-5

[25] Garg R, Jain M. RNA-Seq for Transcriptome Analysis in Non-model Plants. In: Rose RJ, editor. *Legume Genomics: Methods and Protocols*. Totowa, NJ: Humana Press; 2013. pp. 43-58

[26] Trinotate: Transcriptome Functional Annotation and Analysis [Internet]. Available from: https://trinotate.github.io/

[27] Macas J, Neumann P, Navrátilová A. Repetitive DNA in the pea (*Pisum sativum* L.) genome: Comprehensive characterization using 454 sequencing and comparison to soybean and *Medicago truncatula*. BMC Genomics. 2007;**8**:427. DOI: 10.1186/1471-2164-8-427

[28] Yurkov A, Jacobi L, Gapeeva N, Stepanova G, Shishova M. Development of arbuscular mycorrhiza in highly responsive and mycotrophic host plant-black medick (*Medicago lupulina* L.). Russian Journal of Developmental Biology. 2015;**46**:263-275. DOI: 10.1134/S1062360415050082

[29] Yurkov AP, Jacobi LM. Selection of mycorrhizal mutants in black medic (*Medicago lupulina*) [in Russian]. Natural and Technical Sciences. 2011;**6**:127-134

[30] Franssen SU, Shrestha RP, Bräutigam A, Bornberg-Bauer E, Weber AP. Comprehensive transcriptome analysis of the highly complex *Pisum sativum* genome using next generation sequencing. BMC Genomics. 2011;**12**:227. DOI: 10.1186/1471-2164-12-227

[31] Sudheesh S, Sawbridge TI, Cogan NO, Kennedy P, Forster JW, Kaur S. De novo assembly and characterisation of the field pea transcriptome using RNA-Seq. BMC Genomics. 2015;**16**:611. DOI: 10.1186/s12864-015-1815-7

[32] Liu N, Zhang G, Xu S, Mao W, Hu Q, Gong Y. Comparative transcriptomic analyses of vegetable and grain pea (*Pisum sativum* L.) seed development. Frontiers in Plant Science. 2015;**6**:1039. DOI: 10.3389/fpls.2015.01039

[33] Duarte J, Rivière N, Baranger A, Aubert G, Burstin J, Cornet L, et al. Transcriptome sequencing for high throughput SNP development and genetic mapping in pea. BMC Genomics. 2014;**15**:126. DOI: 10.1186/1471-2164-15-126

[34] MIRA—Sequence Assembler and Sequence Mapping for Whole Genome Shotgun and EST/RNASeq Sequencing Data [Internet]. Available from: https://sourceforge.net/projects/mira-assembler/

[35] Sindhu A, Ramsay L, Sanderson LA, Stonehouse R, Li R, Condie J, et al. Gene-based SNP discovery and genetic mapping in pea. Theoretical and Applied Genetics. 2014;**127**:2225-2241. DOI: 10.1007/s00122-014-2375-y

[36] Zhukov VA, Zhernakov AI, Kulaeva OA, Ershov NI, Borisov AY, Tikhonovich IA. De novo assembly of the pea (*Pisum sativum* L.) nodule transcriptome. International Journal of Genomics. 2015;**2015**:695947. DOI: 10.1155/2015/695947

[37] Grabherr MG, Haas BJ, Yassour M, Levin JZ, Thompson DA, Amit I, et al. Trinity: Reconstructing a full-length transcriptome without a genome from RNA-Seq data. Nature Biotechnology. 2011;**29**:644. DOI: 10.1038/nbt.1883

[38] Shtark O, Kumari S, Singh R, Sulima A, Akhtemova G, Zhukov V, et al. Advances and prospects for development of multi-component microbial inoculant for legumes. Legume Perspectives. 2015;**8**:40-44. DOI: 10.13140/RG.2.1.1634.0247

[39] Alves-Carvalho S, Aubert G, Carrère S, Cruaud C, Brochot AL, Jacquin F, et al. Full-length de novo assembly of RNA-seq data in pea (Pisum sativum L.) provides a gene expression atlas and gives insights into root nodulation in this species. The Plant Journal. 2015;**84**:1-19. DOI: 10.1186/s13059-016-0881-8

[40] Tikhonovich IA, Kliukova MS, Kulaeva OA, Zhernakov AI, Zhukov VA. The Process of Bacteroid Differentiation in Pea (*Pisum sativum* L.) is Controlled by Symbiotic Genes that Regulate the Expression of the NCR Gene Family. In: Book of Abstracts 12th European Nitrogen Fixation Conference; 25-28 August 2016; Budapest, Hungary; 2016. p. 232

[41] Pertea M, Kim D, Pertea GM, Leek JT, Salzberg SL. Transcript-level expression analysis of RNA-seq experiments with HISAT, StringTie and Ballgown. Nature Protocols. 2016;**11**:1650-1667. DOI: 10.1038/nprot.2016.095

[42] Tisserant E, Malbreil M, Kuo A, Kohler A, Symeonidi A, Balestrini R, et al. Genome of an arbuscular mycorrhizal fungus provides insight into the oldest plant symbiosis. Proceedings of the National Academy of Sciences. 2013;**110**:20117-20122. DOI: 10.1073/pnas.1313452110

[43] INRA GlomusDB, the Glomus Intraradices Genome Database Version 2.0. [Internet]. Available from: http://mycor.nancy.inra.fr/IMGC/GlomusGenome/index3.html

[44] Simão FA, Waterhouse RM, Ioannidis P, Kriventseva EV, Zdobnov EM. BUSCO: Assessing genome assembly and annotation completeness with single-copy orthologs. Bioinformatics. 2015;**31**:3210-3212. DOI: 10.1093/bioinformatics/btv351

[45] Küster H, Hohnjec N, Krajinski F, El Yahyaoui F, Manthey K, Gouzy J, et al. Construction and validation of cDNA-based Mt6k-RIT macro- and microarrays to explore root endosymbioses in the model legume Medicago truncatula. Journal of Biotechnology. 2004;**108**:95-113. DOI: 10.1016/j.jbiotec.2003.11.011

[46] Fondevilla S, Küster H, Krajinski F, Cubero JI, Rubiales D. Identification of genes differentially expressed in a resistant reaction to *Mycosphaerella pinodes* in pea using microarray technology. BMC Genomics. 2011;**12**:28. DOI: 10.1186/1471-2164-12-28

[47] Chen H, Osuna D, Colville L, Lorenzo O, Graeber K, Kuester H, et al. Transcriptome-wide mapping of pea seed ageing reveals a pivotal role for genes related to oxidative stress and programmed cell death. PLoS One. 2013;**8**:e78471. DOI: 10.1371/journal.pone.0078471

[48] The Pea RNA-Seq Gene Atlas [Internet]. 2015. Available from: http://bios.dijon.inra.fr/FATAL/cgi/pscam.cgi

[49] Zawada AM, Rogacev KS, Müller S, Rotter B, Winter P, Fliser D, et al. Massive analysis of cDNA Ends (MACE) and miRNA expression profiling identifies proatherogenic pathways in chronic kidney disease. Epigenetics. 2014;**9**:161-172. DOI: 10.4161/epi.26931

[50] Borisov AY, Rozov S, Tsyganov V, Morzhina E, Lebsky V, Tikhonovich I. Sequential functioning of *Sym-13* and *Sym-31*, two genes affecting symbiosome development in root nodules of pea (*Pisum sativum* L.). Molecular and General Genetics MGG. 1997;**254**:592-598

[51] Afonin A, Sulima A, Zhernakov A, Zhukov V. Draft genome of the strain RCAM1026 *Rhizobium leguminosarum* bv. *viciae*. Genomics Data. 2016;**11**:85-86. DOI: 10.1016/j.gdata.2016.12.003

[52] Robinson MD, Mccarthy DJ, Smyth GK. edgeR: A bioconductor package for differential expression analysis of digital gene expression data. Bioinformatics. 2010;**26**:139-140. DOI: 10.1093/bioinformatics/btp616

[53] Xie C, Mao X, Huang J, Ding Y, Wu J, Dong S, et al. KOBAS 2.0: A web server for annotation and identification of enriched pathways and diseases. Nucleic Acids Research. 2011;**39**:W316-W322. DOI: 10.1093/nar/gkr483

[54] Beaudet L, Bédard J, Breton B, Mercuri RJ, Budarf ML. Homogeneous assays for single-nucleotide polymorphism typing using AlphaScreen. Genome Research. 2001;**11**:600-608. DOI: 10.1101/gr.1725501

[55] Xiao W, Oefner PJ. Denaturing high-performance liquid chromatography: A review. Human Mutation. 2001;**17**:439-474. DOI: 10.1002/humu.1130

[56] Davey JW, Blaxter ML. RAD-Seq: Next-generation population genetics. Briefings in Functional Genomics. 2010;**9**:416-423. DOI: 10.1093/bfgp/elq031

[57] Boutet G, Carvalho SA, Falque M, Peterlongo P, Lhuillier E, Bouchez O, et al. SNP discovery and genetic mapping using genotyping by sequencing of whole genome genomic DNA from a pea RIL population. BMC Genomics. 2016;**17**:121. DOI: 10.1186/s12864-016-2447-2

[58] Yang T, Fang L, Zhang X, Hu J, Bao S, Hao J, et al. High-throughput development of SSR markers from pea (*Pisum sativum* L.) based on next generation sequencing of a purified chinese commercial variety. PLoS One. 2015;**10**:e0139775. DOI: 10.1371/journal.pone.0139775

[59] Zhernakov A, Rotter B, Winter P, Borisov A, Tikhonovich I, Zhukov V. Massive analysis of cDNA ends (MACE) for transcript-based marker design in pea (*Pisum sativum* L.). Genomics Data. 2017;**11**:75-76. DOI: 10.1016/j.gdata.2016.12.004

[60] Leonforte A, Sudheesh S, Cogan NO, Salisbury PA, Nicolas ME, Materne M, et al. SNP marker discovery, linkage map construction and identification of QTLs for enhanced salinity tolerance in field pea (*Pisum sativum* L.). BMC Plant Biology. 2013;**13**:161

[61] Deulvot C, Charrel H, Marty A, Jacquin F, Donnadieu C, Lejeune-Hénaut I, et al. Highly-multiplexed SNP genotyping for genetic mapping and germplasm diversity studies in pea. BMC Genomics. 2010;**11**:468. DOI: 10.1186/1471-2164-11-468

[62] Shtark OY, Borisov AY, Zhukov VA, Tikhonovich IA. Mutually beneficial legume symbioses with soil microbes and their potential for plant production. Symbiosis. 2012;**58**:51-62. DOI: 10.1007/s13199-013-0226-2

[63] Young ND, Udvardi M. Translating *Medicago truncatula* genomics to crop legumes. Current Opinion in Plant Biology. 2009;**12**:193-201. DOI: 10.1016/j.pbi.2008.11.005

Chapter 10

Transcriptome Analysis in Chickpea (*Cicer arietinum* L.): Applications in Study of Gene Expression, Non-Coding RNA Prediction, and Molecular Marker Development

Chandra Kant, Vimal Pandey, Subodh Verma,
Manish Tiwari, Santosh Kumar and Sabhyata Bhatia

Additional information is available at the end of the chapter

http://dx.doi.org/10.5772/intechopen.69884

Abstract

Extensive analyses of transcriptome have been carried out in chickpea, which is the third most important legume valued as a source of dietary protein and micronutrients. Over the last two decades, several laboratories have used a wide range of techniques encompassing expressed sequence tag (EST) analysis, serial analysis of gene expression (SAGE), microarray and next-generation sequencing (NGS) technologies for analysing the chickpea transcriptomes. However, chickpea transcriptome analysis witnessed significant progress with the advent of the NGS platforms. Gene expression analyses using NGS platforms were carried out in the vegetative and reproductive tissues such as shoot, root, mature leaf, flower bud, young pod, seed and nodule by various groups which resulted in identification of several tissue-specific transcripts. Some laboratories have utilized transcriptomics to explore the response of chickpea to abiotic and biotic stresses such as drought, salinity, heat, cold, *Fusarium oxysporum* and *Ascochyta rabiei* differentially expressed genes and also established crosstalk between biotic and abiotic stress responses. Transcriptome analysis has been utilized extensively to identify non-coding RNAs such as miRNAs and long intergenic non-coding (LINC) RNAs. Transcriptome analysis has facilitated the development of molecular markers such as simple sequence repeats (SSRs), single-nucleotide polymorphisms (SNPs) and potential intron polymorphisms (PIPs) that are being used to expedite the chickpea breeding programmes. The available chickpea transcriptomes will continue to serve as the foundation for devising strategies for chickpea improvement.

Keywords: transcriptome, chickpea, next-generation sequencing (NGS), gene expression, molecular markers

1. Introduction

Chickpea (*Cicer arietinum* L.) is a diploid (2*n* = 16), self-pollinated plant which is grown in the cool season and has a genome size of 738 Mb [1]. It is the third most produced pulse crop in the world (13.73 million tons) after beans (26.52 million tons) and green pea (17.43 million tons) (FAOSTAT 2014). It is considered to be an ideal crop for the semiarid and arid regions as it exhibits an extensive tap root system. Chickpea seeds are an excellent source of nutrition as they contain ≈40% carbohydrates, ≈6% oil and 20–30% protein and good source of minerals and trace elements such as calcium, magnesium, phosphorus, iron and zinc [2]. Moreover, chickpea contributes to improvement of soil fertility since it has the capability to establish symbiotic association with *Mesorhizobium ciceri* that helps in fixing atmospheric nitrogen to the reduced nitrogen (NH_3). Chickpea, through symbiotic nitrogen fixation (SNF), can fulfil up to 80% of its nitrogen requirement [3]. All these qualities make chickpea an economically important crop as it is an affordable source that can fulfil the dietary protein requirement of the masses.

2. Challenges in chickpea production

The world average of chickpea productivity is 982.1 kg/ha (FAOSTAT 2014); however, a simulated study showed that potential productivity of chickpea in rain-fed situations ranged from 1390 to 4590 kg/ha [4]. There is a huge yield gap of 408–3608 kg/ha. A number of biotic and abiotic factors affect chickpea plant growth and, therefore, are responsible for poor productivity.

Chickpea is mostly raised on conserved soil moisture under rain-fed conditions [5]. Therefore, drought stress generally affects the crop at terminal stage [6] and leads to productivity loss of up to 50% [7]. Drought reduces overall biomass, reproductive growth and seed yield and increases flower abortion, pod abscission and number of empty pods [8]. Soil salinity affects productivity by delaying the flowering leading to decrease in reproductive success of chickpea [9]. Since chickpea is a cool season crop, high temperatures adversely affect the development of the plant [10]. Chander [11] reported a decline in yield of chickpea by about 301 kg/ha per 1°C increase in mean seasonal temperature in India [12, 13]. Biotic factors also adversely affect the yield of chickpea crop. *Fusarium* wilt, caused by *Fusarium oxysporum* f.sp. *ciceri*; *Ascochyta* blight, caused by *Ascochyta rabiei* and *Botrytis* grey mould, caused by *Botrytis cinerea* mainly affect the leaves of chickpea, whereas *Pythium ultimum* causes root and seed rot and is common in the areas where the chickpea growing season is cool and humid [14, 15]. A number of other fungi, such as *Alternaria* sp., *Ascochyta pisi*, *Uromyces* sp., *Botrytis* sp., *Phytophthora medicaginis* and so on, cause considerable damage to chickpea crops. Pod borer (*Helicoverpa armigera* Hubner) is the major pest affecting chickpea worldwide [15–17]. Therefore, improvement in yield, nutritional quality and stress tolerance are the major targets of chickpea research and breeding programmes which may be facilitated by detailed understanding of biological processes occurring in tissue-specific and developmental pathways. Moreover, responses to various stresses at molecular level also need to be elucidated in detail.

3. Legume genomics

With the advent of next-generation sequencing technologies, there has been a rapid increase in the efficiency of DNA and RNA sequencing and decrease in the cost involved. *Leguminosae* is a very important family known due to the economic and nutritional value of its members [18]. The recent years have witnessed a spurt in the number of studies utilizing genomic approaches to understand the biology of several agronomic traits in legumes.

The advances in DNA sequencing have led to whole genome sequencing of important legumes such as *Glycine max* [19], *Medicago truncatula* [20], *Lotus japonicus* [21], *Cajanus cajan* [22], *Phaseolus vulgaris* [23], diploid ancestors of peanut *Arachis duranensis* and *Arachis ipaensis* [24] and *C. arietinum* [1, 25]. Moreover, whole genome resequencing has been carried out for soybean [26, 27], *Medicago* [28] and chickpea [1] in order to understand the genetic variability, evolution and domestication in greater depth. Simultaneously, in order to unravel the functional aspects of legume biology, several NGS-based studies of transcriptomes were carried out. These studies have made significant contributions towards understanding of gene expression, alternative splicing events and small RNA identification. Gene expression atlases have been developed for soybean [29, 30], *Medicago* [31], *L. japonicus* [32] and pigeon pea [33]. Moreover, in chickpea a number of transcriptome studies have been performed. These include exploring the overall transcriptome of various tissues [34–37], specifically understanding of the development of flower [38], seed [39] and root nodule [40]. Transcriptome analysis of chickpea under different abiotic and biotic stresses such as drought, desiccation, salinity, cold and *Fusarium* wilt has also been carried out [41–43].

Next-generation sequencing (NGS)-based plant genomics has also assisted in understanding of genetic variation within and between species mostly through identification of single-nucleotide polymorphisms (SNPs). In chickpea, a number of studies have been performed to identify SNPs and utilized for various applications such as construction of linkage maps, synteny analysis, anchoring of whole genome sequencing and quantitative trait loci (QTL) analysis [44–49]. A CicArVarDB has also been developed which includes SNP and InDel variations in chickpea [50].

4. Transcriptome

A cell undergoing a functional or developmental process has a specific set of genes undergoing transcription at a particular time and is collectively called the 'transcriptome'. Thus, a transcriptome represents up to an extant physical, biochemical and developmental status of a cell. A transcriptome represents a pool of protein coding as well as nonprotein-coding RNAs; moreover, there may be the presence of variants of genes originating from alternative splicing and RNA editing, making the transcriptome more complex than a genome. Study of transcriptome may reveal information regarding spatial and temporal expression patterns of genes, and therefore it is possible to generate global expression profiles of genes representing developmental stages of an organism [34].

5. Methods for transcriptome analysis

Transcriptome analysis was initiated with the generation of expressed sequence tags (ESTs) that are 200–800 nucleotide long cDNA sequences, synthesised from mRNA through reverse transcription. ESTs represent the expressed part of an organism's genome and hence are an excellent resource for the study of gene expression at a genome-wide level. Conventionally, EST resources have been developed through Sanger sequencing. Although this process is used to generate and sequence longer fragments of cDNA, it is tedious and labour intensive and offers poor coverage of the transcriptome. These limitations of EST-based transcriptome analysis inspired scientists to develop microarray and other tag-based methods for gene expression analysis. Therefore, tools such as microarrays and serial analysis of gene expression (SAGE) continued to be used for several years for analysis of global gene expression patterns. However, with the advent of NGS and the simultaneous development of in silico analytical tools, global genome and transcriptome analysis has become a standard practice for deriving information to relate genotype to phenotype. However, it is not possible to sequence the transcripts to the full length due to technological limitations. Transcriptome analysis is based on the principle that the depth of coverage of a sequence is proportional to the level of expression of the corresponding gene. Therefore, by mapping and counting the sequenced reads onto the given transcript, expression can be measured, thereby translating sequence information to some biologically significant information. A host of NGS technologies such as sequencing by synthesis (Illumina Inc., USA), SOLiD (ThermoFisher Scientific) and pyrosequencing (454 biosciences/Roche) has provided unprecedented opportunities for high-throughput functional genomic research [51–53]. Moreover, a number of technologies for transcriptome sequencing are emerging such as The Ion Torrent (ThermoFisher Scientific), single-molecule real time (SMRT) (Pacific Biosciences, USA) and Nanopore (Oxford Nanopore Technologies, UK).

6. Using transcriptome analysis for studying biological processes in chickpea

Extensive transcriptome analysis has been carried out in chickpea in order to gain insights into the numerous biological processes. Techniques, such as EST sequencing, SAGE and most importantly the NGS, have been used to analyse the transcriptomes of root, shoot, flower, seed and nodule tissues in order to understand the tissue-specific development and function. Several groups undertook EST sequencing, and till date (March 2017) 53,333 chickpea ESTs are reported in the NCBI database. In another earlier study of the root transcriptome, an EST library was constructed by subtractive suppressive hybridization (SSH) of two related chickpea varieties, ICC 4958 and Annigeri, as they show different root traits. Sequences of more than 2800 ESTs were reported and used to develop the 'Chickpea Root Expressed Sequence Tag Database' [54].

A major advancement in transcriptome analysis for understanding developmental and biological processes occurred with the advent of the NGS platform. Several large-scale NGS-based transcriptome analyses were carried out in chickpea [34–36]. In one of the first NGS-based

studies, the Illumina sequencing of transcriptome of chickpea genotype ICC 4958 root and shoot followed by de novo assembly resulted in generation of 53,409 transcripts. Of these 34,676 transcripts were annotated, and 6577 transcripts were identified as transcription factors (TFs) belonging to 57 families. Another study by Garg et al. reported the Roche/454-based transcriptomes of 'shoot', 'root', 'mature leaf', 'flower bud' and 'young pod' of chickpea genotype ICC 4958 [34]. These sequence reads generated by the Roche/454 platform were merged with the Illumina reads from the previous study, and a hybrid assembly was generated [34], which resulted in 34,760 tentative consensus (TC) transcripts. Of these, 1851 transcripts were annotated as transcription factors belonging to 84 families. This analysis also led to the identification of 1132, 695, 513, 408 and 126 TCs specifically expressed in flower bud, young pod, shoot, root and mature leaf, respectively. The complete data were integrated leading to the development of the 'Chickpea Transcriptome Data Base' (CTDB) which provides a searchable interface to the chickpea transcriptome data [34]. Further, transcriptome analysis of the wild progenitor of chickpea, i.e. *Cicer reticulatum* PI489777, was also performed by Jhanwar et al. [37]. Moreover, transcriptomes of the kabuli, desi and wild chickpeas were compared [55] and used to create an improved version of the Chickpea Transcriptome Data Base V2.0 [56].

Flower development is an important and specialized process that takes place in angiosperms. Hence, in order to gain insights into the molecular mechanisms responsible for flower development in chickpea, transcriptome analysis was carried out using the Illumina sequencing platform [38]. Transcriptome sequencing of eight successive developing stages of flower (flower buds at sizes 4, 6, 8 and 8–10 mm and flowers with closed petals, partially opened petals, opened and faded petals and senescing petals) along with young leaf, germinating seedling and shoot apical meristem was carried out. Differential expression analysis revealed 1572 genes to be differentially expressed in at least one stage of flower development. A number of 1118 genes (908 upregulated and 201 downregulated) and 966 genes (857 upregulated and 109 downregulated) were found to be differentially regulated in flower bud and flower developmental stages, respectively [38]. The majority of the differentially expressed genes were found to be involved in various flower developmental pathways such as floral organ identity; development of corolla, androecium and gynoecium and gametophyte development. Moreover, genes related to cell wall development and transport were also found to be differentially expressed. In addition, 111 TF genes were found differentially expressed in floral bud and flower.

Chickpea is most valued for its seeds since they serve as a source of protein, especially for vegetarian population. Therefore, a thorough understanding of the transcriptional flux during seed development is important in order to get insights into the biological processes that define the seed. Towards this, an NGS-based deep transcriptome analysis of chickpea seed at four developmental stages, i.e. 10 days after anthesis (DAA), 20 DAA, 30 DAA and 40 DAA, was carried out [39]. The transcriptome was sequenced using the 454 pyrosequencing on the GS-FLX Titanium platform followed by its assembly into 51,099 transcripts. A gene ontology enrichment of seed-specific genes revealed genes related to reproductive structure development, fruit development and embryonic and post-embryonic development to be highly represented. Many metabolic pathways such as proteolysis, lipid metabolic process, regulation of RNA metabolic

process, regulation of transcription, terpenoid metabolic process and gibberellin metabolic processes were also found to be significantly represented [39]. In another study, sequencing of ESTs from the chickpea embryo resulted in identification of 1480 unigenes expressed during embryo development [57]. The analysis also identified 12 genes encoding for F-box proteins, of which 2 F-box genes (*CarFbox_PP2* and *CarF-box_LysM*) were predicted to be involved in seed development [57].

Another important distinctive feature of chickpea is its ability to form symbiotic relationship with *M. ciceri* which results in the formation of specialized structures called root nodules. These are formed by the host plant and protect the oxygen-sensitive, bacterial nitrogen fixing machinery. It is a complex phenomenon and a detailed understanding of the molecular pathways governing that the process of nodule development and nitrogen fixation would certainly help plant scientists in developing sustainable farming strategies for chickpea. Towards this, a DeepSuperSAGE-based transcriptome analysis led to the identification of 71 genes being differentially expressed in root nodules [58]. Further, in order to understand the root nodulation in greater depth, a deep transcriptome analysis of the chickpea root nodule at different developing stages was carried out using the 454 pyrosequencing [40]. Sequencing of transcriptomes of uninfected root and three developing stages of nodules followed by reference-based assembly resulted in 83,405 transcripts. Of these 3760 were found to be differentially expressed in at least one of the stages of nodule when compared to uninfected root. Also, 1606 transcripts were identified as transcription factors, of which 171 TFs were found to be differentially expressed during nodulation.

7. Using transcriptome analysis for study of stress response in chickpea

Transcriptome analysis has been utilized exclusively to study different abiotic and biotic stress responses in chickpea. Drought and salinity are the major factors that limit the growth and productivity of the plants. Terminal drought is thought to be a major constraint affecting productivity of chickpea as it can lower the yield of chickpea by about 50% [59]. Cold stress also affects susceptible chickpea mainly at the reproductive stage where it leads to pollen sterility and flower abortion [60]. Thus, it is important to study the response of chickpea under these stress conditions in order to devise strategies for development of stress-tolerant chickpea. Earlier studies based on EST sequencing, SAGE and microarray provided preliminary evidence for drought responses of chickpea at transcriptome level [61–66]. An EST sequencing-based study of drought and salinity stress in chickpea resulted in generation of 20,162 ESTs, of which 105 were found to have differential expression during one of the stresses [65]. In another comparison between ESTs generated from chickpea, ICC 4958 (drought tolerant) and ICC 1882 (drought resistant) varieties resulted in identification of 5494 drought-responsive ESTs [61]. A microarray-based transcriptome analysis of root and leaf of chickpea under drought stress resulted in identification of 4815 differentially expressed genes. Approximately 2623 and 3969 genes were found to be differentially expressed, whereas 88 and 52 genes were found to be specifically expressed during drought stress in root and leaf tissues, respectively [66]. Another microarray analysis in chickpea revealed 109, 210 and 386

genes to be differentially expressed in drought, cold and high-salinity stresses, respectively [62]. A SuperSAGE-based transcriptome analysis of chickpea drought stressed and control tissues gave rise to 17,493 unique transcripts (UniTags) of which 7532 were differentially expressed in drought stress [63]. Another SuperSAGE followed by 454 sequencing of root nodule transcriptome of salt-tolerant variety INRAT-93 identified 363 and 106 genes to be upregulated and downregulated, respectively, in root and nodule tissues [64].

The more global view of stress response in chickpea was provided by the study of Garg et al. [41] in which the transcriptome of chickpea root and shoot under desiccation, salinity and cold stress was analysed. The Illumina sequencing-based transcriptome and comparison revealed 11,640 transcripts to be differentially expressed during at least one of the stresses. Seven hundred forty-five transcription factors (TFs) were also found to be differentially regulated in at least one stress condition. Moreover 3536 unannotated genes from the chickpea transcriptome were also identified [41]. A more detailed transcriptome analysis of drought-tolerant (ICC 4958), drought-sensitive (ICC 1882), salinity-tolerant (JG 62) and salinity-sensitive (ICCV2) chickpea varieties resulted in identification of 18,462 transcripts representing 13,964 unique loci in at least one sample/stress condition. The study also revealed 4954 and 5545 genes exclusively regulated in drought-tolerant and salinity-tolerant varieties. A number of 775 TFs encoding genes belonging to 80 families were also found differentially regulated in stress conditions. Members of the bHLH, WRKY, NAC, AP2-EREBP and MYB were found among the top differentially expressed TFs in stress condition [42]. In order to understand the effect of cold stress, AFLP-based transcript profiling (cDNA-AFLP) approach was used [67], which showed that in cold-tolerant chickpea, 102 transcript-derived fragments (TDFs) were differentially expressed during cold stress. Moreover, transcriptome analysis of cold-tolerant chickpea ICC 16349 using cDNA differential display (DDRT-PCR) resulted in identification of 127 ESTs as differentially expressed in anthers during cold stress conditions.

Ascochyta blight caused by *A. rabiei* and *Fusarium* wilt caused by *F. oxysporum* are major fungal diseases of chickpea. In order to understand the response of chickpea to *A. rabiei*, an EST library sequencing of blight-resistant chickpea variety ICC 3996 infected with *A. rabiei* was performed by Coram and Pang [68]. The study reported 516 genes of which 4% were related to defense and found to encode for lignin and phytoalexin biosynthesis enzymes, pathogenesis-related proteins, signalling proteins and putative-defensive proteins [68]. For further identification of resistance-related genes, transcriptome analysis of four genotypes, *C. arietinum* ICC 3996, *C. arietinum* Lasseter, *C. arietinum* FLIP94-508C and *Cicer echinospermum* ILWC245, was performed using 756 featured microarrays. The study revealed 97 genes to be differentially expressed upon infection with *A. rabiei*. A comparison between resistant and susceptible varieties identified many genes such as pathogenesis-related proteins, SNAKIN2 antimicrobial peptide, proline-rich protein, disease resistance response protein DRRG49-C, environmental stress-inducible protein, leucine-zipper protein, polymorphic antigen membrane protein and Ca-binding protein, which might be responsible for imparting resistance to the tolerant varieties [69]. On the other hand, in order to identify genes involved in wilt resistance in chickpea, EST sequencing followed by microarray analysis of chickpea wilt susceptible genotype (JG-62) and resistant genotype (WR-315) was performed after infecting them with *F. oxysporum*

ciceri. The analysis resulted in identification of 257 differentially expressed genes associated with the early signalling pathway [70]. In order to understand the differential response of susceptible and tolerant/resistant chickpea varieties to *F. oxysporum*, transcriptomes of wilt susceptible (JG62) and wilt-tolerant/wilt-resistant (ICCV2, K850 and WR315) chickpea varieties were analysed using the Illumina platform. Comparison among the transcriptomes led to identification of 303 polymorphic SSRs, 14,462 SNPs and 1864 insertions/deletions (InDels). Moreover, a large number of SNPs and/or InDels were found to be present in defence-related genes [43].

In order to identify common genes between biotic and abiotic responses in chickpea, Mantri et al. [71] performed microarray analysis of chickpea ICC 3996 under three abiotic stresses (drought, cold and high salinity) and biotic stress (infection with *A. rabiei*). This analysis revealed 46, 54, 266 and 51 genes to be differentially regulated in drought, cold, high salinity and *A. rabiei* stresses, respectively. *A. rabiei* stress response was found to be more similar to that of high-salinity stress [71].

8. Transcriptome analysis for non-coding RNA studies in chickpea

Non-coding RNAs usually act as regulatory elements that have a decisive role in fine regulation of gene activity. Non-coding transcripts comprise of small and long non-coding RNAs. Small non-coding RNAs regulate diverse developmental processes by controlling gene expression at transcriptional and post-transcriptional level [72, 73]. MicroRNAs (miRNAs) constitute the major class of small non-coding RNAs and are 20–24 nucleotides long key regulatory elements. They are highly conserved and play an important part in various developmental processes in plants such as leaf development, flowering, formation and maintenance of the shoot, floral and axillary meristems, establishment of organ polarity, root nodule symbiosis, vegetative to reproductive phase transition and response to biotic and abiotic stresses [73–77]. In chickpea, small RNA libraries were sequenced from normal tissues and those under different stress conditions [78–80]. Small RNA sequence data were filtered and processed for miRNA prediction using miRDeep pipeline resulting in identification of distinct conserved miRNAs from shoot (302, including Cat-miR156b-5p, Cat-miR156j.1, Cat-miR159.1, Cat-miR169b-5p), root (280, including Cat-miR156c.1, Cat-miR169n, Cat-miR171k-3p), mature leaf (248, including Cat-miR156k, Cat-miR172d.2, Cat-NovmiR319b, Cat-miR167a, Cat-miR167d.2), stem (268, including Cat-miR172c-3p, Cat-miR159.3, Cat-NovmiR319d, Cat-miR171k-3p), flower bud (247, Cat-miR319g.2, Cat-miR167c.2, Cat-miR167d.1, Cat-miR171b-3p.2), flower (293, Cat-miR159.4, Cat-miR159e, Cat-miR171m) and young pod (274, Cat-miR172d.1, Cat-NovmiR159a, Cat-miR167-5p). By ab initio prediction, a total of 109, 76, 123, 100, 106, 98 and 120 novel candidate miRNAs were identified from the above tissues, respectively. Overall 618 miRNAs were identified from all the tissues with the maximum being 373 miRNAs from the shoot and minimum 303 from flower buds. Of the 618 miRNAs predicted, 158 were present in all the tissues, and 29% of the miRNAs were found to be tissue specific. Of the 618 miRNAs, 421 were clustered to 73 miRNA families, and 197 could not find similarity to any miRNA family and were termed putative novel. Chickpea miRNAs targeted a wide range of transcripts involved

in diverse cellular processes including protein turnover and modification, metabolism, transcriptional regulation and signal transduction [78]. A similar kind of study performed in leaf and flower tissue resulted in the prediction of 96 highly conserved miRNAs belonging to 38 miRNA families and 20 novel miRNAs belonging to 17 miRNA families in chickpea [80]. In addition to identification of miRNA from different tissues, studies were also conducted for characterization of miRNA in response to different biotic and abiotic stresses. In one such kind of study, three libraries were sequenced for small RNA identification [79]. Libraries were constructed from fungal-infected (*F. oxysporum* f.sp. *ciceris*), salt-treated and untreated seedlings of chickpea and were sequenced using the Illumina GAIIx platform. The analysis identified 122 conserved miRNAs belonging to 25 different families along with 59 novel miRNAs. miR156, miR396 and miR319 were upregulated in response to salt stress. miR156 and miR396 expression was found to be 1.5 times upregulated in both wilt and salt stresses, indicating a common mechanism implied by chickpea involving these miRNAs to cope up with both the stresses. miR530 was found to be significantly upregulated during wilt stress and may be involved in defence to fungal infection. Three legume-specific miRNAs, miR2111, miR2118 and miR5213, were also indicated to play a critical role in defence to pathogen attack. Targets of miR2111 include F-box protein and TIR (Toll/Interleukin-1 Receptor) domain-containing NBS-LRR disease-resistance proteins, and miR2118 and miR5213 also target the same class of R genes. Interestingly, miR2118 is upregulated following wilt infection and downregulated following salt stress [79].

Long intergenic non-coding (linc) RNAs belong to a class of non-coding transcripts which have a length of at least 200bp lacking coding potential and are transcribed from intergenic region of protein coding genes [81, 82]. Linc RNAs control gene regulation at transcriptional and post-transcriptional level by mechanisms including chromatin modification, promoter binding complex attachment and shielding mRNA degradation by acting as sponge against miRNA [83–85]. RNA-seq data from 11 different tissues of chickpea were used for mining linc-RNA [86]. RNA-seq data were processed using TopHat2 and Cufflinks program using chickpea genome as the reference. From 32,984 transcripts obtained, 5782 putative intergenic transcripts were extracted out and subjected to the optimized pipeline for identification of linc-RNA. After removing potential coding transcripts and transcripts having similarity to protein domains, finally a total of 2248 transcripts were retained as putative chickpea linc-RNAs. About 79%, i.e. 1790 linc-RNAs, could be assigned a putative function. Through expression profiling it was evident that a large number of linc-RNAs have tissue-specific expression in distinct tissues. Along with this several linc-RNAs were found to be targets of miRNAs and were involved in various developmental and reproductive processes [86].

9. Expanding transcriptome data to aid development of molecular markers

A DNA-based molecular marker is a DNA sequence with an identifiable location on the genome that can be transmitted from one generation to the next following the standard laws

of inheritance [87]. Recent years have witnessed an immense interest in generation and utilization of molecular markers, as they provide the essential tools for a variety of genomic applications such as QTL mapping, map-based cloning, marker-assisted breeding, association mapping and genetic diversity assessment. These approaches can be applied to understand the genomic architecture of the crop and can expand the efficiency of breeding programmes, thereby aiding to expedite agricultural research. The advent of NGS has enabled the exploration of thousands of markers across entire genomes and transcriptomes. Although transcriptomics has been majorly used for gene expression analysis, it has also been utilized to identify molecular markers such as SSRs and SNPs especially in the genic regions. Such gene-based markers located in coding regions of the genes greatly enhance the opportunity of precise mapping of genes linked to important traits. Transcriptome sequencing offers another advantage for those crops in which a reference genome is not available. To identify SSRs from transcriptome data, several bioinformatics tools have been developed such as MISA (MIcroSAtellite identification tool) (pgrc.ipk-gatersleben.de/misa/), RISA (Rapid Identification of SSRs and Analysis of primers) (http://sol.kribb.re.kr/RISA/) and RepeatAnalyzer [88]. In chickpea, initially a large number of molecular markers were derived from ESTs. Buhariwalla et al. [89] reported 106 EST-based markers developed from an EST library of root tissue from chickpea. In another study by Choudhary et al. [90], 2131 ESTs were utilized for development of 246 EST-SSR markers. Apart from SSRs, several types of markers such as ESTPs, PIPs and EST-SNPs were developed in chickpea using transcriptome data. For instance, Choudhary et al. [91] reported 125 EST-SSRs, 109 ESTPs, 102 SNPs and 151 ITPs. Gupta et al. [57] reported 367 novel EST-derived functional markers which included 187 EST-SSRs, 130 potential intron polymorphisms (PIPs) and 50 expressed sequence tag polymorphisms (ESTPs). In another study, 71 gene-based SNP markers were developed utilizing candidate chickpea transcripts [92]. However, currently transcriptomic resources can be easily generated by high-throughput NGS technologies and utilized to identify molecular markers very rapidly and cost-effectively. Hiremath et al. [36] utilizing the Roche platform generated about 3000 gene-based markers from a large subset of transcripts derived from different chickpea tissues. Currently, SNPs are the markers of choice and are preferred over the SSRs and other markers because of their genome-wide presence and amenability to high-throughput genotyping. Theoretically, SNP calling may be defined as the process of identifying a single-nucleotide variation from an accession read that differs from the existing reference genome or a de novo assembly at similar nucleotide position. Read assembly files generated by mapping programs such as BWA, Bowtie and SOAP are used to perform SNP calling. Bioinformatics tools such as HaploSNPer [93], SAMtools [94, 95], POLYBAYES [96], SNVer [97] and SOAPsnp [98] have been designed to detect the variations in the NGS data. Comparison of transcriptome datasets from contrasting genotypes could help derive SNPs. To date, several studies have been carried out using NGS technology-based transcriptome sequencing to generate large sets of molecular markers in various crop species including chickpea. For instance, a report by Garg et al. [35] facilitated identification of 4816 SSRs from the de novo assembly of the chickpea transcriptome. In another study, sequencing the transcriptome of *C. reticulatum* (PI489777), the wild relative of chickpea, by GS-FLX 454 technology, generated a total of 4072 SSRs and 36,446 SNPs.

Likewise, Agarwal et al. (2012) sequenced the transcriptome of ICCV2 and identified 5409 SSRs. Amongst these, 130 and 493 SSRs were found to be polymorphic after comparing with the transcriptome of *desi* and *wild* chickpea. In addition to the SSRs, a total of 1986 and 37,954 SNPs were also identified between the desi, kabuli and wild genotypes. Similarly, in another study, 51,632 genic SNPs were identified by 454 transcriptome sequencing of *C. arietinum* and *C. reticulatum* genotypes [99]. In a recent study, Srivastava et al. [100] identified 11,621 differentially expressed genes in root vs shoot tissues using RNA sequencing of a wild perennial *Cicer microphyllum* and integrated above transcriptome profiling with high-resolution QTL mapping in order to identify drought-responsive root-specific genes. The transcriptomic resources, therefore, clearly have remarkable potential to expedite the development of large numbers of molecular markers which can be used in genomic-assisted breeding for developing improved varieties of chickpea.

10. Future perspectives

The last few years have witnessed legume genomics attaining new heights as genomes, and transcriptomes of many model legumes (*M. truncatula, L. japonicus*) and crop legumes (*G. max, C. cajan, P. vulgaris, Arachis hypogaea, Vignas,* etc.) were sequenced. Transcriptomes of both types of cultivated chickpea (desi and kabuli) and its wild progenitor (*C. reticulatum*) have also been sequenced. Several studies have been carried out to analyse the transcriptome of chickpea which have led to genome-wide determination of transcript levels in various tissues and developmental pathways as well as during biotic and abiotic stresses. This comprehensive analysis of the chickpea transcriptome has advanced the understanding of the molecular mechanisms underlying several critical biological pathways in chickpea. Moreover, analyses of the non-coding RNAs have revealed potential regulators of important pathways affecting the overall development and stress tolerance in chickpea. Further, transcriptome analysis has also facilitated the development of large sets of genic molecular markers such as SSRs and SNPs that will serve as excellent tools for advancing the chickpea breeding programmes. Overall, the transcriptome sequencing of chickpea has not only provided a deep insight into the gene space and quantitation of gene expression but also an opportunity to isolate genes of interest and functional markers for use in chickpea improvement.

Author details

Chandra Kant, Vimal Pandey, Subodh Verma, Manish Tiwari, Santosh Kumar and Sabhyata Bhatia*

*Address all correspondence to: sabhyatabhatia@nipgr.ac.in

National Institute of Plant Genome Research, New Delhi, India

References

[1] Varshney RK, Song C, Saxena RK, Azam S, Yu S, Sharpe AG, et al. Draft genome sequence of chickpea (*Cicer arietinum*) provides a resource for trait improvement. Nature Biotechnology. 2013;**31**(3):240-246

[2] Jukanti AK, Gaur PM, Gowda CLL, Chibbar RN. Nutritional quality and health benefits of chickpea (*Cicer arietinum* L.): A review. British Journal of Nutrition. 2012;**108**(S1):S11-S26

[3] Dixon RA, Sumner LW. Legume natural products: Understanding and manipulating complex pathways for human and animal health. Plant Physiology. 2003;**131**(3):878-885

[4] Singh P, Vijaya D, Srinivas K, Wani SP. Potential productivity, yield gap, and water balance of soybean-chickpea sequential system at selected benchmark sites in India. Global Theme 3: Water, Soil, and Agrobiodiversity Management for Ecosystem Health. Report No. 1. Patancheru, Andhra Pradesh, India: International Crops Research Institute for the Semi-Arid Tropics. 2002.

[5] Leport L, Turner NC, French RJ, Barr MD, Duda R, Davies SL, et al. Physiological responses of chickpea genotypes to terminal drought in a Mediterranean-type environment. European Journal of Agronomy. 1999;**11**(3-4):279-291

[6] Johansen C, Krishnamurthy L, Saxena NP, Sethi SC. Genotypic variation in moisture response of chickpea grown under line-source sprinklers in a semi-arid tropical environment. Field Crops Research. 1994;**37**(2):103-112

[7] Varshney RK, Thudi M, Nayak SP, Gaur PM, Kashiwagi J, Krishnamurthy L. Genetic dissection of drought tolerance in chickpea (*Cicer arietinum* L.). Theoretical and Applied Genetics. 2014;127:445-462

[8] Pang J, Turner NC, Khan T, Du Y-L, Xiong J-L, Colmer TD, et al. Response of chickpea (*Cicer arietinum* L.) to terminal drought: Leaf stomatal conductance, pod abscisic acid concentration, and seed set. Journal of Experimental Botany. 2017; 68(8):1973-1985

[9] Pushpavalli R, Quealy J, Colmer TD, Turner NC, Siddique KHM, Rao MV, et al. Salt stress delayed flowering and reduced reproductive success of chickpea (*Cicer arietinum* L.), a response associated with Na^+ accumulation in leaves. Journal of Agronomy and Crop Science. 2016;**202**(2):125-138

[10] Summerfeld R, Virmani S, Roberts E, Ellis R. Adaptation of chickpea to agroclimatic constraints. Chickpea in the Nineties: proceedings of the Second International Workshop on Chickpea Improvement. ICRISAT, Patancheru, India. 1990:61-72

[11] Kalra N, Chakraborty D, Sharma A, Rai HK, Jolly M, Chander S, et al. Effect of increasing temperature on yield of some winter crops in northwest India. Current Science. 2008;94(1):82-88

[12] Singh D, Peters D, Singh P, Singh M. Diurnal patterns of canopy photosynthesis, evapotranspiration and water use efficiency in chickpea (*Cicer arietinum* L.) under field conditions. Photosynthesis Research. 1987;**11**(1):61-69

[13] Summerfield R, Hadley P, Roberts E, Minchin F, Rawsthorne S. Sensitivity of chickpeas (*Cicer arietinum*) to hot temperatures during the reproductive period. Experimental Agriculture. 1984;**20**(01):77-93

[14] Kaiser WJ. Epidemiology of *Ascochyta rabiei*. In: Singh KB, Saxena MC, editors. Disease Resistance Breeding in Chickpea. Aleppo, Syria: ICARDA; 1992. pp. 117-134

[15] Smithson JB, Thompson JA, Summerfield RJ. Chickpea (*Cicer arietinum* L.). In: Summerfield RJ, Roberts EH, editors. Grain Legume Crops. London, UK: Collins; 1985. pp. 312-390

[16] Duke JA. Handbook of Legumes of World Economic Importance. New York: Plenum Press; 1981. pp. 52-57

[17] Van Emden HF, Ball SL, Rao MR. Pest disease and weed problems in pea lentil and faba bean and chickpea. In: Summerfield RJ, editor. World Crops: Cool Season Food Legumes. Dordrecht, The Netherlands: Kluwer Academic Publishers; 1988. pp. 519-534

[18] Graham PH, Vance CP. Legumes: Importance and constraints to greater use. Plant Physiology. 2003;**131**(3):872-877

[19] Schmutz J, Cannon SB, Schlueter J, Ma J, Mitros T, Nelson W, et al. Genome sequence of the palaeopolyploid soybean. Nature. 2010;**463**(7278):178-183

[20] Young ND, Debelle F, Oldroyd GED, Geurts R, Cannon SB, Udvardi MK, et al. The Medicago genome provides insight into the evolution of rhizobial symbioses. Nature. 2011;**480**(7378):520-524

[21] Sato S, Nakamura Y, Kaneko T, Asamizu E, Kato T, Nakao M, et al. Genome structure of the legume, *Lotus japonicus*. DNA Research. 2008;**15**(4):227-239

[22] Varshney RK, Chen W, Li Y, Bharti AK, Saxena RK, Schlueter JA, et al. Draft genome sequence of pigeon pea (*Cajanus cajan*), an orphan legume crop of resource-poor farmers. Nature Biotechnology. 2012;**30**(1):83-89

[23] Schmutz J, McClean PE, Mamidi S, Wu GA, Cannon SB, Grimwood J, et al. A reference genome for common bean and genome-wide analysis of dual domestications. Nature Genetics. 2014;**46**(7):707-713

[24] Bertioli DJ, Cannon SB, Froenicke L, Huang G, Farmer AD, Cannon EKS, et al. The genome sequences of *Arachis duranensis* and *Arachis ipaensis*, the diploid ancestors of cultivated peanut. Nature Genetics. 2016;**48**(4):438-446

[25] Jain M, Misra G, Patel RK, Priya P, Jhanwar S, Khan AW, et al. A draft genome sequence of the pulse crop chickpea (*Cicer arietinum* L.). The Plant Journal. 2013;**74**(5):715-729

[26] Kim MY, Lee S, Van K, Kim TH, Jeong SC, Choi IY, et al. Whole-genome sequencing and intensive analysis of the undomesticated soybean (*Glycine soja* Sieb. and Zucc.) genome. Proceedings of the National Academy of Sciences of the United States of America. 2010;**107**(51):22032-22037

[27] Lam HM, Xu X, Liu X, Chen W, Yang G, Wong FL, et al. Resequencing of 31 wild and cultivated soybean genomes identifies patterns of genetic diversity and selection. Nature Genetics. 2010;**42**(12):1053-1059

[28] Branca A, Paape TD, Zhou P, Briskine R, Farmer AD, Mudge J, et al. Whole-genome nucleotide diversity, recombination, and linkage disequilibrium in the model legume *Medicago truncatula*. Proceedings of the National Academy of Sciences of the United States of America. 2011;**108**(42):E864-E870

[29] Libault M, Farmer A, Joshi T, Takahashi K, Langley RJ, Franklin LD, et al. An integrated transcriptome atlas of the crop model *Glycine max*, and its use in comparative analyses in plants. The Plant Journal: For Cell and Molecular Biology. 2010;**63**(1):86-99

[30] Severin AJ, Woody JL, Bolon YT, Joseph B, Diers BW, Farmer AD, et al. RNA-Seq Atlas of *Glycine max*: A guide to the soybean transcriptome. BMC Plant Biology. 2010;**10**:160

[31] Benedito VA, Torres-Jerez I, Murray JD, Andriankaja A, Allen S, Kakar K, et al. A gene expression atlas of the model legume *Medicago truncatula*. The Plant Journal: For Cell and Molecular Biology. 2008;**55**(3):504-513

[32] Verdier J, Torres-Jerez I, Wang M, Andriankaja A, Allen SN, He J, et al. Establishment of the *Lotus japonicus* Gene Expression Atlas (LjGEA) and its use to explore legume seed maturation. The Plant Journal: For Cell and Molecular Biology. 2013;**74**(2):351-362

[33] Pazhamala LT, Purohit S, Saxena RK, Garg V, Krishnamurthy L, Verdier J, et al. Gene expression atlas of pigeon pea and its application to gain insights into genes associated with pollen fertility implicated in seed formation. Journal of Experimental Botany. 2017; 68(8):2037-2054

[34] Garg R, Patel RK, Jhanwar S, Priya P, Bhattacharjee A, Yadav G, et al. Gene discovery and tissue-specific transcriptome analysis in chickpea with massively parallel pyrosequencing and web resource development. Plant Physiology. 2011;**156**(4):1661-1678

[35] Garg R, Patel RK, Tyagi AK, Jain M. De novo assembly of chickpea transcriptome using short reads for gene discovery and marker identification. DNA Research. 2011;**18**(1):53-63

[36] Hiremath PJ, Farmer A, Cannon SB, Woodward J, Kudapa H, Tuteja R, et al. Large-scale transcriptome analysis in chickpea (*Cicer arietinum* L.), an orphan legume crop of the semi-arid tropics of Asia and Africa. Plant Biotechnology Journal. 2011;**9**(8):922-931

[37] Jhanwar S, Priya P, Garg R, Parida SK, Tyagi AK, Jain M. Transcriptome sequencing of wild chickpea as a rich resource for marker development. Plant Biotechnology Journal. 2012;**10**(6):690-702

[38] Singh VK, Garg R, Jain M. A global view of transcriptome dynamics during flower development in chickpea by deep sequencing. Plant Biotechnology Journal. 2013;**11**(6):691-701

[39] Pradhan S, Bandhiwal N, Shah N, Kant C, Gaur R, Bhatia S. Global transcriptome analysis of developing chickpea (*Cicer arietinum* L.) seeds. Frontiers in Plant Science. 2014;**5**:698

[40] Kant C, Pradhan S, Bhatia S. Dissecting the root nodule transcriptome of chickpea (*Cicer arietinum* L.). PLoS One. 2016;**11**(6):e0157908

[41] Garg R, Bhattacharjee A, Jain M. Genome-scale transcriptomic insights into molecular aspects of abiotic stress responses in chickpea. Plant Molecular Biology Reporter. 2015;**33**(3):388-400

[42] Garg R, Shankar R, Thakkar B, Kudapa H, Krishnamurthy L, Mantri N, et al. Transcriptome analyses reveal genotype- and developmental stage-specific molecular responses to drought and salinity stresses in chickpea. Scientific Reports. 2016;**6**:19228

[43] Jain M, Pole AK, Singh VK, Ravikumar RL, Garg R. Discovery of molecular markers for Fusarium wilt via transcriptome sequencing of chickpea cultivars. Molecular Breeding. 2015;**35**(10):198

[44] Bajaj D, Upadhyaya HD, Khan Y, Das S, Badoni S, Shree T, et al. A combinatorial approach of comprehensive QTL-based comparative genome mapping and transcript profiling identified a seed weight-regulating candidate gene in chickpea. Scientific Reports. 2015;**5**:9264

[45] Das S, Upadhyaya HD, Bajaj D, Kujur A, Badoni S, Laxmi, et al. Deploying QTL-seq for rapid delineation of a potential candidate gene underlying major trait-associated QTL in chickpea. DNA Research. 2015;**22**(3):193-203

[46] Gaur R, Jeena G, Shah N, Gupta S, Pradhan S, Tyagi AK, et al. High density linkage mapping of genomic and transcriptomic SNPs for synteny analysis and anchoring the genome sequence of chickpea. Scientific Reports. 2015;**5**:13387

[47] Kale SM, Jaganathan D, Ruperao P, Chen C, Punna R, Kudapa H, et al. Prioritization of candidate genes in "QTL-hotspot" region for drought tolerance in chickpea (*Cicer arietinum* L.). Scientific Reports. 2015;**5**:15296

[48] Kujur A, Upadhyaya HD, Bajaj D, Gowda CLL, Sharma S, Tyagi AK, et al. Identification of candidate genes and natural allelic variants for QTLs governing plant height in chickpea. Scientific Reports. 2016;**6**:27968

[49] Pushpavalli R, Krishnamurthy L, Thudi M, Gaur PM, Rao MV, Siddique KH, et al. Two key genomic regions harbour QTLs for salinity tolerance in ICCV 2 × JG 11 derived chickpea (*Cicer arietinum* L.) recombinant inbred lines. BMC Plant Biology. 2015;**15**(1):124

[50] Doddamani D, Khan AW, Katta MAVSK, Agarwal G, Thudi M, Ruperao P, et al. CicArVarDB: SNP and InDel database for advancing genetics research and breeding applications in chickpea. Database. 2015;**2015**:bav078-bav

[51] Mardis ER. Next-generation DNA sequencing methods. Annual Review of Genomics and Human Genetics. 2008;**9**:387-402

[52] Morozova O, Marra MA. Applications of next-generation sequencing technologies in functional genomics. Genomics. 2008;**92**(5):255-264

[53] Schuster SC. Next-generation sequencing transforms today's biology. Nature Methods. 2008;**5**(1):16-18

[54] Jayashree B, Buhariwalla HK, Shinde S, Crouch JH. A legume genomics resource: The Chickpea Root Expressed Sequence Tag Database. Electronic Journal of Biotechnology. 2005;8(2):128-133

[55] Agarwal G, Jhanwar S, Priya P, Singh VK, Saxena MS, Parida SK, et al. Comparative analysis of kabuli chickpea transcriptome with desi and wild chickpea provides a rich resource for development of functional markers. PLoS One. 2012;**7**(12):e52443

[56] Verma M, Kumar V, Patel RK, Garg R, Jain M. CTDB: An integrated chickpea transcriptome database for functional and applied genomics. PLoS One. 2015;**10**(8):e0136880

[57] Gupta S, Garg V, Bhatia S. A new set of ESTs from chickpea (*Cicer arietinum* L.) embryo reveals two novel F-box genes, CarF-box_PP2 and CarF-box_LysM, with potential roles in seed development. PLoS One. 2015;**10**(3):e0121100

[58] Afonso-Grunz F, Molina C, Hoffmeier K, Rycak L, Kudapa H, Varshney RK, et al. Genome-based analysis of the transcriptome from mature chickpea root nodules. Frontiers in Plant Science. 2014;**5**:325

[59] Ahmad F, Gaur P, Croser J. Chickpea (*Cicer arietinum* L.). In: Singh R, Jauhar P, editors. Genetic Resources, Chromosome Engineering and Crop Improvement—Grain Legumes. USA: CRC Press; 2005. pp. 185-214

[60] Sharma KD, Nayyar H. Cold stress alters transcription in meiotic anthers of cold tolerant chickpea (*Cicer arietinum* L.). BMC Research Notes. 2014;**7**:717

[61] Deokar AA, Kondawar V, Jain PK, Karuppayil SM, Raju NL, Vadez V, et al. Comparative analysis of expressed sequence tags (ESTs) between drought-tolerant and -susceptible genotypes of chickpea under terminal drought stress. BMC Plant Biology. 2011;**11**(1):70

[62] Mantri NL, Ford R, Coram TE, Pang EC. Transcriptional profiling of chickpea genes differentially regulated in response to high-salinity, cold and drought. BMC Genomics. 2007;**8**:303

[63] Molina C, Rotter B, Horres R, Udupa SM, Besser B, Bellarmino L, et al. SuperSAGE: The drought stress-responsive transcriptome of chickpea roots. BMC Genomics. 2008;**9**:553

[64] Molina C, Zaman-Allah M, Khan F, Fatnassi N, Horres R, Rotter B, et al. The salt-responsive transcriptome of chickpea roots and nodules via deepSuperSAGE. BMC Plant Biology. 2011;**11**:31

[65] Varshney RK, Hiremath PJ, Lekha P, Kashiwagi J, Balaji J, Deokar AA, et al. A comprehensive resource of drought- and salinity- responsive ESTs for gene discovery and marker development in chickpea (*Cicer arietinum* L.). BMC Genomics. 2009;**10**:523

[66] Wang X, Liu Y, Jia Y, Gu H, Ma H, Yu T, et al. Transcriptional responses to drought stress in root and leaf of chickpea seedling. Molecular Biology Reports. 2012;**39**(8):8147-8158

[67] Dinari A, Niazi A, Afsharifar AR, Ramezani A. Identification of upregulated genes under cold stress in cold-tolerant chickpea using the cDNA-AFLP approach. PLoS One. 2013;**8**(1):e52757

[68] Coram TE, Pang ECK. Isolation and analysis of candidate ascochyta blight defence genes in chickpea. Part I. Generation and analysis of an expressed sequence tag (EST) library. Physiological and Molecular Plant Pathology. 2005;**66**(5):192-200

[69] Coram TE, Pang EC. Expression profiling of chickpea genes differentially regulated during a resistance response to *Ascochyta rabiei*. Plant Biotechnology Journal. 2006;**4**(6):647-666

[70] Ashraf N, Ghai D, Barman P, Basu S, Gangisetty N, Mandal MK, et al. Comparative analyses of genotype dependent expressed sequence tags and stress-responsive transcriptome of chickpea wilt illustrate predicted and unexpected genes and novel regulators of plant immunity. BMC Genomics. 2009;**10**(1):415

[71] Mantri NL, Ford R, Coram TE, Pang ECK. Evidence of unique and shared responses to major biotic and abiotic stresses in chickpea. Environmental and Experimental Botany. 2010;**69**(3):286-292

[72] Bartel DP. MicroRNAs: Genomics, biogenesis, mechanism, and function. Cell. 2004; **116**(2):281-297

[73] Jones-Rhoades MW, Bartel DP, Bartel B. MicroRNAS and their regulatory roles in plants. Annual Review of Plant Biology. 2006;**57**:19-53

[74] Dezulian T, Palatnik JF, Huson D, Weigel D. Conservation and divergence of microRNA families in plants. Genome Biology. 2005;**6**(11):P13

[75] Rogers K, Chen X. Biogenesis, turnover, and mode of action of plant microRNAs. Plant Cell. 2013;**25**(7):2383-2399

[76] Simon SA, Meyers BC, Sherrier DJ. MicroRNAs in the rhizobia legume symbiosis. Plant Physiology. 2009;**151**(3):1002-1008

[77] Sunkar R. MicroRNAs with macro-effects on plant stress responses. Seminars in Cell & Developmental Biology. 2010;**21**(8):805-811

[78] Jain M, Chevala VV, Garg R. Genome-wide discovery and differential regulation of conserved and novel microRNAs in chickpea via deep sequencing. Journal of Experimental Botany. 2014;**65**(20):5945-5958

[79] Kohli D, Joshi G, Deokar AA, Bhardwaj AR, Agarwal M, Katiyar-Agarwal S, et al. Identification and characterization of Wilt and salt stress-responsive microRNAs in chickpea through high-throughput sequencing. PLoS One. 2014;**9**(10):e108851

[80] Srivastava S, Zheng Y, Kudapa H, Jagadeeswaran G, Hivrale V, Varshney RK, et al. High throughput sequencing of small RNA component of leaves and inflorescence revealed conserved and novel miRNAs as well as phasiRNA loci in chickpea. Plant Science. 2015;**235**:46-57

[81] Guttman M, Amit I, Garber M, French C, Lin MF, Feldser D, et al. Chromatin signature reveals over a thousand highly conserved large non-coding RNAs in mammals. Nature. 2009;**458**(7235):223-227

[82] Ulitsky I, Bartel DP. lincRNAs: Genomics, evolution, and mechanisms. Cell. 2013;**154**(1): 26-46

[83] Cabili MN, Trapnell C, Goff L, Koziol M, Tazon-Vega B, Regev A, et al. Integrative annotation of human large intergenic noncoding RNAs reveals global properties and specific subclasses. Genes & Development. 2011;**25**(18):1915-1927

[84] Imig J, Brunschweiger A, Brummer A, Guennewig B, Mittal N, Kishore S, et al. miR-CLIP capture of a miRNA targetome uncovers a lincRNA H19-miR-106a interaction. Nature Chemical Biology. 2015;**11**(2):107-114

[85] Rinn JL, Chang HY. Genome regulation by long noncoding RNAs. Annual Review of Biochemistry. 2012;**81**:145-166

[86] Khemka N, Singh VK, Garg R, Jain M. Genome-wide analysis of long intergenic noncoding RNAs in chickpea and their potential role in flower development. Scientific Reports. 2016;**6**:33297

[87] Semagn K, Bjørnstad Å, Ndjiondjop M. Principles, requirements and prospects of genetic mapping in plants. African Journal of Biotechnology. 2006;**5**(25):2569-2587

[88] Catanese HN, Brayton KA, Gebremedhin AH. RepeatAnalyzer: A tool for analysing and managing short-sequence repeat data. BMC Genomics. 2016;**17**(1):422

[89] Buhariwalla HK, Jayashree B, Eshwar K, Crouch JH. Development of ESTs from chickpea roots and their use in diversity analysis of the *Cicer* genus. BMC Plant Biology. 2005;**5**(1):16

[90] Choudhary S, Sethy NK, Shokeen B, Bhatia S. Development of chickpea EST-SSR markers and analysis of allelic variation across related species. Theoretical and Applied Genetics. 2009;**118**(3):591-608

[91] Choudhary S, Gaur R, Gupta S. EST-derived genic molecular markers: Development and utilization for generating an advanced transcript map of chickpea. Theoretical and Applied Genetics. 2012;**124**(8):1449-1462

[92] Nayak SN, Zhu H, Varghese N, Datta S, Choi H-K, Horres R, et al. Integration of novel SSR and gene-based SNP marker loci in the chickpea genetic map and establishment of new anchor points with *Medicago truncatula* genome. Theoretical and Applied Genetics. 2010;**120**(7):1415-1441

[93] Tang J, Leunissen JA, Voorrips RE, van der Linden CG, Vosman B. HaploSNPer: A web-based allele and SNP detection tool. BMC Genetics. 2008;**9**:23

[94] Li H. A statistical framework for SNP calling, mutation discovery, association mapping and population genetical parameter estimation from sequencing data. Bioinformatics. 2011;**27**(21):2987-2993

[95] Li H, Handsaker B, Wysoker A, Fennell T, Ruan J, Homer N, et al. The sequence alignment/map format and SAMtools. Bioinformatics. 2009;**25**(16):2078-2079

[96] Marth GT, Korf I, Yandell MD, Yeh RT, Gu Z, Zakeri H, et al. A general approach to single-nucleotide polymorphism discovery. Nature Genetics. 1999;**23**(4):452-456

[97] Wei Z, Wang W, Hu P, Lyon GJ, Hakonarson H. SNVer: A statistical tool for variant calling in analysis of pooled or individual next-generation sequencing data. Nucleic Acids Research. 2011;**39**(19):e132

[98] Li R, Li Y, Fang X, Yang H, Wang J, Kristiansen K, et al. SNP detection for massively parallel whole-genome resequencing. Genome Research. 2009;**19**(6):1124-1132

[99] Deokar AA, Ramsay L, Sharpe AG, Diapari M, Sindhu A, Bett K, et al. Genome wide SNP identification in chickpea for use in development of a high density genetic map and improvement of chickpea reference genome assembly. BMC Genomics. 2014;**15**(1):708

[100] Srivastava R, Bajaj D, Malik A, Singh M, Parida SK. Transcriptome landscape of perennial wild *Cicer microphyllum* uncovers functionally relevant molecular tags regulating agronomic traits in chickpea. Scientific Reports. 2016; 6:33616

Chapter 11

Comprehensive Network Analysis of Cancer Stem Cell Signalling through Systematic Integration of Post-Translational Modification Dynamics

Hiroko Kozuka-Hata and Masaaki Oyama

Additional information is available at the end of the chapter

http://dx.doi.org/10.5772/intechopen.69647

Abstract

Post-translational modifications, such as phosphorylation, acetylation and ubiquitination, are widely known to play various important roles in cellular signalling. Recent significant advances in mass spectrometry-based proteomics technology enable us not only to comprehensively identify expressed proteins but also to unveil their post-translational modifications with high sensitivity. In our advanced proteome bioinformatics frameworks, statistical network analyses of large-scale information on various post-translational modification dynamics were conducted to define the key machinery for cancer stem cell properties. The bioinformatical approaches using IPA (ingenuity pathway analysis), NetworKIN and a newly developed platform named PTMapper (post-translational modification mapper) allowed us to perform network-wide prediction of upstream interactors/kinases with the related information on the diseases and functions, leading to systematic finding of novel drug candidates to regulate aberrant signalling in cancer stem cells. In this chapter, we apply patient-derived glioblastoma stem cells as a representative model of cancer stem cells to introduce some useful platforms for statistical and mathematical network analyses based on the large-scale phosphoproteome data.

Keywords: glioblastoma stem cells, signal transduction, proteomics, post-translational modification, network analysis

1. Introduction

Glioblastoma (GBM) is known to be the most common and aggressive brain tumour in adults. Despite the enormous efforts to overcome this tumour for many years, the median survival for GBM patients remains around only 1 year [1]. GBM is characterized by high invasiveness

and intratumoral heterogeneity (ITH) [2, 3]. Up to date, it is known that GBM-ITH contributes to the resistance to chemotherapy, radiation and surgical resection. Since functional diversity is the main feature of multilineage differentiation of cancer stem cells (CSCs) [4, 5], glioblastoma stem cells (GSCs) were thought to be major therapeutic targets of GBM. Furthermore, post-translational modifications (PTMs) of GSCs are reported to tightly regulate highly tumourigenic potential of GSCs through aberrant signalling [6, 7]. Therefore, it is important to comprehensively elucidate PTM-based GSC signalling networks for developing the effective treatment of GBM.

Advanced nanoscale liquid chromatography-tandem mass spectrometry (nanoLC-MS/MS) enables us to identify and quantify thousands of proteins in a single experiment [8]. Moreover, using the nanoLC-MS/MS system coupled to the high-affinity enrichment methods of the peptides with PTMs, we can also acquire in-depth biological information on PTM dynamics. In this chapter, we introduce high-resolution shotgun proteomics technology for large-scale PTM determination in combination with statistical bioinformatics platforms such as IPA [9], NetworKIN [10, 11] and PTMapper [12].

2. System-wide proteomic analysis of PTM dynamics

PTMs are widely known to play crucial roles in cell fate control, such as proliferation, differentiation and apoptosis. More than 500 kinds of PTMs regarding eukaryotes and prokaryotes have been registered with Unimod, a comprehensive database of protein modifications for mass spectrometry [13]. Recent technological advances in mass spectrometry-based proteomics in combination with appropriate enrichment techniques for each PTM enable us to perform comprehensive identification and quantification of PTMs [14]. Here, we introduce biochemical purification methods for highly sensitive detection of the representative PTMs: phosphorylation, acetylation and ubiquitination (**Figure 1**).

2.1. Phosphorylation

Protein phosphorylation is recognized as one of the most important and well-studied PTMs and regulates a variety of biological processes by transmitting diverse external signals [15, 16]. About as many as 280,000 phosphorylation sites have already been registered in PhosphoSitePlus, a knowledgebase containing non-redundant mammalian PTMs [17]. Titanium dioxide (TiO_2), which has very high affinity for phosphorylated peptides, is widely used for large-scale phosphoproteome analysis [18, 19].

2.2. Acetylation

Lysine acetylation plays a key role in modulating transcriptional regulation through the coordinated function of histone acetyltransferases (HATs) and histone deacetylases (HDACs) [20]. The stabilization of p53, one of the most important transcription factors, is reported to greatly depend on lysine acetylation [21]. Thousands of lysine acetylation sites can be identified using an antibody against acetyl-lysine in combination with a high-resolution mass spectrometry system [22, 23].

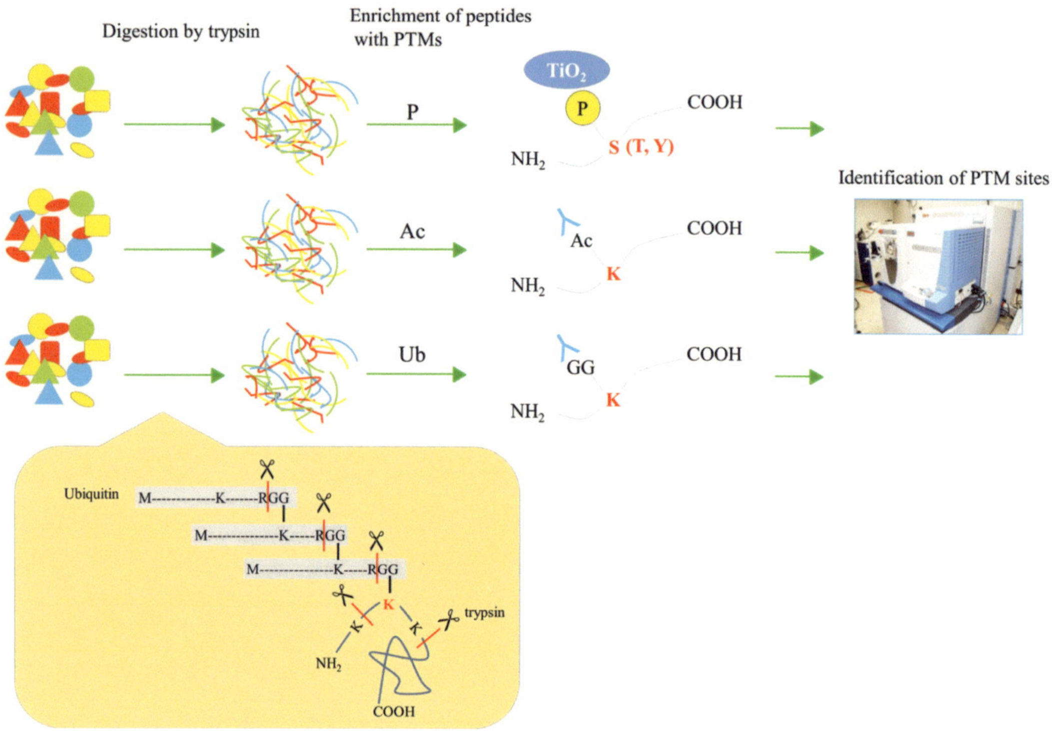

Figure 1. Strategy for mass spectrometry-based identification of peptides modified with phosphorylation, acetylation and ubiquitination. Regarding ubiquitinated lysine residues, Gly-Gly remnants are generated from the C-terminal of ubiquitin as a consequence of tryptic digestion. PTMs: post-translational modifications, P: phosphorylation, Ac: acetylation, Ub: ubiquitination, TiO_2: titanium dioxide.

2.3. Ubiquitination

The ubiquitin system transmits protein degradation signal to proteasome as well as regulates multiple cellular functions such as cell-cycle progression, DNA repair and transcriptional regulation. Dysfunction of this system leads to various pathological conditions [24]. Ubiquitination sites are detected as diglycine (Gly-Gly) remnants on the modified lysine residues, which are generated by tryptic digestion of ubiquitinated proteins [25, 26].

3. Systematic characterization of the phosphoproteome dynamics in GSCs

The quantitative information on the phosphoproteome dynamics can provide us with systematic description of the key machinery for cellular signalling. In this section, we introduce two examples of global phosphoproteome analyses of GSCs using SILAC (stable isotope labelling by amino acids in cell culture)-based quantitative technique [27, 28] (**Figure 2**). One was carried out using epidermal growth factor (EGF) to elucidate the mechanism for stemness maintenance of GSCs [29], whereas the other was conducted through serum-induced differentiation of GSCs to unveil the key pathways responsible for disrupting stemness characteristics [30].

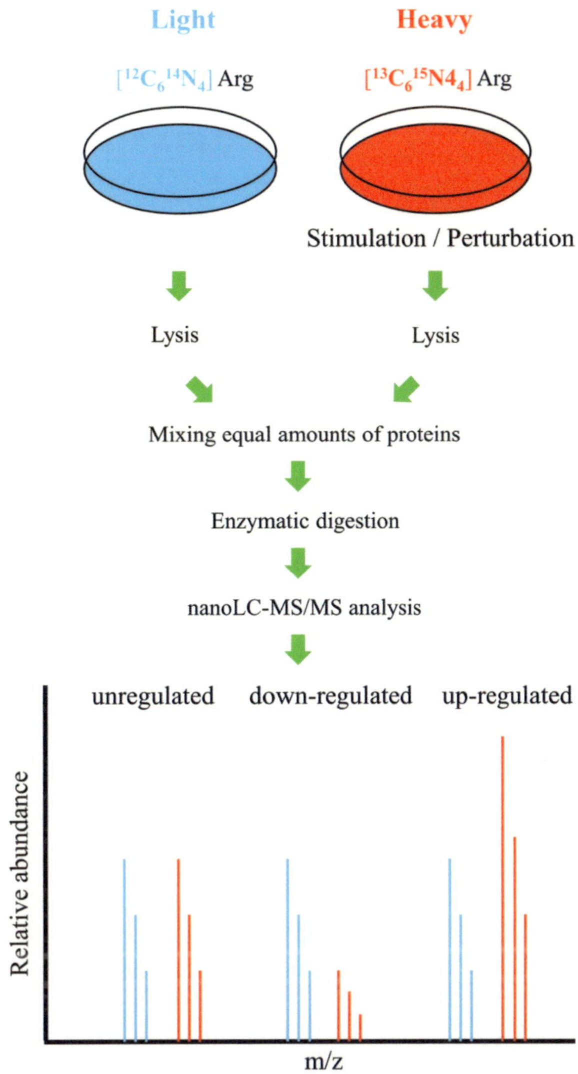

Figure 2. Schematic workflow for quantitative proteome analysis using SILAC, a representative relative quantitation technique based on metabolic labelling of specific amino acids such as arginine. Two populations of GSCs were cultured in the media supplemented with $^{12}C_6{}^{14}N_4$-Arg (light) or $^{13}C_6{}^{15}N_4$-Arg (heavy), respectively. After one of the two cell populations was stimulated/perturbed, both of the cells were lysed, equally combined and enzymatically digested to perform nanoLC-MS/MS analyses. The intensity of each mass peak is used for relative quantitation of each peptide with high accuracy.

3.1. Global quantitative phosphoproteome analyses of EGF-stimulated GSCs

EGF is known to be essential for maintenance and growth of GSCs [31]. The quantitative phosphoproteomic analysis of EGF-stimulated GSCs was performed to acquire network-wide information on the molecules related to stemness maintenance. As a result, a total of 6073 phosphopeptides from 2282 phosphorylated proteins were identified, leading to quantitative classification of 516 upregulated and 275 downregulated phosphorylation sites [29].

3.1.1. *IPA-based network analysis*

IPA canonical pathway analysis was then performed using SILAC-based quantitative phosphoproteome data on EGF-stimulated GSCs [29] (**Figure 3**). Protein synthesis-related pathways (EIF2 signalling, mTOR signalling) and cell cycle regulation-related pathways (cyclins and cell cycle regulation, cell cycle: G1/S checkpoint regulation, cell cycle: G2/M DNA damage checkpoint regulation) were extracted with statistical significance (-log (p-value) > 5).

3.1.2. *Upstream kinase prediction analysis*

Protein phosphorylation is known to be controlled by specific kinases depending on consensus sequence motifs of substrates [32]. The motif-x algorithm [33, 34] is applicable to statistical extraction of significant consensus sequence motifs from the large-scale phosphoproteome data on EGF-stimulated GSCs (**Figure 4(A)** and **(B)**).

NetworKIN [10, 11] is designed to predict upstream kinases based on the sequence motifs around the functionally regulated phosphorylation sites through construction of the related protein-protein interaction (PPI) networks using STRING [35]. The NetworKIN algorithm enables further interpretation of the results obtained from the motif-x analyses (**Figure 4 (C)**).

3.2. Global quantitative phosphoproteome analyses of serum-induced GSCs

CSCs are regarded as one of the most clinically important cell populations in causing tumour heterogeneity, which is responsible for the resistance to chemotherapy [36]. As recent studies have demonstrated that non-CSCs can also readily acquire CSC-like characteristics [37], it is very important to figure out the detailed mechanisms underlying CSC differentiation and

(A) (B)

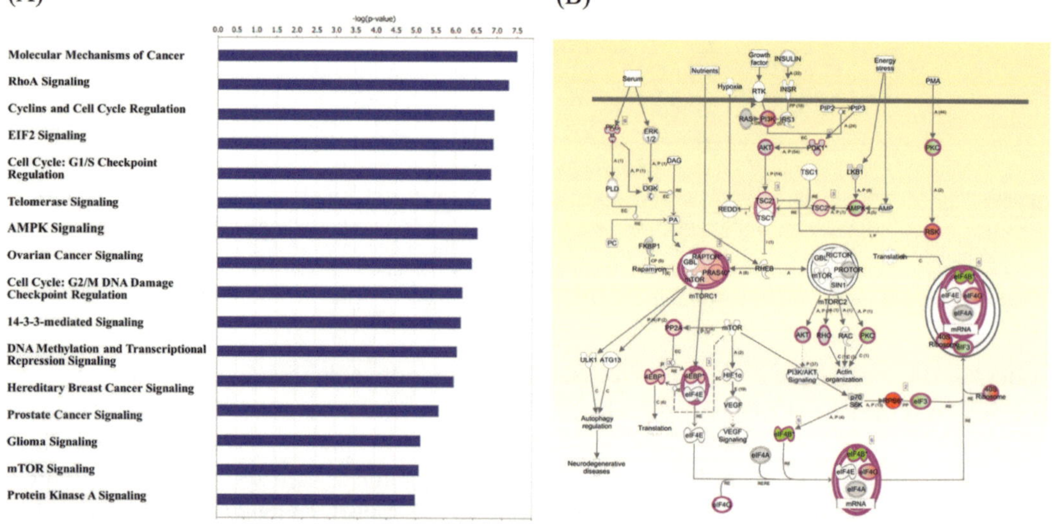

Figure 3. IPA-based pathway analysis of the quantitative phosphoproteome data on EGF-stimulated GSCs. (A) The significant canonical pathways across the entire dataset (-log (p-value) > 5). (B) The mTOR signalling pathway is representatively depicted with the predicted information on the biological activities related to this pathway.

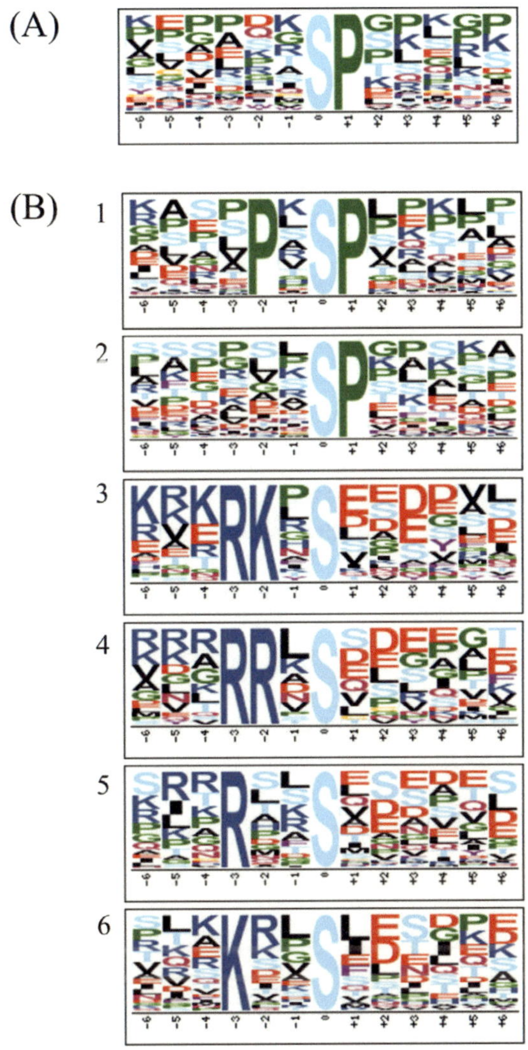

(C)

Predicted Kinase	Down	Up					
		1	2	3	4	5	6
1433beta					1		
1433epsilon					1		
1433eta					1		
1433gamma					1		
1433theta					1		
1433zeta					1		
ATM						1	1
ATR							1
AuroraA					1		
BRCA1					1		
CDK1	4	13	12				
CDK2	1	1	3				
CDK4					1	1	
CDK5	3	1	1				
CK1delta		1		1			
CK2a2							1
CK2alpha				1			2
CLK1			1				
CLK2					1		
CLK3					1		
CaMKIIalpha				1	1		1
CaMKIIbeta					1	1	1
CaMKIIdelta				1	1	2	1
CaMKIIgamma					1	2	1
CaMKIV					1		
DMPK1		1				1	
DNAPK						1	1
EIF2AK2			1				
GRK2				1			
GSK3alpha	1		2				
GSK3beta	2		7				
HIPK2			1	1			
MAPK1	5	8	5				
MAPK10			1				
MAPK11			1				
MAPK13	1		2				
MAPK3	6	6	6				
MAPK7	2	1	1				
MAPK8			1				
NLK			1				
PAK1					1	2	2
PAK2				1	1	1	2
PAK3					1		1
PDHK1							1
PIN1	1						
PKAalpha					2		
PKAbeta						1	1
PKAgamma						1	
PKBalpha						4	1
PKBbeta						1	
PKCalpha	1						2
PKCbeta	1		1	1	1	1	4
PKCepsilon	1						1
PKCzeta	1						1
PKD1						1	1
Piml				1			2
RSK1							1
RSK2				1			
TGFbR2						4	1
TTK					2		
p70S6K				1	1	1	

Figure 4. Phosphorylation site-oriented network analysis of the quantitative phosphoproteome data on EGF-stimulated GSCs. The consensus sequence motifs surrounding the quantitatively regulated phosphorylation sites regarding (A) downregulation and (B) upregulation can be described as a result of the motif-x analyses. (C) The numerical distribution of the putative kinases predicted by NetworKIN. The colour of cells reflects the number of the predicted kinases for each consensus sequence as described in (A) and (B).

understand the principle of their heterogeneity. Serum-induced phosphoproteome dynamics in GSCs was measured to systematically elucidate the regulatory nodes for stemness alteration over the entire signalling networks [30]. Among 2876 phosphorylation sites on 1584 proteins identified, 732 phosphorylation sites on 419 proteins were found to be regulated through serum-induced differentiation. The integrative network analyses of the quantitative phosphoproteome data using various bioinformatical tools including IPA and NetworKIN indicated that transforming growth factor-β receptor type-2 (TGFBR2) might be one of the crucial upstream regulators concerning GSC alteration (**Figure 5**).

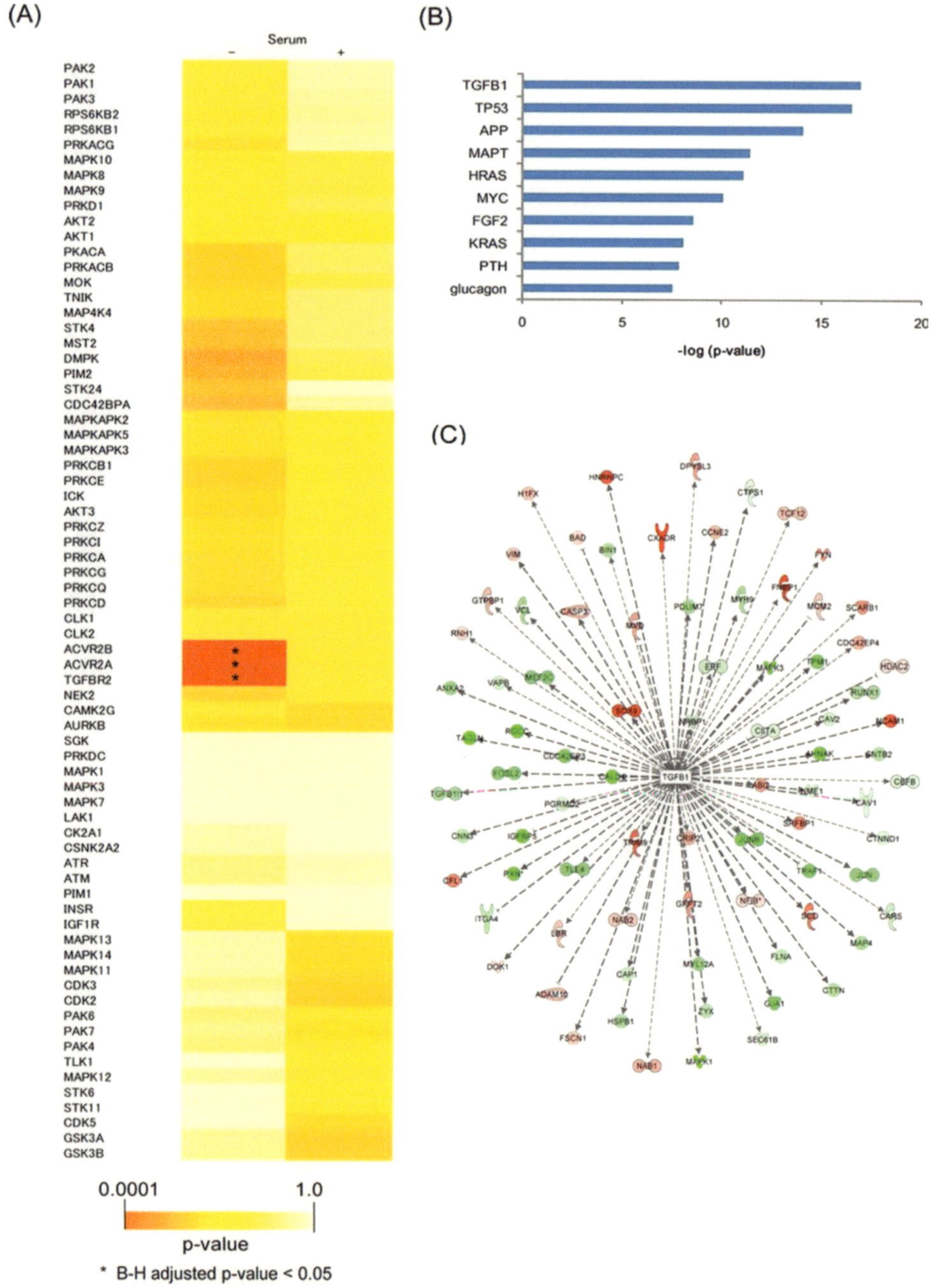

Figure 5. Upstream kinase/regulator analyses based on the regulated phosphoproteome data on serum-induced GSCs. (A) Heatmap of the over-representation p-values calculated for each predicted kinase using PhosphoSiteAnalyzer, a bioinformatical platform for the NetworKIN prediction results from the phosphoproteome data [38]. The subset 'serum (−)' indicates SILAC ratio > 2.0, whereas 'serum (+)' shows SILAC ratio < 0.5. TGFBR2 and ACVR2A/B-specific phosphorylation sites were predicted to be significantly enriched in the 'serum (−)' subset (adjusted p-value < 0.05). (B) Upstream regulator analysis by IPA. The top 10 upstream regulators relevant to the regulated phosphoproteome are shown with the corresponding score (−log [p-value]). (C) IPA-based description of TGF-β1 and the target molecules in the phosphoproteome data. Dashed lines represent indirect interactions caused by TGF-β1, adapted from Ref. [30].

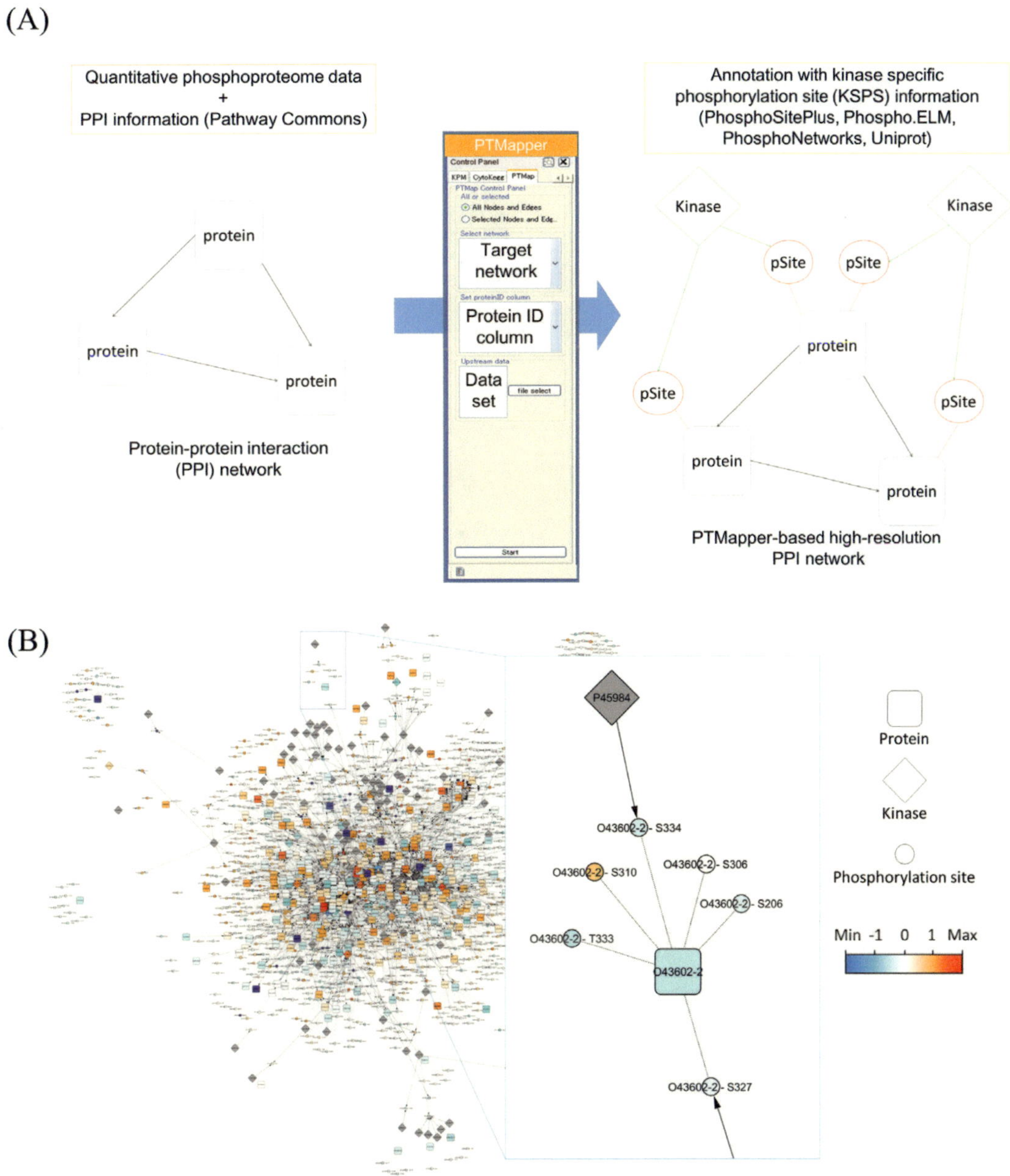

Figure 6. Construction of phosphorylation-oriented PPI networks via PTMapper. (A) Workflow for the visualization of kinase-phosphorylation site relationships in PPI networks via PTMapper. Phosphorylation sites are connected with the parental protein nodes in PPI networks and the upstream kinases are then added to the phosphorylation sites. (B) Phosphorylation site-oriented networks constructed from the phosphoproteome data on EGF-stimulated glioblastoma stem cells. The solid arrows represent functionally directed protein-protein interactions or kinase-substrate interactions, whereas the dotted lines show the linkages of proteins and their phosphorylation sites, adapted from Ref. [12].

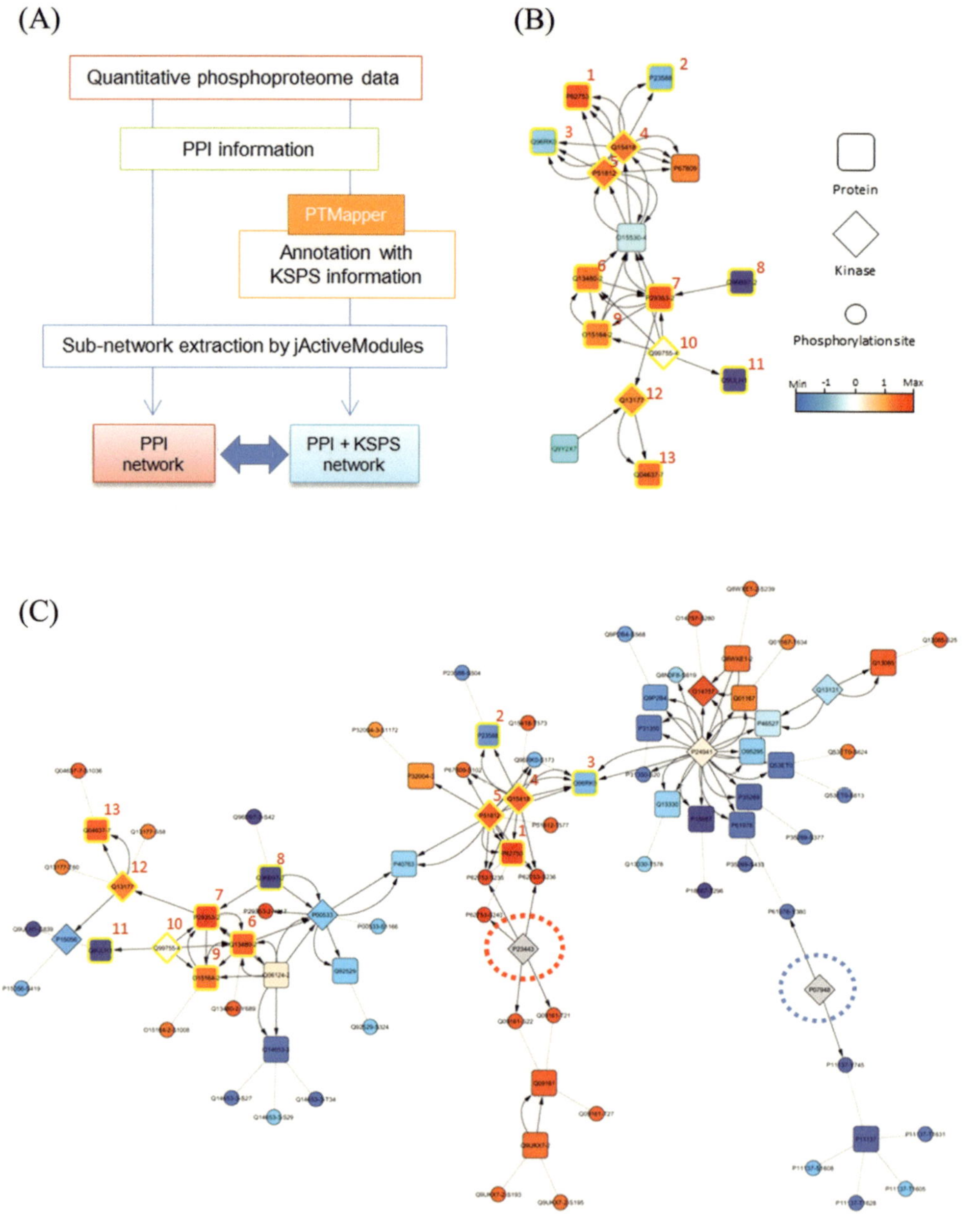

Figure 7. Comparison of the sub-networks extracted from EGF-dependent phosphorylation dynamics of glioblastoma stem cells. (A) Schematic procedure for the evaluation of PTMapper-based network construction. (B) The most significantly regulated sub-networks extracted from the conventional protein interaction network. (C) The phosphorylation site-oriented network generated via PTMapper. The nodes surrounded by the border with the upper-right numbers indicate the common molecules in the two types of the sub-networks. The solid arrows represent functionally directed protein-protein interactions or kinase-substrate interactions, whereas the dotted lines show the linkages of proteins and their phosphorylation sites. The dashed circles indicate p70S6K and Lyn, adapted from Ref. [12].

4. Development of advanced bioinformatical platforms for complicated kinase-substrate interaction networks

Although shotgun proteomics strategy based on advanced nanoLC-MS/MS system can provide us with large-scale information on various kinds of PTMs, there are only a few PTM-based network analysis tools available compared to conventional protein-protein interaction (PPI). Recently, CEASAR: connecting enzymes and substrates at amino acid resolution [39] and PhosphoPath [40] were developed to visualize kinase-substrate interactions in a phosphorylation site-oriented manner. CEASAR was designed to provide a high-resolution map of kinase-phosphorylation networks based on functional protein microarrays and bioinformatics analysis. On the other hand, PhosphoPath was developed as a Cytoscape app [41] to visualize both quantitative proteome and phosphoproteome data using PPI information extracted from BioGRID [42] and PhosphoSitePlus [17]. Recently, we also have developed a Cytoscape-based bioinformatical platform named 'post-translational modification mapper (PTMapper)' to visualize kinase-substrate interactions regarding multiple phosphorylation sites on signalling molecules (**Figure 6**) [12]. The kinase-phosphorylation site interaction dataset for this platform was integratively generated from PhosphoSitePlus [17], Phospho.ELM [43], PhosphoNetworks [44] and Uniprot KB [45], leading to construction of phosphorylation site-oriented PPI networks using Pathway Commons [46]. We applied this platform to extract crucial kinase-substrate interactions from the quantitative phosphoproteome data on EGF-stimulated GSCs [29]. As a result, p70S6K and Lyn were significantly extracted as key regulators (**Figure 7**).

5. Perspectives and conclusions

The bioinformatical description of GSC signalling dynamics based on the global quantitative phosphoproteome data led to network-wide extraction of critical molecules and their related pathways for defining stemness characteristics. Further integrative description of multiple PTM dynamics in GSCs will deepen our understanding of the nature of their cell signalling complexity at the network level. We believe that shotgun proteomics-based quantitative analyses of cancer stem cell signalling networks in combination with various statistical and mathematical platforms will pave the way to establish new directions towards systematic evaluation of drug targets in a cell-type specific manner.

Acknowledgements

We thank Dr. Yuta Narushima for his technical support. We are also thankful to all the members of Medical Proteomics Laboratory, The Institute of Medical Science, The University of Tokyo. This work was supported by grants-in-aid for scientific research on innovative areas (integrative understanding of biological signalling networks based on mathematical science) and grant-in-aid for scientific research (C).

Author details

Hiroko Kozuka-Hata and Masaaki Oyama*

*Address all correspondence to: moyama@ims.u-tokyo.ac.jp

Medical Proteomics Laboratory, The Institute of Medical Science, The University of Tokyo, Minato-ku, Tokyo, Japan

References

[1] Furnari FB, et al. Malignant astrocytic glioma: Genetics, biology, and paths to treatment. Genes & Development. 2007;**21**(21):2683-2710. DOI: 10.1101/gad.1596707

[2] Kreso A, Dick JE. Evolution of the cancer stem cell model. Cell Stem Cell. 2014;**14**(3): 275-291. DOI: 10.1016/j.stem.2014.02.006

[3] Burrell RA, McGranahan N, Bartek J, Swanton C. The causes and consequences of genetic heterogeneity in cancer evolution. Nature. 2013;**501**(7467):338-345. DOI: 10.1038/nature12625

[4] Vescovi AL, Galli R, Reynolds BA. Brain tumour stem cells. Nature Reviews Cancer. 2006;**6**(6):425-436. DOI: 10.1038/nrc1889

[5] Qazi MA, Vora P, Venugopal C, Sidhu SS, Moffat J, Swanton C, Singh SK. Intratumoral heterogeneity: Pathways to treatment resistance and relapse in human glioblastoma. Annals of Oncology. 2017. DOI: 10.1093/annonc/mdx169

[6] Takebe N, Harris PJ, Warren RQ, Ivy SP. Targeting cancer stem cells by inhibiting Wnt, Notch, and Hedgehog pathways. Nature Reviews Clinical Oncology. 2011;**8**(2):97-106. DOI: 10.1038/nrclinonc.2010.196

[7] Wurdak H, et al. An RNAi screen identifies TRRAP as a regulator of brain tumor-initiating cell differentiation. Cell Stem Cell. 2010;**6**(1):37-47. DOI: 10.1016/j.stem.2009.11.002

[8] Aebersold R, Mann M. Mass spectrometry-based proteomics. Nature. 2003;**422**(6928): 198-207. DOI: 10.1038/nature01511

[9] Krämer A, Green J, Pollard Jr J, Tugendreich S. Causal analysis approaches in ingenuity pathway analysis. Bioinformatics. 2014;**30**(4):523-530. DOI: 10.1093/bioinformatics/btt703. Available from: https://apps.ingenuity.com/

[10] Horn H, et al. KinomeXplorer: An integrated platform for kinome biology studies. Nature Methods. 2014;**11**(6):603-604. DOI: 10.1038/nmeth.2968. Available from: http://networkin.info/

[11] Linding R, et al. Systematic discovery of in vivo phosphorylation networks. Cell. 2007;**129**(7):1415-1426. DOI: 10.1016/j.cell.2007.05.052

[12] Narushima Y, Kozuka-Hata H, Tsumoto K, Inoue J, Oyama M. Quantitative phosphoproteomics-based molecular network description for high-resolution kinase-substrate interactome analysis. Bioinformatics. 2016;**32**(14):2083-2088. DOI: 10.1093/bioinformatics/btw164. Available from: https://www.github.com/y-narushima/PTMapper/

[13] Creasy DM, Cottrell JS. Unimod: Protein modifications for mass spectrometry. Proteomics. 2004;**4**(6):1534-1536. DOI: 10.1002/pmic.200300744. Available from: http://www.unimod.org/

[14] Mann M, Jensen ON. Proteomic analysis of post-translational modifications. Nature Biotechnology. 2003;**21**(3):255-261. DOI: 10.1038/nbt0303-255

[15] Hunter T. Protein kinases and phosphatases: The yin and yang of protein phosphorylation and signalling. Cell. 1995;**80**(2):225-236

[16] Hunter T. Signalling--2000 and beyond. Cell. 2000;**100**(1):113-127

[17] Hornbeck PV, et al. PhosphoSitePlus, 2014: Mutations, PTMs and recalibrations. Nucleic Acids Research. 2015;**43**(Database issue):D512-D520. DOI: 10.1093/nar/gku1267. Available from: http://www.phosphosite.org/

[18] Larsen MR, Thingholm TE, Jensen ON, Roepstorff P, Jørgensen TJ. Highly selective enrichment of phosphorylated peptides from peptide mixtures using titanium dioxide microcolumns. Molecular & Cellular Proteomics. 2005;**4**(7):873-886. DOI: 10.1074/mcp.T500007-MCP200

[19] Olsen JV, et al. Global, in vivo, and site-specific phosphorylation dynamics in signaling networks. Cell. 2006;**127**(3):635-648. DOI: 10.1016/j.cell.2006.09.026

[20] Kouzarides T. Acetylation: A regulatory modification to rival phosphorylation? EMBO Journal. 2000;**19**(6):1176-1179. DOI: 10.1093/emboj/19.6.1176

[21] Yang XJ, Seto E. Lysine acetylation: Codified crosstalk with other posttranslational modifications. Molecular Cell. 2008;**31**(4):449-461. DOI: 10.1016/j.molcel.2008.07.002

[22] Kim SC, et al. Substrate and functional diversity of lysine acetylation revealed by a proteomics survey. Molecular Cell. 2006;**23**(4):607-618. DOI: 10.1016/j.molcel.2006.06.026

[23] Choudhary C, et al. Lysine acetylation targets protein complexes and co-regulates major cellular functions. Science. 2009;**325**(5942):834-840. DOI: 10.1126/science.1175371

[24] Hershko A, Ciechanover A. The ubiquitin system. Annual Review of Biochemistry. 1998;**67**:425-479. DOI: 10.1146/annurev.biochem.67.1.425

[25] Xu G, Paige JS, Jaffrey SR. Global analysis of lysine ubiquitination by ubiquitin remnant immunoaffinity profiling. Nature Biotechnology. 2010;**28**(8):868-873. DOI: 10.1038/nbt.1654

[26] Wagner SA, et al. A proteome-wide, quantitative survey of in vivo ubiquitylation sites reveals widespread regulatory roles. Molecular & Cellular Proteomics. 2011;**10**(10):M111.013284. DOI: 10.1074/mcp.M111.013284

[27] Ong SE, et al. Stable isotope labelling by amino acids in cell culture, SILAC, as a simple and accurate approach to expression proteomics. Molecular & Cellular Proteomics. 2002;**1**(5):376-386

[28] Blagoev B, et al. A proteomics strategy to elucidate functional protein-protein interactions applied to EGF signaling. Nature Biotechnology. 2003;**21**(3):315-318. DOI: 10.1038/nbt790

[29] Kozuka-Hata, et al. Phosphoproteome of human glioblastoma initiating cells reveals novel signaling regulators encoded by the transcriptome. PLoS One. 2012;**7**(8):e43398. DOI: 10.1371/journal.pone.0043398

[30] Narushima Y, et al. Integrative network analysis combined with quantitative phosphoproteomics reveals transforming growth Factor-beta receptor type-2 (TGFBR2) as a novel regulator of glioblastoma stem cell properties. Molecular & Cellular Proteomics. 2016;**15**(3):1017-1031. DOI: 10.1074/mcp.M115.049999

[31] Pollard SM, et al. Glioma stem cell lines expanded in adherent culture have tumor-specific phenotypes and are suitable for chemical and genetic screens. Cell Stem Cell. 2009;**4**(6):568-580. DOI: 10.1016/j.stem.2009.03.014

[32] Seet BT, Dikic I, Zhou MM, Pawson T. Reading protein modifications with interaction domains. Nature Reviews Molecular Cell Biology. 2006;**7**(7):473-483. DOI: 10.1038/nrm1960

[33] Schwartz D, Gygi SP. An iterative statistical approach to the identification of protein phosphorylation motifs from large-scale data sets. Nature Biotechnology. 2005;**23**(11):1391-1398. DOI: 10.1038/nbt1146. Available from: http://motif-x.med.harvard.edu/

[34] Chou MF, Schwartz D. Biological sequence motif discovery using motif-x. Current Protocols in Bioinformatics. 2011;**13**(13):15-24. DOI: 10.1002/0471250953.bi1315s35

[35] Szklarczyk D, et al. The STRING database in 2017: Quality-controlled protein-protein association networks, made broadly accessible. Nucleic Acids Research. 2017;**45**(D1):D362-D368. DOI: 10.1093/nar/gkw937. Available from: http://string-db.org/

[36] Meacham CE, Morrison SJ. Tumour heterogeneity and cancer cell plasticity. Nature. 2013;**501**(7467):328-337. DOI: 10.1038/nature12624

[37] Chaffer CL, et al. Poised chromatin at the ZEB1 promoter enables breast cancer cell plasticity and enhances tumorigenicity. Cell. 2013;**154**(1):61-74. DOI: 10.1016/j.cell.2013.06.005

[38] Bennetzen MV, Cox J, Mann M, Andersen JS. PhosphoSiteAnalyzer: A bioinformatic platform for deciphering phosphoproteomes using kinase predictions retrieved from NetworKIN. Journal of Proteome Research. 2012;**11**(6):3480-3486. DOI: 10.1021/pr300016e. Available from: http://phosphosite.sourceforge.net

[39] Newman RH, et al. Construction of human activity-based phosphorylation networks. Molecular Systems Biology. 2013;**9**:655. DOI: 10.1038/msb.2013.12

[40] Raaijmakers LM, et al. PhosphoPath: Visualization of Phosphosite-centric dynamics in temporal molecular networks. Journal of Proteome Research. 2015;**14**(10):4332-4341. DOI: 10.1021/acs.jproteome.5b00529. Available from: https://github.com/linseyr/PhosphoPath/

[41] Shannon P, et al. Cytoscape: A software environment for integrated models of biomolecular interaction networks. Genome Research. 2003;**13**(11):2498-2504. DOI: 10.1101/gr.1239303. Available from: http://www.cytoscape.org/

[42] Chatr-Aryamontri A, et al. The BioGRID interaction database: 2015 update. Nucleic Acids Research. 2015;**43**(Database issue):D470-D478. DOI: 10.1093/nar/gku1204. Available from: https://thebiogrid.org/

[43] Dinkel H, et al. Phospho.ELM: A database of phosphorylation sites--update 2011. Nucleic Acids Research. 2011;**39**(Database issue):D261-D267. DOI: 10.1093/nar/gkq1104. Available from: http://phospho.elm.eu.org/

[44] Hu J, et al. PhosphoNetworks: A database for human phosphorylation networks. Bioinformatics. 2014;**30**(1):141-142. DOI: 10.1093/bioinformatics/btt627. Available from: http://www.phosphonetworks.org/

[45] Magrane M, et al. UniProt Knowledgebase: A hub of integrated protein data. Database (Oxford). 2011;bar009. DOI: 10.1093/database/bar009. Available from: http://www.uniprot.org/

[46] Cerami EG, et al. Pathway commons, a web resource for biological pathway data. Nucleic Acids Research. 2011;**39**(Database issue):D685-D690. DOI: 10.1093/nar/gkq1039. Available from: http://www.pathwaycommons.org/

Chapter 12

Epitranscriptomics for Biomedical Discovery

Min Xiong, Daniel P. Heruth, Xun Jiang,
Shamima Islam, Li Qin Zhang, Ding-You Li and
Shui Q. Ye

Additional information is available at the end of the chapter

http://dx.doi.org/10.5772/intechopen.69033

Abstract

Epitranscriptomics is a newly burgeoning field pertaining to the complete delineation and elucidation of chemical modifications of nucleotides found within all classes of RNA that do not involve a change in the ribonucleotide sequence. More than 140 diverse and distinct nucleotide modifications have been identified in RNA, dwarfing the number of nucleotide modifications found in DNA. The majority of epitranscriptomic modifications have been identified in ribosomal RNA (rRNA), transfer RNA (tRNA), and small nuclear RNA (snRNA). However, in total, the knowledge of the occurrence, and specifically the function, of RNA modifications remains scarce. Recently, the rapid advancement of next-generation sequencing and mass spectrometry technologies have allowed for the identification and functional characterization of nucleotide modifications in both protein-coding and non-coding RNA on a global, transcriptome scale. In this chapter, we will introduce the concepts of nucleotide modification, summarize transcriptome-wide RNA modification mapping techniques, highlight recent studies exploring the functions of RNA modifications and their association to disease, and finally offer insight into the future progression of epitranscriptomics.

Keywords: epitranscriptomics, RNA modifications, gene expression

1. Introduction

RNA has been shown to play critical roles in regulating cellular functions. Comparative transcriptomics between mammals has revealed that ~66% of human genomic DNA is transcribed. Remarkably, only ~2% of the transcriptional production is protein-coding messenger RNA (mRNA), while ~98% encompasses a wide variety of non-coding RNA (ncRNA) molecules [1, 2]. ncRNAs have been classified functionally as either housekeeping or regulatory. The

housekeeping ncRNA genes include ribosomal RNA (rRNA), transfer RNA (tRNA), and small nuclear RNA (snRNA), while examples of regulatory ncRNAs are microRNA (miRNA) and long non-coding RNA (lncRNA) [3–5]. The complexity of RNA is further complicated by numerous post-transcriptional modifications which alter the chemical structure of the nucleotides without changing the nucleotide sequence. Similar to the field of epigenetics which investigates the modifications of DNA and histone proteins, the study of chemical modifications of RNA is called epitranscriptomics [6, 7]. More than 140 chemically diverse and distinct modified nucleotides have been identified in both mRNA and ncRNA, including N^6-methyladenosine (m^6A), 5-methyl cytidine (m^5C), pseudouridine (Ψ), adenosine (A) to inosine (I), and N^1-methyladenosine (m^1A). These modifications have been identified mostly in the housekeeping ncRNAs [3, 4, 8]; however, chemical modifications have also been detected in mRNA and the regulatory ncRNAs [9–11]. Unfortunately, the knowledge about the occurrence and function of RNA modifications at transcriptome level remains scarce. Recently, the interest in RNA modifications and their functions have gained momentum owing mainly to the application of novel modifications to next-generation sequencing (NGS) and mass spectrometry technologies, which have allowed transcriptome-wide detection of distinct RNA modifications [12, 13]. Accurate regulation of the transcriptome is critical for gene expression and its subsequent control of cellular functions, including metabolism, proliferation, differentiation, and development. Thus, alterations in transcriptome regulation can disrupt cellular functions and lead to disease. Accumulating evidence has identified and functionally characterized several distinct types of chemical modifications of RNA nucleotides in both protein-coding and ncRNAs, further advancing the burgeoning field of epitranscriptomics. In this chapter, we will first provide an overview of RNA modifications and then synopsize several transcriptome-wide RNA modification mapping techniques such as m^6A-seq, m^5C-seq, pseudouridine-seq, and NAD captureSeq. Next, we will highlight novel insights into the potential functions of RNA modifications and their disease relevance as revealed and facilitated by epitranscriptomic profiling. Finally, we will offer our perspective on how the field will progress or evolve in the near future.

2. An overview of post-transcriptional modifications of RNA

The process of mRNA maturation involving 5'-capping, splicing, and polyadenylation has been well studied [14]. However, the more subtle post-transcriptional modifications of epitranscriptomics, also termed RNA-epigenetics, are now just fully coming to light. The post-transcriptional modifications found in RNA are often called marks because they mark a region of RNA that potentially contributes to the regulation of cellular processes, including gene expression, protein translation, or RNA stability. Like mRNA maturation, enzymes are required to catalyze the reactions, which chemically modify RNA nucleotides. The most common post-transcriptional RNA modification, Ψ, was also the first to be discovered [15]. Originally discovered in rRNA and tRNA, Ψ modifications are also present in mRNA [16, 17]. Site-specific isomerization of uridine (U) to Ψ (5-ribosyluracil) is irreversibly catalyzed via Ψ synthases. The family of Ψ synthases (PUS) consists of enzymes which can either function independently or those that require H/ACA ribonucleotide complexes [18]. Compared to

U, Ψ contains an extra imino group (>C=NH), which serves as an additional hydrogen bond donor, while the carbon-carbon (C—C) glycosidic bond linking the sugar to the base is more stable than the carbon-nitrogen (C—N) found in U. These two chemical changes confer rigidity to the sugar-phosphate backbone and enhances local base stacking [19].

The most common internal modification in eukaryotic mRNA is m^6A [20]. Unlike Ψ, m^6A modifications are reversible, suggesting that the modifications are involved in regulatory switches. Methyltransferases (METTL3, METTL14, and WTAP), termed writers, catalyze the methylation of adenosine [21–23], whereas demethylases (FTO and ALKBH5), termed erasers, remove the methyl group [24, 25]. The m^6A marks are recognized by YTH domain proteins, termed readers, which regulate mRNA processing and metabolism [26, 27].

An additional class of nucleotide modifications, termed RNA editing, creates an irreversible change in the nucleotide sequence. These modifications include insertions, deletions, and base substitutions and occur in all classes of RNA. When they occur in mRNA, the amino acid sequence of the protein will be altered relative to the sequence encoded by genomic DNA. RNA editing by deamination results in adenosine (A) to inosine (I) and cytosine (C) to uridine (U). A-to-I editing is an abundant class of RNA modifications found throughout metazoans [28]. The conversion of A-to-I residues by base deamination results in the synthesis of distinct proteins, which creates functional diversity and serves to enhance the response to rapid environmental changes [29]. RNA editing by deamination is mediated by two major classes of enzymes; the first class is a group of tissue-specific and context-dependent adenosine deaminases called ADARs [30–32]. The ADAR enzyme class (adenosine deaminases acting on RNA) catalyzes hydrolytic deamination of A-to-I in double-stranded regions of RNA secondary structure [33]. The second class of enzymes, the vertebrate-specific apolipoprotein B mRNA editing catalytic polypeptide-like (APOBEC) family, promotes C-to-U editing by cytosine deamination [34]. APOBEC1, the first-discovered member of the APOBEC family, was characterized as the zinc-dependent cytidine deaminase which catalyzed a C-to-U modification, resulting in an in-frame stop codon in APOB mRNA [35].

3. NGS-based RNA modification techniques

The first transcriptome-wide and NGS-based approach for mapping m^6A modifications demonstrated the feasibility of identifying RNA modifications across the entire transcriptome and established the field of epitranscriptomics [6]. The most important aspects of NGS-based techniques are the ability to map modifications on a global scale at the single nucleotide resolution and that the modified nucleotides are analyzed within the context of the surrounding gene sequence. These features insure that the nucleotide modifications are accurately assigned to the appropriate RNA and not falsely attributed to homologous genes or RNA contaminates [6]. Now, several high-throughput NGS-based technologies, including RNA-seq, have been established to profile and quantitate RNA modifications (m^6A, $m6^Am$, m^5C, m^1A, A-to-I, Ψ, and NAD cap). These RNA-seq-based methodologies can be divided into two classes: immunoprecipitation-based and chemical-based methods. **Table 1** lists six representative NGS-based detection methods of RNA modifications.

Method	Modification	Strategies
m^6A-seq [26], MeRIP-seq [36], m^6A-LAICIC-seq [37]	m^6A, m^6Am	Methyl-RNA immunoprecipitation and UV cross-linking
m^1A-ID-seq [39]	m^1A	Methyl-RNA immunoprecipitation and the inherent ability of m^1A to stall reverse transcription
Bisulfite sequencing [40]	m^5C	Chemical conversion of modified nucleotides
ICE-seq [42]	A-to-I editing	Cyanoethylation of RNA combined with reverse transcription
Pseudo-seq [16], Ψ-seq [17]	ψ	Chemical modification to terminate reverse transcription in the pseudouridylated site
NAD captureSeq [43]	NAD	Chemoenzymatic capture

Table 1. NGS-based methods to profile transcriptome-wide RNA modifications.

RNA immunoprecipitation (RIP)-based methods use an RNA modification-specific antibody or an enzyme-specific antibody to capture modified RNA followed by RNA-seq. m^6A-seq [26], methylated RIP-seq (MeRIP-seq) [36] and m^6A-level, and isoform-characterization sequencing (m^6A-LAIC-seq) [37] combine RNA-seq with RIP specific for m^6A methylation. **Figure 1A** displays a typical m^6A-seq workflow. RIP is performed using an anti-m^6A antibody to enrich m^6A-modified RNAs followed by cDNA library preparation and high throughput NGS sequencing and finally analysis to identify the occurrence and consensus motif (RRACU) of global m^6A modifications. A modified RIP approach, called m^6A individual-nucleotide-resolution by cross-linking and immunoprecipitation (miCLIP), uses ultraviolet light-induced antibody RNA cross-linking to induce site-specific mutations at m^6A marks. These mutational signatures block reverse transcription and facilitate the detection of m^6A marks at single-nucleotide resolution [38]. As illustrated in **Figure 1B**, m^1A-ID-seq, which combines m^1A

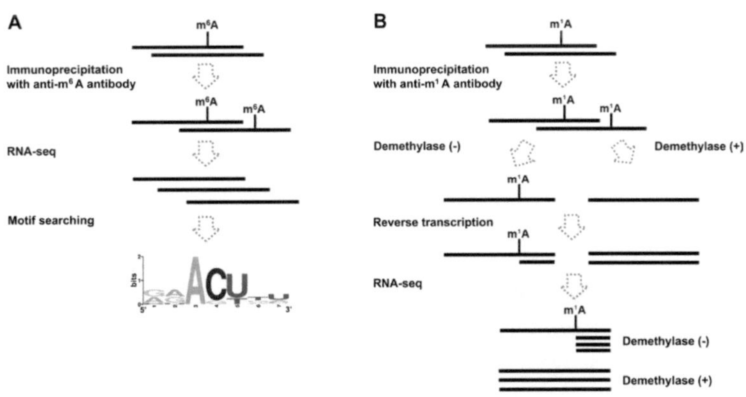

Figure 1. Immunoprecipitation-based strategies to detect RNA modifications. (A) m^6A-seq workflow: RNA immunoprecipitation is done using anti-m^6A antibody to enrich m^6A-modified RNAs followed by cDNA library preparation and high throughput NGS sequencing before occurrence and consensus motif (RRACU) of global m^6A modifications are analyzed. (B) m^1A-ID-seq workflow: RNA immunoprecipitation is carried out using anti-m^1A antibody to enrich m^1A-modified RNAs, which are then subjected to either the demethylase (−) treatment or the demethylase (+). Reverse transcription is stopped at m^1A site in demethylase (−) group while extended in the demethylase (+) group. After NGS, m^1A site can be identified by comparing the data of the demethylase (−) group to those of the demethylase (+) group.

http://dx.doi.org/10.5772/intechopen.69033

immunoprecipitation and the m[1]A residue to cause truncated reverse transcription products, has been applied successfully for the transcriptome-wide characterizations of m[1]A [39].

Chemical-based methods rely on the misincorporation of nucleotide or nucleotide conversion to truncate or stop RNA products during reverse transcription. RNA bisulfite conversion followed by high-throughput sequencing (BS-seq, **Figure 2A**) is a chemical conversion method based on converting unmodified cytosine residues to uracil and keeping m[5]C residues unchanged by bisulfite treatment. BS-seq is the only method currently available for the detection of site-specific endogenous m[5]C [40, 41]. Inosine chemical erasing (ICE) uses nucleotide switching to detect A-to-I modifications [42]. Inosine ribonucleotides are

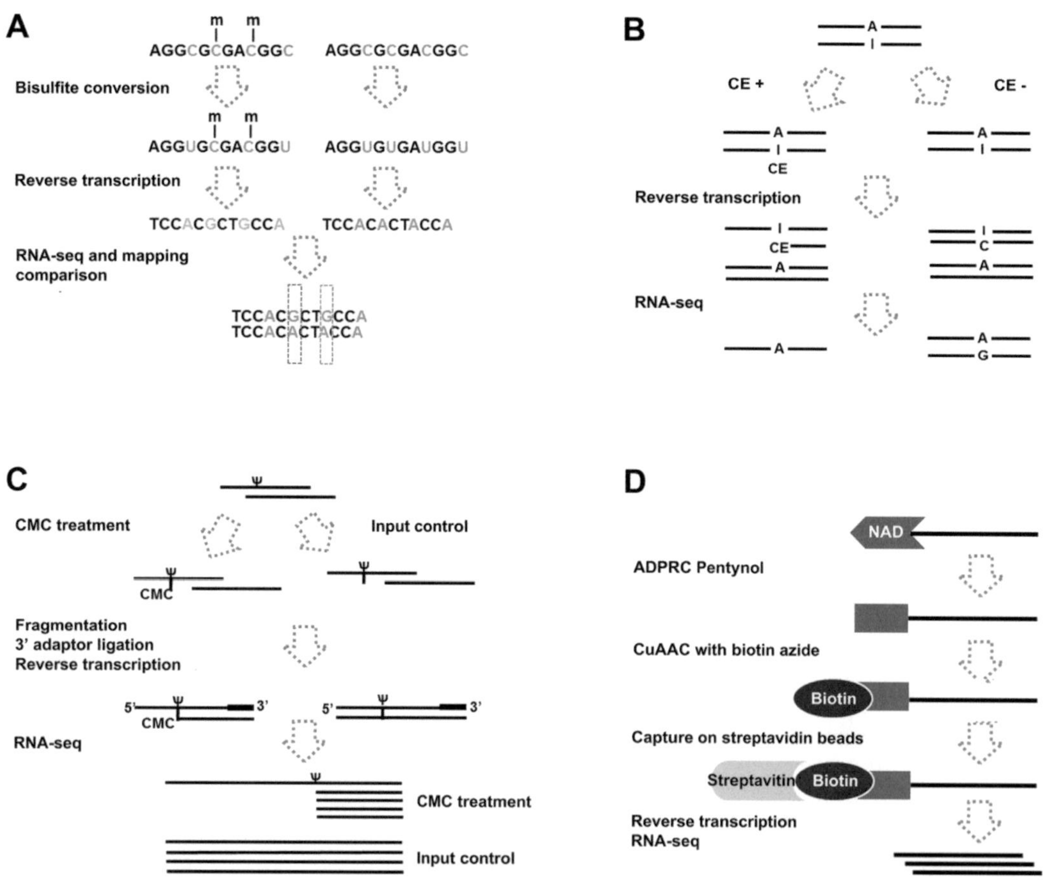

Figure 2. Chemical-based strategies to detect RNA modification. (A) BS-seq: Bisulfite selectively converts cytosine, not m[5]C, into uracil, subsequent to reverse transcription and RNA-seq processes. After comparison with reference genome or control, m[5]C residues are identified as cytosine, whereas unmethylated cytosine as thymine. (B) ICE-seq: The acrylonitrile can cyanoethylate inosine into N1-cyanoethylinosine (ce[1]I). Reverse transcription will transcript inosine into cytidine but arrest at the ce[1]I site after the CE treatment. cDNA library, sequencing, reads mapping, and analysis will detect A-to-I sites. (C) Ψ-seq: The reagent CMC followed by incubation at alkaline pH leads to hydrolysis of U-CMC adducts, which are less stable than Ψ-CMC. Reverse transcription in Ψ-CMC sample will stop at Ψ site. Following RNA-seq and reads mapping will detect Ψ sites with increased transcript termination in the CMC-treated sample. (D) NAD captureSeq: ADPRC enzyme catalyzes a transglycosylation reaction of NAD with pentynol, which are bound by CuAAC with biotin azide. The RNA with NAD is captured by streptavidin beads before being readied for cDNA library preparation and sequenced for identifying NAD-capped RNAs.

cyanoethylated with acrylonitrile to form N^1-cyanoethylinosine (ce^{1}I). Subsequently, the Watson-Crick base pairing of I with C is inhibited by the newly formed N^1-cyanoethyl group of ce^{1}I. Thus, cyanoethylation of I blocks cDNA synthesis by preventing extension of the cDNA that bears a cytosine (C) corresponding to the editing site during reverse transcription. However, I will be replaced by guanosine (G) [42] (**Figure 2B**). To detect RNA pseudouridylation, several groups developed Pseudo-seq (Ψ-seq). RNA is treated with N_3-[N-cyclohexyl-N'-β-(4-methylmorpholinium) ethylcarbodiimide-Ψ (N_3-CMC-Ψ)], which binds covalently to U, G, and Ψ residues and then exposed to alkaline pH to reduce stable U-CMC and G-CMC adducts. Reverse transcription will pause at the remaining intact Ψ-CMC sites, allowing for the mapping of Ψ-modifications [16, 17] (**Figure 2C**). Comparison of mapping reads from CMC-treated samples versus non-treated controls, Ψ will be detected as the sites with an increased proportion of reads supporting reverse transcription termination. NAD captureSeq (**Figure 2D**) requires the chemo-enzymatic modification of NAD which is capping the 5' end of RNA. The first step, the transglycosylation of NAD, is catalyzed by ADP-ribosyl cyclase (ADPRC) from *Aplysia californica* in the presence of an alkynyl alcohol. In the second step, the modified NAD is biotinylated by a copper-catalyzed azide-alkyne cycloaddition. Thirdly, the biotin-linked RNA is captured on streptavidin beads and processed further for cDNA library preparation and NGS. The NAD-biotin-captured sequences are then identified by comparison with the control samples which were not subjected to the first step of chemo-enzymatic biotinylation [43].

4. Physiological functions of RNA modifications

Although we do not have full knowledge on the effects of RNA modification on physiological function, there is increasing evidence that they play critical roles in the regulation of gene expression, cellular functions, and development. Disruptions of RNA modification mechanisms have also been associated with disease. We present here a few examples, which demonstrate the importance of RNA modification on physiological function.

As stated earlier, m^6A modifications are commonly found throughout eukaryotes, as demonstrated by multiple m^6A-seq studies. Human m^6A-seq analyses revealed 12,769 putative m^6A sites within 6990 and 250 protein-coding and non-coding transcripts, respectively [26], whereas, in mice, 4513 m^6A peaks were identified in 3376 and 66 protein-coding and non-coding transcripts, respectively [26]. The m^6A consensus motif, RRACU, was identified with a median distance from m^6A peaks of 24 nucleotides [26]. Interestingly, the majority of m^6A sites were conserved between both mouse and human transcriptomes and enriched further within long internal exons and around stop codons, suggesting strong evolutionary selection [26, 36]. m^6A-LAIC-seq showed that methylated transcripts utilized proximal alternative polyadenylation (APA) sites, which resulted in shorter 3′ untranslated regions, whereas non-methylated transcripts tended to use distal APA sites [37]. This observation correlated with the finding that m^6A-modified transcripts had both significantly shorter RNA half lives and slightly lower translational efficiencies than unmarked transcripts [44].

In vitro and in vivo genetic depletion of the m^{6}A writer, *Mettl3*, in both mouse and human, led to the absence of m^{6}A modification within *Nanog* mRNA which encodes a pluripotency factor. The absence of m^{6}A marks extended Nanog expression throughout differentiation and inhibited embryonic stem cell exit from self-renewal towards lineage differentiation [44]. m^{6}A-seq in mouse naïve embryonic stem cells (ESCs), 11-day-old embryoid bodies (EBs), and mouse embryonic fibroblasts (MEFs) revealed m^{6}A marks in naïve pluripotency-promoting genes reduced mRNA stability of key pluripotency-promoting transcripts and facilitated differentiation [45]. These findings suggest that m^{6}A modification provides the flexibility of the stem cell transcriptome required to differentiate into different lineages [44]. NANOG is also important in both the maintenance and specification of cancer stem cells which can metastasize and form primary tumors. The exposure of breast cancer cells to hypoxia induced the expression of the eraser ALKBH5 which resulted in m^{6}A demethylation in the 3' UTR of *NANOG* mRNA and the increased half life of *NANOG* mRNA, thereby promoting the breast cancer stem cell (BCSC) phenotype [46]. The m^{6}A reader YTHDF2 protects the 5′ UTR of stress-induced transcripts from demethylation. Cap-independent translation initiation was enhanced by 5′ UTR methylation [47]. m^{6}A modification is critical for the regulation of HIV-1 replication and HIV-1's effect on the host immune system [48]. HIV-1 viral infection induced m^{6}A modification in both host and viral mRNAs. HIV-1 coding, non-coding, and splicing regulatory regions contained a total of 14 m^{6}A methylation peaks. In addition, methylation of two highly conserved m^{6}A target sites in the HIV-1 rev response element (RRE) stem loop II region enriched the binding of the HIV-1 rev protein to the RRE in vivo and enhanced nuclear export of HIV-1 RNA [48]. The long non-coding RNA X-inactive specific transcript (XIST) regulates transcriptional silencing of genes on the X chromosome. XIST is heavily modified with at least 78 m^{6}A sites. Knockdown of METTL3 leads to decreased XIST m^{6}A marks and impairs XIST-mediated gene silencing [49].

The tRNA T-loop at position 58 commonly contains a m^{1}A modification [50], along with position 9 of metazoan mitochondrial tRNAs [51] and eukaryotic rRNAs [52]. Initiator tRNA^{Met} contains fully modified m^{1}A 58 which stabilizes its tertiary structure. Hypomodification of tRNA m^{1}A 58 affects the association with polysomes and the subsequent efficiency of translation [53, 54]. m^{1}A modifications in tRNA function in response to environmental stress [55], whereas m^{1}A-modified rRNA regulates ribosome biogenesis [52]. m^{1}A-ID-seq demonstrated that m^{1}A methylation regulated the dynamic response to stimuli and identified 901 m^{1}A peaks enriched within the 5' UTR near the start codons of 600 distinct protein-coding and non-coding RNAs [39].

m^{5}C sites have been detected in several eukaryotic tRNA, Rrna, and mRNA. m^{5}C marks stabilize the secondary structure of tRNA, alter aminoacylation and codon recognition [56], and regulate translational fidelity [57]. A low level of internal m^{5}C was found in mRNA cap structures in mammalian- and virus-infected mammalian cells [58, 59]. BS-seq identified 10,275 sites in protein-coding and non-coding RNAs [41]. m^{5}C marks in mRNAs were enriched near argonaute-binding sites within the 3' UTR [41].

A-to-I editing sites are distributed through human mRNA, including exons, introns. and 5' and 3' UTRs [60]. Alu repeat elements contain the highest frequency of A-to-I editing sites

among the untranslated regions of the genome [61]. Intronic editing mediated by ADAR1 contributes to the maintenance of mature mRNA by protecting it against unfavorable processing of the Alu sequence and by degradation of aberrant transcripts by nonsense-mediated decay (NMD) [42]. A-to-I RNA editing is diminished in brain tissue from patients with Alzheimer's disease relative to controls [62]. The reduction occurs predominantly in the hippocampus and to a lesser extent in the temporal and frontal lobes. These alterations result in decreased levels of protein recoding, the process of changing the amino acid sequence by A-to-I editing, in Alzheimer's disease [62]. The APOBEC3 family of cytidine deaminases has been associated with mutations in cancer genomes in several types of cancer. Accumulated data linking mutations in oncogenes and tumor suppressor genes with APOBEC3B activity are providing evidence that cytidine deaminase-induced mutagenesis is activated in tumorigenesis, thus providing novel therapeutic targets [63].

Pseudo-seq revealed that mRNA Ψ marks mRNA are regulated in response to stimuli, such as serum starvation in human cells and nutrient deprivation in yeast. The observations indicate that Ψ triggers a rapid regulatory mechanism to rewire the genetic code through inducible mRNA [16]. Pseudouridylation of rRNA and telomerase RNA component (TERC) were also found to be reduced in dyskeratosis congenita patients [17]. Furthermore, missense mutations in pseudouridine synthase 1 (PUS1) may lead to deficient pseudouridylation of mitochondrial tRNAs in mitochondrial myopathy and sideroblastic anemia (MLASA) patients [64].

NAD captureSeq identified NAD as a 5' RNA cap in a subset of regulatory RNAs in bacteria [43] and subsequently proposed that this type of capping may be common across all of life [65]. It is safe to predict that investigation of the roles and mechanisms of 5' NAD caps in eukaryotes will draw increasing attention in the biomedical field. This is due to mainly two reasons. First, the chemical modification of the 5' end of RNA is critical for RNA processing, localization, stability, translational efficiency, and epitranscriptomic regulation of gene expression [66]. Second, NAD is both a co-substrate for enzymes, such as the sirtuins and poly(adenosine diphosphate-ribose) polymerases, and a critical electron-carrying coenzyme for enzymes that catalyze oxidation-reduction reactions. NAD is involved in nearly all physiological processes. For example, cellular NAD^+ levels are modulated during aging, and the use and production of NAD^+ usage has been associated with prolonged health and life spans [67]. Regulation of NAD-mediated RNA capping and hence gene expression will undoubtedly enrich our understanding of NAD's expanding roles in normal physiology and disease pathogenesis.

5. Perspective

Although rapid advances have been made in the past few years in epitranscriptomics, more work is needed in this field. To date, more than 140 different RNA modifications have been identified. However, there are only a few reliable high-throughput techniques available to determine the global occurrence of a particular RNA modification. Thus, there is a need for the development of more high-throughput techniques to characterize the full spectra of RNA modifications. It is also important to pursue the comprehensive

http://dx.doi.org/10.5772/intechopen.69033

identification and characterization of the enzymes responsible for RNA modification since several of these enzymes have been shown to play important roles in development and disease. It is essential to decipher all functions and disease involvements of all RNA modifications. Development of additional technologies to alter RNA modifications, including the engineering of RNA-modifying enzymes with modified substrate specificity and activity via the CRISPR-Cas 9 system, will open the door to new types of detection and analysis pipelines. With further technological development, we will be able to elucidate the sequence-specific signatures in RNA that direct modifications and then better relate these RNA marks to their corresponding biological functions. Finally, the advancement of current approaches, coupled with new technologies, will allow for the development of new therapies and therapeutic targets for human diseases associated with deficient RNA modification.

Author details

Min Xiong[1], Daniel P. Heruth[1], Xun Jiang[2], Shamima Islam[1], Li Qin Zhang[1], Ding-You Li[3] and Shui Q. Ye[1,4*]

*Address all correspondence to: sqye@cmh.edu

1 Division of Experimental and Translational Genetics, The Children's Mercy Hospital, MO, USA

2 Department of Pediatrics, Tangdu Hospital, Fourth Military Medical University, Xian, China

3 Division of Pediatric Gastroenterology, University of Missouri Kansas City School of Medicine, MO, USA

4 Department of Biomedical and Health Informatics, University of Missouri Kansas City School of Medicine, MO, USA

References

[1] Djebali S, et al. Landscape of transcription in human cells. Nature. 2012;**489**(7414):101-108

[2] Maeda N, et al. Transcript annotation in FANTOM3: Mouse gene catalog based on physical cDNAs. PLoS Genetics. 2006;**2**(4):e62

[3] Kirchner S, Ignatova Z. Emerging roles of tRNA in adaptive translation, signalling dynamics and disease. Nature Reviews Genetics. 2015;**16**(2):98-112

[4] Sato H, Kamiya M. Deleterious effect of prednisolone on the attachment of *Taenia crassiceps* cysticerci to the intestine of gerbils. Nihon Juigaku Zasshi. 1989;**51**(5):1099-1101

[5] Fatica A, Bozzoni I. Long non-coding RNAs: New players in cell differentiation and development. Nature Reviews Genetics. 2014;**15**(1):7-21

[6] Frye M, et al. RNA modifications: What have we learned and where are we headed? Nature Reviews Genetics. 2016;**17**(6):365-372

[7] Dominissini D. Genomics and proteomics. Roadmap to the epitranscriptome. Science. 2014;**346**(6214):1192

[8] Milanowska K, et al. RNApathwaysDB—a database of RNA maturation and decay pathways. Nucleic Acids Research. 2013;**41**(Database issue):D268-D272

[9] Machnicka MA, et al. MODOMICS: A database of RNA modification pathways—2013 update. Nucleic Acids Research. 2013;**41**(Database issue):D262-D267

[10] Zhao BS, Roundtree IA, He C. Post-transcriptional gene regulation by mRNA modifications. Nature Reviews Molecular Cell Biology. 2017;**18**(1):31-42

[11] Saletore Y, et al. The birth of the epitranscriptome: Deciphering the function of RNA modifications. Genome Biology. 2012;**13**(10):175

[12] Nishikura K. A-to-I editing of coding and non-coding RNAs by ADARs. Nature Reviews Molecular Cell Biology. 2016;**17**(2):83-96

[13] Chi KR. The RNA code comes into focus. Nature. 2017;**542**(7642):503-506

[14] Bentley DL. Coupling mRNA processing with transcription in time and space. Nature Reviews Genetics. 2014;**15**(3):163-175

[15] Davis FF, Allen FW. Ribonucleic acids from yeast which contain a fifth nucleotide. Journal of Biological Chemistry. 1957;**227**(2):907-915

[16] Carlile TM, et al. Pseudouridine profiling reveals regulated mRNA pseudouridylation in yeast and human cells. Nature. 2014;**515**(7525):143-146

[17] Schwartz S, et al. Transcriptome-wide mapping reveals widespread dynamic-regulated pseudouridylation of ncRNA and mRNA. Cell. 2014;**159**(1):148-162

[18] Kiss T, Fayet-Lebaron E, Jady BE. Box H/ACA small ribonucleoproteins. Molecular Cell. 2010;**37**(5):597-606

[19] Charette M, Gray MW. Pseudouridine in RNA: What, where, how, and why. IUBMB Life. 2000;**49**(5):341-351

[20] Desrosiers R, Friderici K, Rottman F. Identification of methylated nucleosides in messenger RNA from Novikoff hepatoma cells. Proceedings of the National Academy of Sciences of the United States of America. 1974;**71**(10):3971-3975

[21] Bokar JA, et al. Characterization and partial purification of mRNA N6-adenosine methyltransferase from HeLa cell nuclei. Internal mRNA methylation requires a multisubunit complex. Journal of Biological Chemistry. 1994;**269**(26):17697-17704

[22] Liu J, et al. A METTL3-METTL14 complex mediates mammalian nuclear RNA N6-adenosine methylation. Nature Chemical Biology. 2014;**10**(2):93-95

[23] Wang Y, et al. N6-methyladenosine modification destabilizes developmental regulators in embryonic stem cells. Nature Cell Biology. 2014;**16**(2):191-198

[24] Zheng G, et al. ALKBH5 is a mammalian RNA demethylase that impacts RNA metabolism and mouse fertility. Molecular Cell. 2013;**49**(1):18-29

[25] Fu Y, et al. FTO-mediated formation of N6-hydroxymethyladenosine and N6-formyladenosine in mammalian RNA. Nature Communications. 2013;**4**:1798

[26] Dominissini D, et al. Topology of the human and mouse m6A RNA methylomes revealed by m6A-seq. Nature. 2012;**485**(7397):201-206

[27] Liu N, Pan T. N6-methyladenosine-encoded epitranscriptomics. Nature Structural & Molecular Biology. 2016;**23**(2):98-102

[28] Bass BL. RNA editing by adenosine deaminases that act on RNA. Annual Review of Biochemistry. 2002;**71**:817-846

[29] Nainar S, et al. Evolving insights into RNA modifications and their functional diversity in the brain. Nature Neuroscience. 2016;**19**(10):1292-1298

[30] Paupard MC, et al. Patterns of developmental expression of the RNA editing enzyme rADAR2. Neuroscience. 2000;**95**(3):869-879

[31] Sansam CL, Wells KS, Emeson RB. Modulation of RNA editing by functional nucleolar sequestration of ADAR2. Proceedings of the National Academy of Sciences of the United States of America. 2003;**100**(24):14018-14023

[32] Cattenoz PB, et al. Transcriptome-wide identification of A> I RNA editing sites by inosine specific cleavage. RNA. 2013;**19**(2):257-270

[33] Keegan LP, et al. Adenosine deaminases acting on RNA (ADARs): RNA-editing enzymes. Genome Biology. 2004;**5**(2):209

[34] Smith HC. RNA binding to APOBEC deaminases; not simply a substrate for C to U editing. RNA Biology. 2016. DOI:10.1080/15476286.2016.1259783

[35] Teng B, Burant CF, Davidson NO. Molecular cloning of an apolipoprotein B messenger RNA editing protein. Science. 1993;**260**(5115):1816-1819

[36] Meyer KD, et al. Comprehensive analysis of mRNA methylation reveals enrichment in 3' UTRs and near stop codons. Cell. 2012;**149**(7):1635-1646

[37] Molinie B, et al. m(6)A-LAIC-seq reveals the census and complexity of the m(6)A epitranscriptome. Nature Methods. 2016;**13**(8):692-698

[38] Linder B, et al. Single-nucleotide-resolution mapping of m6A and m6Am throughout the transcriptome. Nature Methods. 2015;**2**(8):767-772

[39] Li X, et al. Transcriptome-wide mapping reveals reversible and dynamic N(1)-methyladenosine methylome. Nature Chemical Biology. 2016;**12**(5):311-316

[40] Schaefer M, et al. RNA cytosine methylation analysis by bisulfite sequencing. Nucleic Acids Research. 2009;**37**(2):e12

[41] Squires JE, et al. Widespread occurrence of 5-methylcytosine in human coding and non-coding RNA. Nucleic Acids Research. 2012;**40**(11):5023-5033

[42] Sakurai M, et al. Inosine cyanoethylation identifies A-to-I RNA editing sites in the human transcriptome. Nature Chemical Biology. 2010;**6**(10):733-740

[43] Cahova H, et al. NAD captureSeq indicates NAD as a bacterial cap for a subset of regulatory RNAs. Nature. 2015;**519**(7543):374-377

[44] Batista PJ, et al. m(6)A RNA modification controls cell fate transition in mammalian embryonic stem cells. Cell Stem Cell. 2014;**15**(6):707-719

[45] Geula S, et al. Stem cells. m6A mRNA methylation facilitates resolution of naive pluripotency toward differentiation. Science. 2015;**347**(6225):1002-1006

[46] Zhang C, et al. Hypoxia induces the breast cancer stem cell phenotype by HIF-dependent and ALKBH5-mediated m(6)A-demethylation of NANOG mRNA. Proceedings of the National Academy of Sciences of the United States of America. 2016;**113**(14):E2047–E2056

[47] Zhou J, et al. Dynamic m(6)A mRNA methylation directs translational control of heat shock response. Nature. 2015;**526**(7574):591-594

[48] Lichinchi G, et al. Dynamics of the human and viral m(6)A RNA methylomes during HIV-1 infection of T cells. Nature Microbiology. 2016;**1**:16011

[49] Patil DP, et al. m6A RNA methylation promotes XIST-mediated transcriptional repression. Nature. 2016;**537**(7620):369-373

[50] Ozanick S, et al. The bipartite structure of the tRNA m1A58 methyltransferase from *S. cerevisiae* is conserved in humans. RNA. 2005;**11**(8):1281-1290

[51] Helm M, et al. The presence of modified nucleotides is required for cloverleaf folding of a human mitochondrial tRNA. Nucleic Acids Research. 1998;**26**(7):1636-1643

[52] Peifer C, et al. Yeast Rrp8p, a novel methyltransferase responsible for m1A 645 base modification of 25S rRNA. Nucleic Acids Research. 2013;**41**(2):1151-1163

[53] Schevitz RW, et al. Crystal structure of a eukaryotic initiator tRNA. Nature. 1979;**278** (5700):188-190

[54] Saikia M, et al. Genome-wide analysis of N1-methyl-adenosine modification in human tRNAs. RNA. 2010;**16**(7):1317-1327

[55] Chan CT, et al. A quantitative systems approach reveals dynamic control of tRNA modifications during cellular stress. PLoS Genetics. 2010;**6**(12):e1001247

[56] Motorin Y, Helm M. tRNA stabilization by modified nucleotides. Biochemistry. 2010;**49** (24):4934-4944

[57] Chow CS, Lamichhane TN, Mahto SK. Expanding the nucleotide repertoire of the ribosome with post-transcriptional modifications. ACS Chemical Biology. 2007;**2**(9):610-619

[58] Sommer S, et al. The methylation of adenovirus-specific nuclear and cytoplasmic RNA. Nucleic Acids Research. 1976;**3**(3):749-765

[59] Dubin DT, Taylor RH. The methylation state of poly A-containing messenger RNA from cultured hamster cells. Nucleic Acids Research. 1975;**2**(10):1653-1668

[60] Levanon EY, et al. Systematic identification of abundant A-to-I editing sites in the human transcriptome. Nature Biotechnology. 2004;**22**(8):1001-1005

[61] Athanasiadis A, Rich A, Maas S. Widespread A-to-I RNA editing of Alu-containing mRNAs in the human transcriptome. PLoS Biology. 2004;**2**(12):e391

[62] Khermesh K, et al. Reduced levels of protein recoding by A-to-I RNA editing in Alzheimer's disease. RNA. 2016;**22**(2):290-302

[63] Kanu N, et al. DNA replication stress mediates APOBEC3 family mutagenesis in breast cancer. Genome Biology. 2016;**17**(1):185

[64] Bykhovskaya Y, et al. Missense mutation in pseudouridine synthase 1 (PUS1) causes mitochondrial myopathy and sideroblastic anemia (MLASA). American Journal of Human Genetics. 2004;**74**(6):1303-1308

[65] Bird JG, et al. The mechanism of RNA 5' capping with NAD^+, NADH and desphospho-CoA. Nature. 2016;**535**(7612):444-447

[66] Jaschke A, et al. Cap-like structures in bacterial RNA and epitranscriptomic modification. Current Opinion in Microbiology. 2016;**30**:44-49

[67] Verdin E. NAD(+) in aging, metabolism, and neurodegeneration. Science. 2015;**350**(6265): 1208-1213

Chapter 13

Application of Next-Generation Sequencing in the Era of Precision Medicine

Michele Araújo Pereira,
Frederico Scott Varella Malta,
Maíra Cristina Menezes Freire and
Patrícia Gonçalves Pereira Couto

Additional information is available at the end of the chapter

http://dx.doi.org/10.5772/intechopen.69337

Abstract

Next-generation sequencing (NGS) technologies represented the next step in the evolution of DNA sequencing, through the generation of thousands to millions of DNA sequences in a short time. The relatively fast emergence and success of NGS in research revolutionized the field of genomics and medical diagnosis. The traditional medicine model of diagnosis has changed to one precision medicine model, leading to a more accurate diagnosis of human diseases and allowing the selection of molecular target drugs for individual treatment. This chapter attempts to review the main features of NGS technique (concepts, data analysis, applications, advances and challenges), starting with a brief history of DNA sequencing followed by a comprehensive description of most used NGS platforms. Further topics will highlight the application of NGS towards routine practice, including variant detection, whole-exome sequencing (WES), whole-genome sequencing (WGS), custom panels (multi-gene), RNA-seq and epigenetic. The potential use of NGS in precision medicine is vast and a better knowledge of this technique is necessary for an efficacious implementation in the clinical workplace. A centralized chapter describing the main NGS aspects in the clinic could help beginners, scientists, researchers and health care professionals, as they will be responsible for translating genomic data into genomic medicine.

Keywords: NGS, precision medicine, diagnostic, exome, panels, diseases, welfare

1. Introduction

Precision medicine is a new way of practising medicine, which has been gaining strength in recent years, is based on the individual characteristics of each patient (genetic, environmental, behavioural) to optimize and customize strategies for prevention, detection and therapy [1, 2]. The molecular knowledge has contributed strongly to the advancement of precision medicine, providing specific strategies for target therapies and diagnosis of patients with cancer, Mendelian diseases and others. Statistics indicated that traditional clinical practices sometimes lead to poor health outcomes and also a waste of medical resources. It is estimated that about 75 billion US dollars per year (30% of health care expenditure) are destined for unnecessary or ineffective treatments in the USA [3].

As a result of the genome project, many molecular tools have been developed and allow medical and scientific groups to improve patient management based on a better understanding of disease biology, providing a more specific and accurate prevention and treatment of diseases [4]. Precision medicine redefines the way traditional medicine is practised. There is a great deal of investment nowadays in prevention using these new technologies, as opposed to old medicine based on treatment since the disease was already evident or irreversible [2].

In recent times, Sanger sequencing, referred to as a 'first-generation' sequencing method, has partly been replaced by 'next-generation' sequencing (NGS) methods [4, 5]. NGS allows identifying biomarkers for early diagnosis as well as for personalized treatments. The emergence of NGS has changed the way clinical research, basic and applied science are done. The NGS allows producing millions of data with a smaller investment [4, 6]. Among the available NGS applications, one of them will be the resequencing of the human genome and the better genetic understanding of various human diseases. A great challenge will be the interpretation of this great number of data and its translation for the medical application [6]. One of the major near-term medical impact of the NGS revolution will be the elucidation of mechanisms of human pathogenesis, leading to improvements in the diagnosis and the selection of treatment and prevention. Thanks to second-generation sequencing technologies, it has become easier to sequence the expressed genes ('transcriptomes'), known exons ('exomes') and complete genomes of patient's samples [7].

This chapter encompasses revised concepts, applications, advances, limitations and the history of technological advances until the emergence of NGS technique in the era of precision medicine, starting with a brief history of DNA sequencing followed by a comprehensive description of most used NGS platforms, sequencing chemistries methodology and general workflows. Further topics will highlight the application of NGS towards routine practice, including variant detection, whole-genome sequencing (WGS), whole-exome sequencing (WES) and multi-gene panels. A centralized chapter describing the main NGS features in the clinic could help beginners, scientists, researchers and health care professionals, as they will be responsible for translating genomic data into genomic medicine.

2. From Sanger to NGS sequencing

In 1908, Garrod introduced his concept 'the inborn error of metabolism' that changed the areas of biochemistry, genetics and medicine [8]. His principal contribution was the understanding about the relationship between gene-enzyme, the molecular basis of genetic diseases. Although today this concept is considered outdated because of discoveries like RNA splicing, RNAi and others, its development allowed the researchers to understand how changes in DNA sequence could cause genetic disease. This finding increased the interest of scientists to know about human DNA sequence and mutations.

The search to know the nucleotide sequence of DNA began in the 1960s with several studies that demonstrated new methods with different strategies [9–13], but it was in 1977 that Sanger developed the method called 'Chain-termination' that became the most used method (first generation) to sequencing DNA (**Figure 1**). The method consisted of the use of dideoxynucleotides (ddNTPs), which are deoxynucleotide analogs (dNTPs) that disrupt DNA synthesis, and the separation of the different DNA fragments in a gel. These special nucleotides were radiolabeled and therefore the sequence could be inferred after the disclosure of gel autoradiography [14]. Numerous modifications have been made in this technique to make the method more efficient, robust and sensitive. Among them are the substitution of nucleotide radiolabeled to fluorescence that allowed the sequencing reaction to occur in one tube [15], the development of the polymerase chain reaction [16], the separation of DNA fragments by capillary electrophoresis [17] and later the development of equipment that allowed the sequencing of

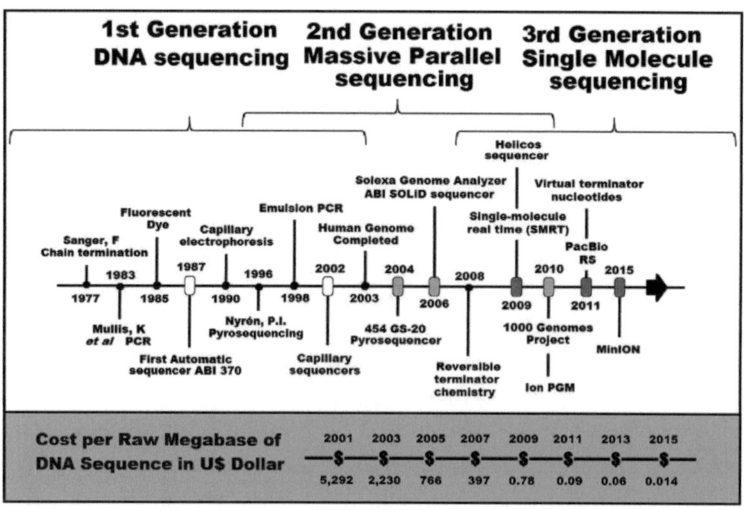

Figure 1. Timeline of DNA sequencing evolution from Sanger to NGS and the cost per raw megabase of DNA sequenced [17]. Equipment of all generations is still being improved and released commercially. Dot: milestones; rectangle: equipments; White: first-generation sequencing; Light gray: second-generation sequencing; Dark gray: third-generation sequencing.

more complex genomes. The most famous sequencing project, the Human Genome Project, produced in 13 years 3 billion of sequenced bases with the estimated cost around $2.7 billion [18]. To date, Sanger is still the gold-standard method in diagnostic tests and although the most recent methods have a much higher processing capacity, confirmation of some findings is made using this method.

The second generation of DNA sequencing can be defined as the era of the parallel massive sequencing on a micro scale. The Pyrosequencing method developed by Nyrén and colleagues in 1996 was the starting point for this generation. This technique differed substantially from previous ones because it did not use radio or fluorescence-labelled nucleotides and there was no need of electrophoretic run. The method is based on the action of two enzymes: ATP sulfurylase and luciferase. ATP sulfurylase converts pyrophosphate released in nucleotide incorporation into an ATP molecule that is used by luciferase substrate. This process releases light signal in proportion to the amount of nucleotides incorporated, and the sequence can be determined according to the serial addition of nucleotides [19]. Later on, this technology was improved and licensed generating the first 'second-generation' equipment, known as 454 (Roche). Among the improvements made, there are the DNA binding in beads through an adapter and the amplification of this DNA in water-in-oil microreactors (emulsion PCR). These changes and the use of microplates that compartmentalized the process and high-definition detection systems dramatically increased the amount of DNA sequenced and defined the second generation [20]. The disadvantage of this technology is related to homopolymer regions because of difficulty in interpreting the signal strength when five or more nucleotides are incorporated in a single wash cycle. Other technologies were then developed, such as that used by Illumina which consists of binding the DNA in a flow-cell through adapters, and the parallel massive amplification occurs in clusters for each DNA strand that was originally bound in the flow-cell, called bridge-amplification. This process generates paired-ends sequences that are an advantage over other methodologies, since they improve the accuracy of mapping, mainly in repetitive regions or where DNA rearrangements or gene fusions occur. The method uses 'reversible terminator chemistry' which is a modified fluorescent dNTP that reversibly blocks DNA synthesis, so the addition of each nucleotide can be synchronized and monitored by a charge-coupled device (CCD) sensor [21]. This is one of the most accurate and with lowest error rate of sequencing methodologies used currently; however, it generally requires higher DNA concentration. Another methodology is based on oligonucleotide ligation sequencing known as SOLiD and developed by Applied Biosystems (now Thermo Fisher Scientific). The method does not do sequencing by synthesis but by ligation of oligonucleotides fluorescence-labelled. Each probe is an octamer, which contains two known nucleotides in the 3′ end followed by six degenerated nucleotides with one of four fluorescent labels linked to the 5′ end. After probe annealing and ligation, fluorescent dye is cleavage and a new probe is ligated. Multiple cycles are performed according to the read length. The template from primer (n) is removed and the second round of sequencing is performed with a primer complementary to the (n-1) position [22]. This method shows good results; however, it is considered slow compared to the others and therefore was replaced by Ion Torrent (Thermo Fisher Scientific) technology. Like 454, the DNA bound in a bead is massively amplified by emulsion PCR and detection occurs in picotiter wells using complementary metal-oxide-semiconductor (CMOS) due to the pH difference caused by the

release of H+ ions in the nucleotide incorporation. This methodology is the first to use a detection method that does not work with light signal [23]. The advantage of this technology is the speed of the process and the low cost of the equipment; however, it has the same problem about the detection of homopolymers. The second generation of the sequencing was marked by the high capacity of the sequencers in the generation of data in a single run and consequently the computational development-like bioinformatics tools to analyse them. The cost of sequencing decreased dramatically at this stage. At the beginning of the first-generation sequencing (2001), the approximate cost per megabase sequenced was $5292.39 and at the end of this phase (2007) was $397.09, while in the second generation the sequencing cost was $102.13 (2008) and at the end (2015) only $0.014 [18], showing a more pronounced decline in this phase (**Figure 1**).

There are some discussions about which technology marked the beginning of the third generation [24–27]. In this review, we will consider the technology of single-molecule sequencing (SMS), which has no need to amplify the DNA. The first technology to use SMS was 'virtual terminators' based on a method very similar to Illumina, but a single DNA molecule is fixed in a flow-cell with 25 channels. The process occurs in cycles where the dNTPs are incorporated and the corresponding fluorescence is captured by a CCD camera. This process generates short readings (25 bp) and it is considered slow and there is a lot of noise in the signal [28]. Despite being the first third-generation sequencing technology, its history was brief because the company Helicos Biosciences filed for Chap. 11 bankruptcy. Another technology developed is the 'single molecule real time' (SMRT) that is commercialized by Pacific Biosciences. The SMRT consists of the immobilization of a single molecule in a chamber called 'zero-mode waveguide (ZMW)' where the incorporation of the fluorescent nucleotides occurs. ZMW allows the incorporation of each nucleotide to be monitored in real time and without interference from other light signals. The reads are very long (40 kb) and allow detecting modified bases [29, 30]. Finally, the technology of 'nanopores' consists of conducting a molecule of DNA or RNA through a biological or not nanopore. The detection occurs due to differences in the current of ions generated by each nucleotide. The reads are incredibly long (500 kb), and the process is extremely fast without the need for special nucleotides. The company Oxford Nanopore Technologies (ONT) is the first company to commercialize sequencers using this technology, including a portable version (MinION) that was used to sequence a mixture of bacteriophage, *Escherichia coli* and *Mus musculus* DNA at the international space station (ISS) [31]. In common, these technologies still have high error rates that are improving with the development of technology. Its main use today is to aid in the assembly of complex regions of the genome where gene fusions, large deletions and insertions and repetitive regions occur. The third generation will further revolutionize precision medicine, enabling sequencing at lower cost and enabling this to occur virtually anywhere.

3. Clinical applications

In recent times, NGS has made possible a better understanding of genetic diseases and became a significant technological advance in the practice of diagnostic and clinical medicine

[32]. NGS allows the analysis of multiple regions of the genome in one single reaction and has been shown to be a cost-effective and an efficient tool in investigating patients with genetic diseases. Genetic data produced via NGS provides significant benefits to medical practice including accurate identification of biomarkers of disease, detecting inherited disorders and identifying genetic factors that can help predict responses to therapies [32, 33]. However, recommendations on clinical implementation of NGS that are still in discussion and that hamper its use in the genetic clinic. A variety of molecular diagnostic test use sequencing technology, such as single- and multi-gene panel tests, cell-free DNA for non-invasive prenatal testing, whole-exome sequencing (WES), whole-genome sequencing (WGS). Considering that the use of NGS as a diagnostic tool is recent, there are challenges including when to order, on whom to order and how to interpret and communicate the results to the patient and family [32]. Therefore, it is necessary to understand the application, strength and limitations of the different approaches to recognize which one is the most suitable for your case. In the following topics, we will emphasize common applications of this technology into clinical practice.

3.1. Multi-gene panels

The traditional approach still holds great value for many disorders. Single-gene testing is indicated when the clinical features for a patient are typical for a particular disorder and the association between the disorder and the specific gene is well established and has the minimal locus heterogeneity [34]. However, many genetic conditions are intractable to diagnostic evaluation, mainly because of the clinical variability and genetic locus heterogeneity, such as cardiomyopathies, epilepsy, congenital muscular dystrophy, X-linked intellectual disability and cancer susceptibility in families with atypical phenotypes [35]. The diagnostic process is exhausted, with clinical assessment followed by sequential laboratory testing, in most cases tests being negative. In cases with unidentified genetic conditions (e.g., developmental delay/ cognitive disability and autism spectrum disorders), the diagnosis rate can vary greatly [36] and a multi-gene panel is more appropriate. In diagnostic of cancer, for example, Tothill and colleagues [37] illustrate the application of these multi-gene panel by analysing samples of patients with cancers of unknown primary (CUP). The clinical management of patients with CUP is hampered by the absence of a definitive site of origin and this kind of NGS analysis could help to define new therapeutic options.

In multi-gene panel tests, many genes associated with a specific phenotype are sequenced and analysed concomitantly, decreasing cost and improving efficiency of genetic diagnostic [37]. The number and which genes will be evaluated for the same or similar indications may vary significantly among different clinical laboratories and several considerations need to be taken for gene inclusion. The majority of authors believe that only genes with a strong disease association should be included since the ability to interpret their findings is much better due to clinical evidence [38]. However, some authors consider including associated genes that have overlapping phenotypes for the purpose of differential diagnosis, or all possible genes that are remotely associated with the phenotype of interest with the objective of a better and faster diagnostic [34]. For cancer diagnostic, multi-gene panel may include high-penetrance genes as well as associated genes with a moderate increase in risk [35].

The transition from single-gene to multi-gene testing should not compromise the sensitivity of the test to identify variants, mainly at genes that are responsible for a significant proportion of the defects (core genes). The sensitivity of NGS does not depend only on horizontal coverage but the vertical coverage is important as well [39]. Additional genes will increase the chance of the diagnostic, but this should not be at cost of missing mutations that would previously have been detected by single-gene testing [38]. Sanger sequencing or other available techniques can help to solve this problem for filling in low-coverage and no-coverage regions.

3.2. Whole-genome and whole-exome sequencing

Whole-genome sequencing (also known as WGS, full-genome sequencing, complete genome sequencing or entire genome sequencing) is the process of determining the complete DNA sequence of an organism's genome at a single time. The major benefit of WGS is completed coverage of the genome, including promoters and regulatory regions. In whole-exome sequencing (WES), all coding regions are sequenced with a relatively deeper depth. Compared to WGS, the major advantage of WES is a significant cost reduction [40].

Human genome comprises ~3×10^9 bp having coding and non-coding sequences. About 3×10^7 bp (1%) (30 Mb) of the genome are the coding sequences [33]. It is estimated that 85% of the disease-causing mutations are located in coding and functional regions of the genome [41, 42]. For this reason, sequencing the complete coding regions (exome) has the power to uncover the causes of large number of rare, mostly monogenic, genetic disorders as well as predisposing variants in common diseases and cancers [33]. In 2009, Choi and colleagues first showed the value of WES in the medical practice by making genetic diagnoses of congenital chloride diarrhoea in patients suspected of Bartter syndrome, a renal salt-wasting disease. WES was conducted on six patients who do not show any mutations in classic genes for Bartter syndrome. Results revealed homozygous deletion in *SLC26A3* gene for all patients, which provided a molecular diagnosis of congenital chloride diarrhoea that was later confirmed on clinical evaluation. This result was the first to show the value of WES in making a clinical diagnosis and several similar studies have followed [43].

There are certain considerations to order WES instead of other NGS tools [32]. Although exomes are supposed to cover all the protein-coding regions of the genome, the average coverage in many platforms tends to be between 85 and 95% [32, 44]. This means that a particular gene of interest that is closely linked to patient's phenotype may not be covered, completely or partially. There are many reasons that include poorly performing capture probes due to high GC content, sequence homology or repetitive sequences. A targeted approach, such as NGS single- or multi-gene panels, on the other hand, has higher or even complete coverage of all the specific genes by filling in the gaps with complementary technologies such as Sanger sequencing or long-range PCR. Besides offering a more comprehensive coverage of the 'known' phenotype-specific gene panels, this targeted approach also allows for deeper coverage of these genes compared to WES, which provides greater confidence in the variants detected. However, all NGS tools are still prone to sequencing artefacts, and Sanger sequencing is recommended to confirm the variants detected before returning the results to the patient [44]. In addition, the patient and their family need to be aware of all the nuances

related to WES and WGS [45]. It is important to let them know that the test may not yield positive results, and it is crucial to clarify that even positive results can offer diagnoses but do not improve prognosis and treatment.

To request an exam that uses the WES technique, one must start collecting as much information as possible about the patient. It is important to have a detailed family history, phenotype condition, symptoms and also, if possible, the inheritance pattern of the suspected disease [46]. With the phenotype and pedigree information, a systematic review of literature and databases should be performed to guide the clinician on which gene(s) are crucial and must be analysed. In cases of genetic heterogeneity, targeted NGS may be the preferred approach. On the other hand, if the disease mechanism is unknown, WES may be the best choice [47].

WES can result in approximately 60,000–100,000 genetic variants that can be classified into pathogenic, benign or with uncertain significance (VUS) [48]. With WES, a single pathogenic variant that is probably the cause of the patient phenotype can be detected in about 20–36%. For the other cases, it is possible to find multiple candidate variants or even no one. If no candidate variants are found, there are many reasons for it that include poor coverage or the mutation residing outside the protein-coding region of the gene, clinical summary with insufficient information or the defect is not due to a simple nucleotide change in a single gene [49–53].

The outcome of an exome should be evaluated by a multidisciplinary team that is involved with each patient's case. A discussion is necessary between physicians, geneticists, and other health professionals about all the clinical and laboratory findings to make a link with phenotype, family history and symptoms. It is necessary to review the WES results, scientific literature and medical information [32]. If more than one candidate variant is detected, this multidisciplinary team must perform further evaluation(s) to determine which of the variant is causing the phenotype. Finally, if the test results are negative, reasons for this should be discussed in the report. As the use of this tool is becoming more frequent and more accessible, it is possible that in the near future new pathogenic variants and genetic syndromes will be described and characterized, which causes these negative results to be reanalysed within a few years [32].

In cases of suspicion of Mendelian disease, the exome sequencing is usually indicated for the detection of rare variants and samples from the patient and his/her parents could be needed. This is usually the standard setting in cases where the Sanger sequencing of the candidate gene gave negative result or so there are multiple genes that must be tested for the condition that would be costly and time consuming. In most cases, the results obtained from WES reach a molecular diagnosis but do not alter the management, treatment or prognosis [32, 54].

Targeted exome sequencing is becoming increasingly popular in oncology for assessing the full sequence of cancer-related genes. Targeted exome sequencing also facilitates sequencing at a greater depth, and thus the identification of subclonal mutations. Alternately, rather than sequencing the full exome sequence, it is possible to look at all the genes reported to be related to cancer in general. Although hotspot mutation testing facilitates large-scale sequencing of many samples, it does limit the knowledge that is acquired through sequencing because it

limits the evaluation to small regions in selected genes. Consequently, small, targeted NGS panels increase the possibility of omitting relevant mutations for which evaluation is not being conducted, thus limiting the clinical knowledge that is gained through WES. WES could highlight novel insights into cancer mechanisms; identification of the DNA sequence of cancer cells in comparison with that of normal cells could help to reach an in-depth understanding of cancer. Using WES, it is also feasible to check germline and somatic mutations in human cancers [33].

Approximately 5–10% of cancers are hereditary. WES allows testing of multiple genes at once and greatly improves the variation detection rate. Many patients with hereditary cancer have tested negative for one specific genetic variation, but with WES, it is easier to find causative mutations. In a study of 300 high-risk breast cancer families, it was found previously undetected mutations in 52 probands and the reduced sequencing costs and turnaround time made the approach even more practical in clinics [55].

To detect familial germline mutations, WGS might be advantageous for WES-negative cases in families with a great chance of carrying a genetic variant [56]. The major technical advantage of WGS is that the specificity is theoretically 100% (average 95–98% in practice, practically without gaps) with a uniform coverage in the regions of interest (ROIs) throughout the input material. Thus, the chance of losing disease-causing variants due to technical errors is much lower with WGS [57–59]. The major challenge in applying this tool on a medical routine is the great costs, the complex pipeline for data analysis and data interpretation. However, in the near future, the costs of NGS should be lowered, studies on genetics over non-coding regions should be improved and more approach will be implemented. With that, WGS should be performed regularly for diagnostic in order to find the causative genetic variants [56].

Under gene panel analysis, about 70–92% of all cases remain negative, depending on the disease. It is expected that important genes will not be contemplated with these tools, making WES and WGS analysis more appropriate to identify genetic variants in cases of familial syndromes. These tools (WES and WGS) have already been reported in identifying several risk genes for various types of cancer such as the *PALB2* and *ATM* genes in pancreatic cancer, the hereditary pheochromocytoma susceptibility gene *MAX* [60] or the hereditary colorectal cancer moderate-risk genes *POLD1* and *POLE* [61].

Nowadays, the clinical utility of WES and WGS as a generic test for mutation discovery for every genetic diagnostic question is not yet appropriate [62] and should be directed to specific patient groups [63]. This limitation is due to the high cost, the need of complex bioinformatics pipelines, large storage capacity and the expected high number of VUS detected.

3.3. RNA-sequencing

A transcriptome represents the complete set of RNA molecules from any genome at any time or condition and RNA plays essential role in several biological processes, including untranslated RNA species such as microRNAs (miRNAs). RNA-sequencing (RNA-seq) consists of an in-depth RNA analysis through NGS technologies and became the state-of-art technique for transcriptomic [64]. A typical RNA-seq experiment consists of a good experimental design,

sample preparation, library construction, sequencing and data analysis. However, due to several experimental options available, a careful planning and cost estimation is necessary before starting. These include number and type of replicates (technical vs. biological), sequencing platform (e.g. Illumina, Ion Torrent), library preparation method (e.g. rRNA depletion or mRNA enrichment; strand-specific or not; single or paired end), throughput, read length, sequencing depth and coverage. RNA-seq best practices can be found in Chap. *RNA-seq: Applications and Best Practices* from this book.

RNA-seq enables detection of novel genes and isoforms, gene fusions, splice and chimeric variants, genomic alterations and gene expression quantification. Although RNA-seq outperforms microarray in transcriptomic analysis [65], its clinical application is still in its infancy and, for instance, will not replace current approaches. RNA-seq is considered a complementary method depending on the needs and resources available, assisting clinicians in making decisions. In clinical practice, RNA measurement has applications across different areas in human health such as therapeutic selection, disease diagnostic and treatment [66].

Clinical diagnosis of infectious disease through RNA-seq is still rare, since quantitative PCR (RT-qPCR) assays are still the most common technique used for viral detection and genotyping. Applications of NGS in virology diagnostic can be used for analysis of patients with unexplained illness, especially during outbreaks and epidemics [67–70]. It also includes the identification of novel pathogens [71–74], viral community characterization [75–77], whole viral genome reconstruction [73, 78, 79], antiviral drug resistance [80–83], epidemiology [84–87] and transcriptomic [88–90]. The use of NGS in virology is increasing the knowledge of viral infection dynamics and their correlation with human health and treatment.

For oncology, RNA-based cancer diagnostics is being used by clinical oncologist to define tumour transcriptome due to its potential to guide treatment and drug therapy [91]. Its application are especially related to gene expression profile and variants, and gene fusions detection. The pathogenicity of gene fusions in cancer is well known. Most gene fusions are correlated with specific tumour subtypes, representing diagnostic biomarkers and leading to novel therapeutic opportunities and benefits [92–94]. Some pharmacological treatments are already in clinical use [94]. Key somatic DNA mutations can also represent cancer biomarkers and can be identified by transcriptomic mapping [95–98].

Gene expression in cancer is still quantified by non-sequencing methods (e.g. RT-qPCR and microarrays) [91]. RNA-seq can measure expression of tumour antigens or immune checkpoint receptors and ligands after a given treatment, giving some answers about patient drug response [91, 99, 100]. Gene expression signatures can also be used for cancer types' classification that directly impact prognosis and treatment definition and response [100].

NGS can also be applied for circulating tumour RNA (ctRNA) discovery. The analysis of ctRNA in plasma is still in its beginning and presents specific challenges. ctRNA degrades faster than circulating tumour DNA (ctDNA) and needs to be purified rapidly or added in preservative solutions (e.g. TRIzol) and freezed at −80°C, not always an accessible technique to many clinical sites [101]. Despite these challenges, ctRNAs represent good biomarkers of early detection of multiple tumour types, such as breast, lung, prostate and colorectal cancers

[101–109]. NGS is a more powerful tool for ctRNA detection; however, RT-qPCR remains more usable for clinical diagnostic applications [110].

3.4. Epigenetics

An emerging field that has a huge impact on medicine and clinical diagnostic is epigenetics. The term was coined by Conrad Waddington in the 1940s and refers to the study of heritable changes in gene activity and expression that do not involve the DNA sequence itself, that is, a change in phenotype without a change in genotype [111, 112]. Additional information about epigenetics history can be found in Ref. [113]. Epigenetics mechanisms represent another layer of gene regulation and NGS allowed to understand the epigenetics status on a large scale and at a single base-resolution, including mainly DNA methylation, histone modification and non-coding RNA (ncRNA)-associated silencing [111, 112].

DNA methylation was the first epigenetic mechanism identified and is the best known and the most frequent in human cancer. It involves covalent modification of cytosine through the addition of a methyl group to cytosines of CpG (cytosine/guanine) islands [111, 112]. This methylation is maintained by DNA methyltransferase (DNMTs) and plays roles for gene transcriptional repression, transposable elements silencing and viral defence [111]. Unmethylated DNA is found in active regions of chromatin, and methylated DNA is found in inactive regions [112].

Post-translational histone modifications are markers for chromatin activity through acetylation and methylation of conserved lysine residues on the amino-terminal tail domains [112]: acetylation is found in active regions of chromatin, whereas hypoacetylation is found in inactive euchromatic or heterochromatic regions [111, 112]. Enzymes involved in this process include histone deacetylases (HDACs), histone acetylases and histone methyltransferases [112]. These and other post-translational histone modification processes (e.g. phosphorylation) result in distinct histone modification patterns that form a 'histone code' [114].

Since epigenetic mechanisms regulate DNA accessibility, perturbations of the cell epigenetic pattern affect gene expression and can give rise to human diseases, that can be inherited or somatically acquired [111, 112]. Prader-Willi, Angelman and Beckwith-Wiedemann syndromes, for example, are the best characterized congenital imprinting disorders [111, 115, 116].

4. Data analysis

Data analysis is a critical step of NGS tests. This analysis consist of a primary analysis, in which the base pairs are called and quality score are generated; a secondary analysis, numerous reads are aligned to the human reference sequence; and a tertiary analysis which consists of variant calling and annotation [117]. Many databases are useful for helping the variant annotation, such as the 1000 Genome Project [118], dbSNP database [119], Clinvar—NCBI [120], LOVD—Leiden Open Variation Database [121], The Cancer Genome Atlas (TCGA) [122] and others. However, information from these sources can contain ambiguous and insufficient information. Variants detected should be reported according to Human Genome Variation

Society (HGVS) recommendations, with information of the human reference genome version and transcript information used to variant description [117]. The reference coding sequence should be preferably from the RefSeq database [123].

All pathogenic, likely pathogenic and VUS variants have to be reported. Secondary or incidental finding (IF) is one significant matter, especially for WES, WGS and multi-gene panels, and its report will depend on local practice [38].

An in-house database containing all relevant variants identified in the laboratory provides an important tool in order to allow for further annotations, which greatly streamline the diagnostic process. Furthermore, an in-house database, linking patients and variants can help when a variant is re-classified. In this case, the laboratory is responsible for re-contacting the clinicians of the patients that are possibly affected by the new status of the variant [38].

4.1. Sanger sequencing validation

Concerning the limitations of technology, the false positive rate for NGS, a second method, as Sanger sequencing, is required to confirm any findings with possible clinical significance. The laboratory must be able to guarantee that report variants are true variants; therefore, it is essential to mention that the variant reports were confirmed by Sanger method. An NGS technology will likely evolve, and within a few years confirmation might prove to be unnecessary [34, 39].

In some cases, mainly in large panels, complementing NGS testing with Sanger sequencing is inevitable. This limitation of NGS is dependent on the platform and on the enrichment methods, once that there are a number of strategies available with advantages and disadvantages. Sanger sequencing can also be used to fill regions that fail to amplify for having sequence complexities, such as sequence homology with pseudo genes, highly repetitive regions, GC-rich content, allelic dropout, or regions that are supported by an insufficient number of reads to call variants confidently [34]. However, in practice, the laboratories can opt to apply different settings for NGS tests. Three kinds of tests of multi-genes panel are identified: (A) the lab informs that more than 99% of interest region are covered, and all the gaps are filled with Sanger sequencing; (B) the lab describes which regions are sequenced and fills some specific gaps (core genes) with Sanger sequencing; and (C) no additional Sanger sequencing is offered [38]. It is essential to mention the horizontal coverage acquired in the test and the limitations of these tests in a disclaimer [39].

5. Challenges

The diversity and rapid evolution of NGS technology causes many challenges associated with data generation, data manipulation and data storage [124]. Some of the major issues with analysis, interpretation, reproducibility and accessibility of NGS data includes: (A) NGS is still too expensive to be accessible by small labs or an individual; (B) data analysis is time-consuming and needs sufficient knowledge of bioinformatics; (C) the short sequencing read lengths supported by NGS is one of the major shortcomings which limit its application,

especially in de novo and highly repetitive regions sequencing; (D) data processing steps or bioinformatics is one major bottleneck for the implementation of NGS; (E) routine analysis of NGS data requires multidisciplinary teams; (F) it is critical to standardize the quality metrics for the NGS data generated. These include validation and comparison among platforms, data reliability, robustness and reproducibility, and quality of assemblers; (G) it is crucial to have a complete knowledge of family and personal history of the patient to help define the ideal analysis method, the analysis of the results obtained, and the post-test counselling and management [124–127].

Despite some challenges, it is hard not to be optimistic about the future of personalized genome sequencing and its potential impact on patient care and the advancement of knowledge of human biology and disease.

5.1. Regulation on NGS tests

With the advancement of gene-sequencing technologies, numerous opportunities have arisen in the genetic diagnostic, preventive medicine and other areas of human health. As a result, several life science companies and clinical laboratories started their activities in this field offering equipment and supplies as well as molecular tests using the new-generation (parallel massive) sequencing methodology. However, most manufacturers do not market IVD products (in vitro diagnostic), but, in general, these products are classified as RUO (research use only). In practice, this difference in the classification of products and reagents represents serious implications on health. Products classified as IVD are regulated and therefore follow technical standards in their production and use, and consequently the efficiency must be guaranteed by the manufacturer. The ISO 13485 [128] is often used to ensure the quality of medical products, but other regulatory agencies such as the US Food and Drug Administration (FDA) may require other tests to prove this product is safe and effective, which is necessary for the product be classified as IVD and be commercialized on the American market. The same applies to the CE-IVD Marking in the European Economic Area (EEA). These requirements are part of an effort to ensure that users of these services and devices do not seek unnecessary treatment, delay their treatment or are exposed to inappropriate therapies. In the case of RUO products, none of these situations can be guaranteed, so the manufacturer will only be obliged to replace the product or its cost if it is performing improperly. In fact, some manufacturers may use standards of good manufacturing practice in the production of RUO equipment and supplies, but rarely perform tests to prove their efficiency in a particular case of diagnostic.

In some cases due to the need to respond quickly to the market, especially in areas where the technological advance exceeds the regulatory capacity, some agencies allow the use of tests developed by clinical laboratories. The regulation in these cases is very simpler and favours the development of new technologies as the case of new-generation sequencing (NGS). However, these tests should also be used with caution, and the laboratories must prove its accuracy, or otherwise there may be the same hazards of products classified as RUO. In 2013, the US FDA agency required to genetic testing company 23andME to suspend the marketing of its products until it receives clearance from the agency. In a letter addressed to one of its

founders, the agency states its concern about the use of one of its tests and the implications on the health of the patient in case of false results.

> Some of the uses for which PGS (Personal Genome Service) is intended are particularly concerning, such as assessments for BRCA-related genetic risk and drug responses (e.g., warfarin sensitivity, clopidogrel response, and 5-fluorouracil toxicity) because of the potential health consequences that could result from false positive or false negative assessments for high-risk indications such as these. For instance, if the BRCA-related risk assessment for breast or ovarian cancer reports is false positive, it could lead to undergo prophylactic surgery, chemoprevention, intensive screening, or other morbidity-inducing actions, while false negative could result in failure to recognize an existing risk that may exist. [129]

This example illustrates the importance of evaluating the analytical characteristics of diagnostic tests as well as the reagents and equipment used to perform these tests. In 2013, Illumina was the first company to get FDA approval for the commercialization of four NGS products. It was the first approval for a system based on NGS technology that will allow other companies to develop their own tests using this technology. In 2014, it was the time of SOPHiA Genetics and Vela Diagnostics companies that obtained the CE-IVD Marking of the first products based on the NGS technology for clinical use.

Since then, the number of products that have the classification of IVD has been increasing; however, it is important to note that the classification of an IVD product depends on local regulations, and therefore products that are classified as IVD in a market may not have this classification in other markets. This is due to the regulatory differences between the agencies and the different requirements from each market. Anyway, it is usual that classification process of these products for clinical use must be complex and sometimes elaborated, especially in areas such as genomics. Therefore, initiatives are needed to make the approval process for these products simpler and more flexible, to make the products available, but that ensures the accuracy and usefully testing.

In 2016, the US FDA agency issued two draft guidelines: 'Use of Standards in FDA's Regulatory Oversight of Next Generation Sequencing (NGS) Based In Vitro Diagnostics (IVDs) Used for Diagnosing Germ line Diseases' and 'Use of Public Human Genetic Variant Databases to Support Clinical Validity for Next Generation Sequencing (NGS)-Based In Vitro Diagnostics'. Both are part of an initiative that aims to contribute to new testing using the NGS technology to reach the public with more speed and quality required by the market and health system.

5.2. Clinical validation

Almost all NGS approaches are still RUO, and validation is necessary before implementation as a diagnostic test. Prior clinical utility, a test must demonstrate analytical and clinical validity. Sensitivity, specificity, robustness, limits of detection, reproducibility, accuracy, precision and concordance between test results and clinical diagnosis should be analysed and measured. The test needs to evaluate patient outcomes and have positive impact on patient care [66, 130]. To assist the usage and implementation of NGS in clinical laboratories, some standards and best practice

guidelines are already available [38, 39, 44, 131–134]. Several NGS validation studies in clinical laboratories have been published and are rich sources of information [135–138]. Improvements in NGS technologies and data analysis require revalidation before implementation.

5.3. Computational infrastructure

The high volume of NGS data generated requires a complex computational infrastructure for processing, analysing and storing the data, including sophisticated data analysis pipelines. Cloud solutions such as Google, Amazon and Microsoft can be an alternative to an in-house computational infrastructure. More user-friendly bioinformatics software are desirable for non-bioinformaticians, such as Google Genomics [139], SOPHiA Genetics [140], IBM Watson [141], Illumina BaseSpace [142], Ion Reporter [143], Galaxy [144], CLC Genomics [145]. The variability of data formats generated during the analysis (e.g. FASTQ, UBAM, BAM/SAM and VCF files) and the laboratory must decide the appropriate data to be stored since the cost of managing, analysing and storing is high [124, 130, 146–149].

5.4. Genomic education

A multidisciplinary team of bioinformaticians, computational biologists, IT technicians, statisticians, molecular biologists, geneticists, genetic counsellors and clinicians is strongly needed and should be properly trained and educated for a successful implementation of NGS into routine diagnostic. Other related areas, such as lawyers, policy-makers, sales representative and investors, also need to be trained. Due to the constant updates of NGS approaches, an ongoing and continuing education about emerging technologies, software, databases and data analysis pipelines that reflect current practice is necessary. Genomic education also needs to be incorporated into medical school curriculum [148, 150].

Author details

Michele Araújo Pereira[1]*, Frederico Scott Varella Malta[1], Maíra Cristina Menezes Freire[2] and Patrícia Gonçalves Pereira Couto[1]

*Address all correspondence to: michele.pereira@hermespardini.com.br

1 Hermes Pardini Group/Federal University of Minas Gerais, Vespasiano, Brazil

2 Progenética Laboratory, Hermes Pardini Group, Rio de Janeiro, Brazil

References

[1] Langreth R, Waldholz M. New era of personalized medicine: Targeting drugs for each unique genetic profile. Oncologist. 1999;**4**(5):426-427

[2] Ginsburg GS, Willard HF. Genomic and personalized medicine: Foundations and applications. Translational Research. 2009;**154**(6):277-287

[3] IOM (Institute of Medicine). The Healthcare Imperative: Lowering Costs and Improving Outcomes: Workshop Series Summary. Washington, DC: The National Academies Press; 2010

[4] Rabbani B, Nakaoka H, Akhondzadeh S, Tekin M, Mahdieh N. Next generation sequencing: Implications in personalized medicine and pharmacogenomics. Molecular BioSystems. 2016;**12**(6):1818-1830

[5] Gonzalez-Garay ML. The road from next-generation sequencing to personalized medicine. Personalized Medicine. 2014;**11**(5):523-544

[6] Vogenberg FR, Isaacson Barash C, Pursel M. Personalized medicine: Part 1: Evolution and development into theranostics. Pharmacy and Therapeutics. 2010;**35**(10):560-576

[7] Wong AHH, Deng CX. Precision medicine for personalized cancer therapy. International Journal of Biological Sciences. 2015;**11**(12):1410-1412

[8] Scriver CR. Garrod's Croonian Lectures (1908) and the charter "Inborn Errors of Metabolism": Albinism, alkaptonuria, cystinuria, and pentosuria at age 100 in 2008. Journal of Inherited Metabolic Disease. 2008;**31**(5):580-598

[9] Holley RW, Apgar J, Everett GA, Madison JT, Marquisee M, Merrill SH, et al. Structure of a ribonucleic acid. Science. 1965;**147**(3664):1462-1465

[10] Sanger F, Brownlee GG, Barrell BG. A two-dimensional fractionation procedure for radioactive nucleotides. Journal of Molecular Biology. 1965;**13**(2):373-398

[11] Min Jou W, Haegeman G, Ysebaert M, Fiers W. Nucleotide sequence of the gene coding for the bacteriophage MS2 coat protein. Nature. 1972;**237**(5350):82-88

[12] Sanger F, Donelson JE, Coulson AR, Kössel H, Fischer D. Use of DNA polymerase I primed by a synthetic oligonucleotide to determine a nucleotide sequence in phage fl DNA. Proceedings of the National Academy of Sciences of the USA. 1973;**70**(4):1209-1213

[13] Padmanabhan R, Jay E, Wu R. Chemical synthesis of a primer and its use in the sequence analysis of the lysozyme gene of bacteriophage T4. Proceedings of the National Academy of Sciences of the USA. 1974;**71**(6):2510-2514

[14] Sanger F, Nicklen S. DNA sequencing with chain-terminating. 1977;**74**(12):5463-5467

[15] Smith LM, Fung S, Hunkapiller MW, Hunkapiller TJ, Hood LE. The synthesis of oligonucleotides containing an aliphatic amino group at the 5′ terminus: Synthesis of fluorescent DNA primers for use in DNA sequence analysis. Nucleic Acids Research. 1985;**13**(7):2399-2412

[16] Saiki RK, Scharf S, Faloona F, Mullis KB, Horn GT, Erlich HA, et al. Enzymatic amplification of beta-globin genomic sequences and restriction site analysis for diagnosis of sickle cell anemia. Science. 1985;**230**(4732):1350-1354

[17] Swerdlow H, Gesteland R. Capillary gel electrophoresis for rapid, high resolution DNA sequencing. Nucleic Acids Research. 1990;**18**(6):1415-1419

[18] Wetterstrand KA. DNA Sequencing Costs. NHGRI Genome Sequencing Program (GSP) [Internet]. Available from: www.genome.gov/sequencingcostsdata [Accessed: 18 January 2017]

[19] Ronaghi M, Karamohamed S, Pettersson B, Uhlén M, Nyrén P. Real-time DNA sequencing using detection of pyrophosphate release. Analytical Biochemistry. 1996;**242**(1): 84-89

[20] Margulies M, Egholm M, Altman WE, Attiya S, Bader JS, Bemben LA, et al. Genome sequencing in microfabricated high-density picolitre reactors. Nature. 2005;**437**(7057): 376-380

[21] Bentley DR, Balasubramanian S, Swerdlow HP, Smith GP, Milton J, Brown CG, et al. Accurate whole human genome sequencing using reversible terminator chemistry. Nature. 2008;**456**(7218):53-59

[22] McKernan KJ, Peckham HE, Costa GL, McLaughlin SF, Fu Y, Tsung EF, et al. Sequence and structural variation in a human genome uncovered by short-read, massively parallel ligation sequencing using two-base encoding. Genome Research. 2009;**19**(9):1527-1541

[23] Rothberg JM, Hinz W, Rearick TM, Schultz J, Mileski W, Davey M, et al. An integrated semiconductor device enabling non-optical genome sequencing. Nature. 2011;**475**(7356): 348-352

[24] Schadt EE, Turner S, Kasarskis A. A window into third-generation sequencing. Human Molecular Genetics. 2010;**19**(R2):R227–R240

[25] Niedringhaus TP, Milanova D, Kerby MB, Snyder MP, Barron AE. Landscape of next-generation sequencing technologies. Analytical Chemistry. 2011;**83**(12):4327-4341

[26] Pareek CS, Smoczynski R, Tretyn A. Sequencing technologies and genome sequencing. Journal of Applied Genetics. 2011;**52**(4):413-435

[27] Gut IG. New sequencing technologies. Clinical and Translational Oncology. 2013;**15**(11): 879-881

[28] Bowers J, Mitchell J, Beer E, Buzby PR, Causey M, Efcavitch JW, et al. Virtual terminator nucleotides for next-generation DNA sequencing. Nature Methods. 2009;**6**(8):593-595

[29] Levene MJ, Korlach J, Turner SW, Foquet M, Craighead HG, Webb WW. Zero-mode waveguides for single-molecule analysis at high concentrations. Science. 2003;**299**(5607): 682-686

[30] Eid J, Fehr A, Gray J, Luong K, Lyle J, Otto G, et al. Real-time DNA sequencing from single polymerase molecules. Science. 2009;**323**(5910):133-138

[31] Castro-Wallace SL, Chiu CY, John KK, Stahl SE, Rubins KH, McIntyre ABR, et al. Nanopore DNA sequencing and genome assembly on the international space station. bioRxiv. 2016;077651

[32] Jamuar SS, Tan EC. Clinical application of next-generation sequencing for Mendelian diseases. Human Genomics. 2015;**9**:10

[33] Rabbani B, Tekin M, Mahdieh N. The promise of whole-exome sequencing in medical genetics. Journal of Human Genetics. 2014;**59**(1):5-15

[34] Xue Y, Ankala A, Wilcox WR, Hegde MR. Solving the molecular diagnostic testing conundrum for Mendelian disorders in the era of next-generation sequencing: Single-gene, gene panel, or exome/genome sequencing. Genetics in Medicine. 2015;**17**(6):444-451

[35] LaDuca H, Stuenkel AJ, Dolinsky JS, Keiles S, Tandy S, Pesaran T, et al. Utilization of multigene panels in hereditary cancer predisposition testing: Analysis of more than 2,000 patients. Genetics in Medicine. 2014;**16**(11):830-837

[36] Shashi V, McConkie-Rosell A, Rosell B, Schoch K, Vellore K, McDonald M, et al. The utility of the traditional medical genetics diagnostic evaluation in the context of next-generation sequencing for undiagnosed genetic disorders. Genetics in Medicine. 2014;**16**(2):176-182

[37] Tothill RW, Li J, Mileshkin L, Doig K, Siganakis T, Cowin P, et al. Massively-parallel sequencing assists the diagnosis and guided treatment of cancers of unknown primary. Journal of Pathology. 2013;**231**(4):413-423

[38] Matthijs G, Souche E, Alders M, Corveleyn A, Eck S, Feenstra I, et al. Guidelines for diagnostic next-generation sequencing. European Journal of Human Genetics. 2016;**24**(10):1515

[39] Weiss MM, Van der Zwaag B, Jongbloed JDH, Vogel MJ, Brüggenwirth HT, Lekanne Deprez RH, et al. Best practice guidelines for the use of next-generation sequencing applications in genome diagnostics: A national collaborative study of Dutch genome diagnostic laboratories. Human Mutation. 2013;**34**(10):1313-1321

[40] Gonzaga-Jauregui C, Lupski JR, Gibbs RA. Human genome sequencing in health and disease. Annual Review of Medicine. 2012;**63**:35-61

[41] Botstein D, Risch N. Discovering genotypes underlying human phenotypes: Past successes for Mendelian disease, future approaches for complex disease. Nature Genetics. 2003;**33**(Suppl):228-237

[42] Majewski J, Schwartzentruber J, Lalonde E, Montpetit A, Jabado N. What can exome sequencing do for you? Journal of Medical Genetics. 2011;**48**(9):580-589

[43] Choi M, Scholl UI, Ji W, Liu T, Tikhonova IR, Zumbo P, et al. Genetic diagnosis by whole exome capture and massively parallel DNA sequencing. Proceedings of the National Academy of Sciences of the USA. 2009;**106**(45):19096-19101

[44] Rehm HL, Bale SJ, Bayrak-Toydemir P, Berg JS, Brown KK, Deignan JL, et al. ACMG clinical laboratory standards for next-generation sequencing. Genetics in Medicine. 2013;**15**(9):733-747

[45] van El CG, Cornel MC, Borry P, Hastings RJ, Fellmann F, Hodgson SV, et al. Whole-genome sequencing in health care. Recommendations of the European Society of Human Genetics. European Journal of Human Genetics. 2013;**21**(Suppl 1):S1-S5

[46] Chial H. Mendelian genetics: Patterns of inheritance and single-gene disorders. Nature Education. 2008;**1**(1):63

[47] Biesecker LG, Green RC. Diagnostic clinical genome and exome sequencing. New England Journal of Medicine. 2014;**371**(12):1170

[48] MacArthur DG, Manolio TA, Dimmock DP, Rehm HL, Shendure J, Abecasis GR, et al. Guidelines for investigating causality of sequence variants in human disease. Nature. 2014;**508**(7497):469-476

[49] Need AC, Shashi V, Hitomi Y, Schoch K, Shianna K V, McDonald MT, et al. Clinical application of exome sequencing in undiagnosed genetic conditions. Journal of Medical Genetics. 2012;**49**(6):353-361

[50] Yang Y, Muzny DM, Reid JG, Bainbridge MN, Willis A, Ward PA, et al. Clinical whole-exome sequencing for the diagnosis of Mendelian disorders. New England Journal of Medicine. 2013;**369**(16):1502-1511

[51] Lee H, Deignan JL, Dorrani N, Strom SP, Kantarci S, Quintero-Rivera F, et al. Clinical exome sequencing for genetic identification of rare Mendelian disorders. Journal of the American Medical Association. 2014;**312**(18):1880-1887

[52] Yang Y, Muzny DM, Xia F, Niu Z, Person R, Ding Y, et al. Molecular findings among patients referred for clinical whole-exome sequencing. Journal of the American Medical Association. 2014;**312**(18):1870

[53] Deciphering Developmental Disorders Study. Large-scale discovery of novel genetic causes of developmental disorders. Nature. 2015;**519**(7542):223-228

[54] ACMG Board of Directors. ACMG policy statement: Updated recommendations regarding analysis and reporting of secondary findings in clinical genome-scale sequencing. Genetics in Medicine. 2015;**17**(1):68-69

[55] Walsh T, Casadei S, Coats KH, Swisher E, Stray SM, Higgins J, et al. Spectrum of mutations in BRCA1, BRCA2, CHEK2, and TP53 in families at high risk of breast cancer. Journal of the American Medical Association. 2006;**295**(12):1379-1388

[56] Kamps R, Brandão RD, Bosch BJ van den, Paulussen ADC, Xanthoulea S, Blok MJ, et al. Next-generation sequencing in oncology: Genetic diagnosis, risk prediction and cancer classification. International Journal of Molecular Sciences. 2017;**18**(2)

[57] Leggett RM, Ramirez-Gonzalez RH, Clavijo BJ, Waite D, Davey RP. Sequencing quality assessment tools to enable data-driven informatics for high throughput genomics. Frontiers in Genetics. 2013;**4**:1-5

[58] Ekblom R, Wolf JBW. A field guide to whole-genome sequencing, assembly and annotation. Evolutionary Applications. 2014;**7**(9):1026-1042

[59] Chrystoja CC, Diamandis EP. Whole genome sequencing as a diagnostic test: Challenges and opportunities. Clinical Chemistry. 2014;**60**(5):724-733

[60] Comino-Méndez I, Gracia-Aznárez FJ, Schiavi F, Landa I, Leandro-García LJ, Letón R, et al. Exome sequencing identifies MAX mutations as a cause of hereditary pheochromocytoma. Nature Genetics. 2011;**43**(7):663-667

[61] Palles C, Cazier JB, Howarth KM, Domingo E, Jones AM, Broderick P, et al. Germline mutations affecting the proofreading domains of POLE and POLD1 predispose to colorectal adenomas and carcinomas. Nature Genetics. 2013;**45**(2):136-144

[62] Snape K, Ruark E, Tarpey P, Renwick A, Turnbull C, Seal S, et al. Predisposition gene identification in common cancers by exome sequencing: Insights from familial breast cancer. Breast Cancer Research and Treatment. 2012;**134**(1):429-433

[63] Fecteau H, Vogel KJ, Hanson K, Morrill-Cornelius S. The evolution of cancer risk assessment in the era of next generation sequencing. Journal of Genetic Counseling. 2014;**23**(4):633-639

[64] Wang Z, Gerstein M, Snyder M. RNA-Seq: A revolutionary tool for transcriptomics. Nature Reviews Genetics. 2009;**10**(1):57-63

[65] Zhang W, Yu Y, Hertwig F, Thierry-Mieg J, Zhang W, Thierry-Mieg D, et al. Comparison of RNA-seq and microarray-based models for clinical endpoint prediction. Genome Biology. 2015;**16**(1):133

[66] Byron SA, Van Keuren-Jensen KR, Engelthaler DM, Carpten JD, Craig DW. Translating RNA sequencing into clinical diagnostics: opportunities and challenges. Nature Reviews Genetics. 2016;**17**(5):257-271

[67] Capobianchi MR, Giombini E, Rozera G. Next-generation sequencing technology in clinical virology. Clinical Microbiology and Infection. 2013;**19**(1):15-22

[68] Barzon L, Lavezzo E, Militello V, Toppo S, Palù G. Applications of next-generation sequencing technologies to diagnostic virology. International Journal of Molecular Sciences. 2011;**12**(12):7861-7884

[69] Quiñones-Mateu ME, Avila S, Reyes-Teran G, Martinez MA. Deep sequencing: Becoming a critical tool in clinical virology. Journal of Clinical Virology. 2014;**61**(1):9-19

[70] Radford AD, Chapman D, Dixon L, Chantrey J, Darby AC, Hall N. Application of next-generation sequencing technologies in virology. Journal of General Virology. 2012;**93**(Pt 9):1853-1868

[71] Datta S, Budhauliya R, Das B, Chatterjee S, Vanlalhmuaka, Veer V. Next-generation sequencing in clinical virology: Discovery of new viruses. World Journal of Virology. 2015;**4**(3):265-276

[72] Tang P, Chiu C. Metagenomics for the discovery of novel human viruses. Future Microbiology. 2010;**5**(2):177-189

[73] Oude Munnink BB, Cotten M, Canuti M, Deijs M, Jebbink MF, van Hemert FJ, et al. A novel astrovirus-like RNA virus detected in human stool. Virus Evolution. 2016;**2**(1):vew005

[74] Naccache SN, Peggs KS, Mattes FM, Phadke R, Garson JA, Grant P, et al. Diagnosis of neuroinvasive astrovirus infection in an immunocompromised adult with encephalitis by unbiased next-generation sequencing. Clinical Infectious Diseases. 2015;**60**(6):919-923

[75] Parker J, Chen J. Application of next generation sequencing for the detection of human viral pathogens in clinical specimens. Journal of Clinical Virology. 2017;**86**:20-26

[76] Strong MJ, Blanchard E, Lin Z, Morris CA, Baddoo M, Taylor CM, et al. A comprehensive next generation sequencing-based virome assessment in brain tissue suggests no major virus - tumor association. Acta Neuropathologica Communications. 2016;**4**(1):71

[77] Reyes A, Haynes M, Hanson N, Angly FE, Heath AC, Rohwer F, et al. Viruses in the faecal microbiota of monozygotic twins and their mothers. Nature. 2010;**466**(7304):334-338

[78] Donald CL, Brennan B, Cumberworth SL, Rezelj VV, Clark JJ, Cordeiro MT, et al. Full genome sequence and sfRNA interferon antagonist activity of Zika virus from Recife, Brazil. Morrison AC, editor. PLoS Neglected Tropical Diseases. 2016;**10**(10):e0005048

[79] Kuroda M, Katano H, Nakajima N, Tobiume M, Ainai A, Sekizuka T, et al. Characterization of quasispecies of Pandemic 2009 influenza a virus (A/H1N1/2009) by de novo sequencing using a next-generation DNA sequencer. Jacobson S, editor. PLoS One. 2010;**5**(4):e10256

[80] Dunn DT, Coughlin K, Cane PA. Genotypic resistance testing in routine clinical care. Current Opinion in HIV and AIDS. 2011;**6**(4):251-257

[81] Quer J, Rodríguez-Frias F, Gregori J, Tabernero D, Soria ME, García-Cehic D, et al. Deep sequencing in the management of hepatitis virus infections. Virus Research. 2016;pii: S0168-1702(16)30456-7

[82] Chen X, Zou X, He J, Zheng J, Chiarella J, Kozal MJ. HIV drug resistance mutations (DRMs) detected by deep sequencing in virologic failure subjects on therapy from Hunan Province, China. Jin X, editor. PLoS One. 2016;**11**(2):e0149215

[83] Lataillade M, Chiarella J, Yang R, Schnittman S, Wirtz V, Uy J, et al. Prevalence and clinical significance of HIV drug resistance mutations by ultra-deep sequencing in antiretroviral-naïve subjects in the CASTLE study. Ndhlovu LC, editor. PLoS One. 2010;**5**(6):e10952

[84] Gire SK, Goba A, Andersen KG, Sealfon RSG, Park DJ, Kanneh L, et al. Genomic surveillance elucidates Ebola virus origin and transmission during the 2014 outbreak. Science. 2014;**345**(6202):1369-1372

[85] Fischer W, Ganusov VV, Giorgi EE, Hraber PT, Keele BF, Leitner T, et al. Transmission of single HIV-1 genomes and dynamics of early immune escape revealed by ultra-deep sequencing. Nixon DF, editor. PLoS One. 2010;**5**(8):e12303

[86] Bull RA, Luciani F, McElroy K, Gaudieri S, Pham ST, Chopra A, et al. Sequential bottlenecks drive viral evolution in early acute hepatitis C virus infection. Ou JJ, editor. PLoS Pathogens. 2011;**7**(9):e1002243

[87] Howard S, Qiu W. Viral small RNAs reveal the genomic variations of three grapevine vein clearing virus quasispecies populations. Virus Research. 2017;**229**:24-27

[88] Zhang Q, Lai MM, Lou YY, Guo BH, Wang HY, Zheng XQ. Transcriptome altered by latent human cytomegalovirus infection on THP-1 cells using RNA-seq. Gene. 2016;**594**(1):144-150

[89] Sijmons S, Van Ranst M, Maes P. Genomic and functional characteristics of human cytomegalovirus revealed by next-generation sequencing. Viruses. 2014;**6**(3):1049-1072

[90] Chen SJ, Chen GH, Chen YH, Liu CY, Chang KP, Chang YS, et al. Characterization of Epstein-Barr virus miRNAome in nasopharyngeal carcinoma by deep sequencing. Jin DY, editor. PLoS One. 2010;**5**(9):e12745

[91] Pedersen G, Kanigan T. Clinical RNA sequencing in oncology: Where are we? Personalized Medicine. 2016;**13**(3):209-213

[92] Maher CA, Kumar-Sinha C, Cao X, Kalyana-Sundaram S, Han B, Jing X, et al. Transcriptome sequencing to detect gene fusions in cancer. Nature. 2009;**458**(7234):97-101

[93] Hessels D, Schalken JA. Recurrent gene fusions in prostate cancer: Their clinical implications and uses. Current Urology Reports. 2013;**14**(3):214-222

[94] Mertens F, Antonescu CR, Mitelman F. Gene fusions in soft tissue tumors: Recurrent and overlapping pathogenetic themes. Genes, Chromosomes and Cancer. 2016;**55**(4):291-310

[95] Heravi-Moussavi A, Anglesio MS, Cheng SWG, Senz J, Yang W, Prentice L, et al. Recurrent somatic DICER1 mutations in nonepithelial ovarian cancers. New England Journal of Medicine. 2012;**366**(3):234-242

[96] Wiegand KC, Shah SP, Al-Agha OM, Zhao Y, Tse K, Zeng T, et al. ARID1A mutations in endometriosis-associated ovarian carcinomas. New England Journal of Medicine. 2010;**363**(16):1532-1543

[97] Shah SP, Köbel M, Senz J, Morin RD, Clarke BA, Wiegand KC, et al. Mutation of FOXL2 in granulosa-cell tumors of the ovary. New England Journal of Medicine. 2009;**360**(26): 2719-2729

[98] Wartman LD. A case of me: Clinical cancer sequencing and the future of precision medicine. Molecular Case Studies. 2015;**1**(1):a000349

[99] Linsley PS, Chaussabel D, Speake C. The relationship of immune cell signatures to patient survival varies within and between tumor types. Haibe-Kains B, editor. PLoS One. 2015;**10**(9):e0138726

[100] Oberg JA, Glade Bender JL, Sulis ML, Pendrick D, Sireci AN, Hsiao SJ, et al. Implementation of next generation sequencing into pediatric hematology-oncology practice: Moving beyond actionable alterations. Genome Medicine. 2016;**8**(1):133

[101] Molina-Vila MA, Mayo-de-las-Casas C, Giménez-Capitán A, Jordana-Ariza N, Garzón M, Balada A, et al. Liquid biopsy in non-small cell lung cancer. Frontiers of Medicine. 2016;**3**

[102] Batth IS, Mitra A, Manier S, Ghobrial IM, Menter D, Kopetz S, et al. Circulating tumor markers: Harmonizing the yin and yang of CTCs and ctDNA for precision medicine. Annals of Oncology. 2017;1;**28**(3):468-477

[103] Chakraborty C, Das S. Profiling cell-free and circulating miRNA: A clinical diagnostic tool for different cancers. Tumor Biology. 2016;**37**(5):5705-5714

[104] Zhao Y, Song Y, Yao L, Song G, Teng C. Circulating microRNAs: Promising biomarkers involved in several cancers and other diseases. DNA and Cell Biology. 2017;**36**(2):77-94

[105] Wang WT, Chen YQ. Circulating miRNAs in cancer: From detection to therapy. Journal of Hematology and Oncology. 2014;**7**(1):86

[106] Zhang L, Xu Y, Jin X, Wang Z, Wu Y, Zhao D, et al. A circulating miRNA signature as a diagnostic biomarker for non-invasive early detection of breast cancer. Breast Cancer Research and Treatment. 2015;**154**(2):423-434

[107] Brase JC, Johannes M, Schlomm T, Fälth M, Haese A, Steuber T, et al. Circulating miRNAs are correlated with tumor progression in prostate cancer. International Journal of Cancer. 2011;**128**(3):608-616

[108] Clancy C, Joyce MR, Kerin MJ. The use of circulating microRNAs as diagnostic biomarkers in colorectal cancer. Cancer Biomarkers. 2015;**15**(2):103-113

[109] Nandagopal L, Sonpavde G. Circulating biomarkers in bladder cancer. Bladder Cancer. 2016;**2**(4):369-379

[110] Pimentel F, Bonilla P, Ravishankar YG, Contag A, Gopal N, LaCour S, et al. Technology in MicroRNA profiling. Journal of Laboratory Automation. 2015;**20**(5):574-588

[111] Egger G, Liang G, Aparicio A, Jones PA. Epigenetics in human disease and prospects for epigenetic therapy. Nature. 2004;**429**(6990):457-463

[112] Rodenhiser D, Mann M. Epigenetics and human disease: Translating basic biology into clinical applications. Canadian Medical Association Journal. 2006;**174**(3):341-348

[113] Skinner MK, Manikkam M, Guerrero-Bosagna C. Epigenetic transgenerational actions of environmental factors in disease etiology. Trends in Endocrinology and Metabolism. 2010;**21**(4):214-222

[114] Strahl BD, Allis CD. The language of covalent histone modifications. Nature. 2000;**403** (6765):41-45

[115] Nicholls RD, Saitoh S, Horsthemke B. Imprinting in Prader-Willi and Angelman syndromes. Trends in Genetics. 1998;**14**(5):194-200

[116] Maher ER, Reik W. Beckwith-Wiedemann syndrome: Imprinting in clusters revisited. Journal of Clinical Investigation. 2000;**105**(3):247-252

[117] Chang F, Li MM. Clinical application of amplicon-based next-generation sequencing in cancer. Cancer Genetics. 2013;**206**(12):413-419

[118] 1000 Genome Project [Internet]. Available from: http://www.internationalgenome.org [Accessed: 6 March 2017]

[119] dbSNP database [Internet]. Available from: https://www.ncbi.nlm.nih.gov/SNP [Accessed: 6 March 2017]

[120] Clinvar – NCBI [Internet]. Available from: https://www.ncbi.nlm.nih.gov/clinvar [Accessed: 6 March 2017]

[121] LOVD – Leiden Open Variation Database [Internet]. Available from: http://www.lovd.nl/3.0/home [Accessed: 6 March 2017]

[122] The Cancer Genome Atlas (TCGA) Research Network [Internet]. Available from: https://cancergenome.nih.gov [Accessed: 18 April 2017]

[123] RefSeq database [Internet]. Available from: https://www.ncbi.nlm.nih.gov/refseq [Accessed: 6 March 2017]

[124] Gullapalli RR, Desai KV, Santana-Santos L, Kant JA, Becich MJ. Next generation sequencing in clinical medicine: Challenges and lessons for pathology and biomedical informatics. Journal of Pathology Informatics. 2012;**3**:40

[125] Shendure J, Ji H. Next-generation DNA sequencing. Nature Biotechnology. 2008;**26**(10): 1135-1145

[126] Raza K, Ahmad S. Principle, analysis, application and challenges of next-generation sequencing: A review. 2016. arXiv:1606.05254 [q-bio.GN]

[127] Stanislaw C, Xue Y, Wilcox WR. Genetic evaluation and testing for hereditary forms of cancer in the era of next-generation sequencing. Cancer Biology and Medicine. 2016;**13**(1):55-67

[128] ISO, E. (2012). 13485: 2012. Medical Devices. Quality management systems. Requirements for regulatory purposes (ISO 13485: 2003). Suomen Standardisoimisliitto SFS ry, (s 57)

[129] Public Health Service Food and Drug Administration. Inspections, Compliance, Enforcement, and Criminal Investigations [Internet]. 2014. Available from: http://www.fda.gov/ICECI/EnforcementActions/WarningLetters/2013/ucm376296.htm [Accessed: 29 January 2017]

[130] Singh RR, Luthra R, Routbort MJ, Patel KP, Medeiros LJ. Implementation of next generation sequencing in clinical molecular diagnostic laboratories: Advantages, challenges and potential. Expert Review of Precision Medicine and Drug Development. 2016;**1**(1):109-120

[131] Strom SP. Current practices and guidelines for clinical next-generation sequencing oncology testing. Cancer Biology and Medicine. 2016;**13**(1):3-11

[132] Gargis AS, Kalman L, Berry MW, Bick DP, Dimmock DP, Hambuch T, et al. Assuring the quality of next-generation sequencing in clinical laboratory practice. Nature Biotechnology. 2012;**30**(11):1033-1036

[133] Aziz N, Zhao Q, Bry L, Driscoll DK, Funke B, Gibson JS, et al. College of American pathologists' laboratory standards for next-generation sequencing clinical tests. Archives of Pathology and Laboratory Medicine. 2015;**139**(4):481-493

[134] Jennings LJ, Arcila ME, Corless C, Kamel-Reid S, Lubin IM, Pfeifer J, et al. Guidelines for validation of next-generation sequencing-based oncology panels: A joint consensus recommendation of the association for molecular pathology and college of American pathologists. Journal of Molecular Diagnostics. 2017;**19**(3):341-365

[135] Lin MT, Mosier SL, Thiess M, Beierl KF, Debeljak M, Tseng LH, et al. Clinical validation of KRAS, BRAF, and EGFR mutation detection using next-generation sequencing. American Journal of Clinical Pathology. 2014;**141**(6):856-866

[136] Singh RR, Patel KP, Routbort MJ, Reddy NG, Barkoh BA, Handal B, et al. Clinical validation of a next-generation sequencing screen for mutational hotspots in 46 cancer-related genes. Journal of Molecular Diagnostics. 2013;**15**(5):607-622

[137] Rathi V, Wright G, Constantin D, Chang S, Pham H, Jones K, et al. Clinical validation of the 50 gene AmpliSeq ™ Cancer Panel V2 for use on a next generation sequencing platform using formalin fixed, paraffin embedded and fine needle aspiration tumour specimens. Pathology. 2017;**49**(1):75-82

[138] Wallace AJ. New challenges for BRCA testing: A view from the diagnostic laboratory. European Journal of Human Genetics. 2016;**24**(S1):10-18

[139] Google Genomics [Internet]. Available from: https://cloud.google.com/genomics [Accessed: 16 April 2017]

[140] SOPHiA Genetics [Internet]. Available from: http://www.sophiagenetics.com [Accessed: 16 April 2017]

[141] IBM Watson [Internet]. Available from: https://www.ibm.com/watson [Accessed: 16 April 2017]

[142] Illumina BaseSpace [Internet]. Available from: https://basespace.illumina.com [Accessed: 16 April 2017]

[143] Ion Reporter [Internet]. Available from: https://ionreporter.thermofisher.com/ir [Accessed: 16 April 2017]

[144] Afgan E, Baker D, van den Beek M, Blankenberg D, Bouvier D, Čech M, et al. The galaxy platform for accessible, reproducible and collaborative biomedical analyses: 2016 update. Nucleic Acids Research. 2016;**44**(W1):W3–W10

[145] CLC Genomics [Internet]. Available from: https://www.qiagenbioinformatics.com/products/clc-genomics-workbench [Accessed: 16 April 2017]

[146] Desai A, Jere A. Next-generation sequencing: Ready for the clinics? Clinical Genetics. 2012;**81**(6):503-510

[147] Sboner A, Mu X, Greenbaum D, Auerbach RK, Gerstein MB. The real cost of sequencing: Higher than you think! Genome Biology. 2011;**12**(8):125